Th**pplied Microbial Physiology**

2

30

The Practical Approach Series

SERIES EDITORS

D. RICKWOOD
Department of Biology, University of Essex,
Wivenhoe Park, Colchester, Essex CO4 3SQ, UK

B. D. HAMES
Department of Biochemistry and Molecular Biology
University of Leeds, Leeds LS2 9JT, UK

★ **indicates new and forthcoming titles**

Affinity Chromatography
★ Affinity Separations
Anaerobic Microbiology
Animal Cell Culture
(2nd edition)
Animal Virus Pathogenesis
Antibodies I and II
★ Antibody Engineering
★ Applied Microbial Physiology
Basic Cell Culture
Behavioural Neuroscience
Biochemical Toxicology
Bioenergetics
Biological Data Analysis
Biological Membranes
Biomechanics—Materials
Biomechanics—Structures and
Systems
Biosensors
★ Calcium-PI signalling
Carbohydrate Analysis
(2nd edition)
Cell–Cell Interactions

The Cell Cycle
Cell Growth and Apoptosis
Cellular Calcium
Cellular Interactions in
Development
Cellular Neurobiology
Clinical Immunology
★ Complement
Crystallization of Nucleic
Acids and Proteins
Cytokines (2nd edition)
The Cytoskeleton
Diagnostic Molecular Pathology
I and II
Directed Mutagenesis
★ DNA and Protein Sequence
Analysis
DNA Cloning 1: Core
Techniques (2nd edition)
DNA Cloning 2: Expression
Systems (2nd edition)
★ DNA Cloning 3: Complex
Genomes (2nd edition)

★ DNA Cloning 4: Mammalian Systems (2nd edition)

Electron Microscopy in Biology

Electron Microscopy in Molecular Biology

Electrophysiology

Enzyme Assays

★ Epithelial Cell Culture

Essential Developmental Biology

Essential Molecular Biology I and II

Experimental Neuroanatomy

★ Extracellular Matrix

Flow Cytometry (2nd edition)

★ Free Radicals

Gas Chromatography

Gel Electrophoresis of Nucleic Acids (2nd edition)

Gel Electrophoresis of Proteins (2nd edition)

Gene Probes 1 and 2

Gene Targeting

Gene Transcription

Glycobiology

Growth Factors

Haemopoiesis

Histocompatibility Testing

HIV Volumes 1 and 2

Human Cytogenetics I and II (2nd edition)

Human Genetic Disease Analysis

★ Immunochemistry 1

★ Immunochemistry 2

Immunocytochemistry

In Situ Hybridization

Iodinated Density Gradient Media

★ Ion Channels

Lipid Analysis

Lipid Modification of Proteins

Lipoprotein Analysis

Liposomes

Mammalian Cell Biotechnology

Medical Bacteriology

Medical Mycology

Medical Parasitology

Medical Virology

★ MHC Volume 1

★ MHC Volume 2

Microcomputers in Biology

Molecular Genetic Analysis of Populations

Molecular Genetics of Yeast

Molecular Imaging in Neuroscience

Molecular Neurobiology

Molecular Plant Pathology I and II

Molecular Virology

Monitoring Neuronal Activity

Mutagenicity Testing

★ Neural Cell Culture

Neural Transplantation

★ Neurochemistry (2nd edition)

Neuronal Cell Lines

NMR of Biological Macromolecules

Non-isotopic Methods in Molecular Biology

Nucleic Acid Hybridization

Nucleic Acid and Protein Sequence Analysis

Oligonucleotides and Analogues

Oligonucleotide Synthesis

PCR 1

PCR 2

Peptide Antigens

Photosynthesis: Energy Transduction

Plant Cell Biology

Plant Cell Culture (2nd edition)

Plant Molecular Biology

Plasmids (2nd edition)

★ Platelets

Pollination Ecology

Postimplantation Mammalian Embryos

Preparative Centrifugation

Prostaglandins and Related Substances

Protein Blotting

Protein Engineering

★ Protein Function (2nd edition)

Protein Phosphorylation

Protein Purification Applications

Protein Purification Methods

Protein Sequencing

★ Protein Structure (2nd edition)

★ Protein Structure Prediction

Protein Targeting

Proteolytic Enzymes

Pulsed Field Gel Electrophoresis

Radioisotopes in Biology

Receptor Biochemistry

Receptor–Ligand Interactions

RNA Processing I and II

★ Subcellular Fractionation

Signal Transduction

Solid Phase Peptide Synthesis

Transcription Factors

Transcription and Translation

Tumour Immunobiology

Virology

Yeast

Applied Microbial Physiology

A Practical Approach

Edited by

P. M. RHODES

*Bioscot Ltd, King's Buildings, West Mains Road,
Edinburgh EH9 3JF, UK*

and

P. F. STANBURY

*Division of Biochemistry and Microbiology, University of Hertfordshire,
Hatfield, Herts AL10 9AB, UK*

◯IRL PRESS
——at——
OXFORD UNIVERSITY PRESS
Oxford New York Tokyo

Oxford University Press, Great Clarendon Street, Oxford OX2 6DP

Oxford   New York
Athens   Auckland   Bangkok   Bogota   Bombay   Buenos Aires
Calcutta   Cape Town   Dar es Salaam   Delhi   Florence   Hong Kong
Istanbul   Karachi   Kuala Lumpur   Madras   Madrid   Melbourne
Mexico City   Nairobi   Paris   Singapore   Taipei   Tokyo   Toronto   Warsaw
and associated companies in
Berlin   Ibadan

Oxford is a trade mark of Oxford University Press

Published in the United States
by Oxford University Press Inc., New York

Users of books in the Practical Approach Series are advised that prudent
laboratory safety procedures should be followed at all times. Oxford
University Press makes no representation, express or implied, in respect of
the accuracy of the material set forth in books in this series and cannot
accept any legal responsibility or liability for any errors or omissions
that may be made.

A catalogue record for this book is available from the British Library

Library of Congress Cataloging in Publication Data
(Data available)
ISBN 0 19 963577 3 (Pbk)
ISBN 0 19 963578 1 (Hbk)

Typeset by Footnote Graphics, Warminster, Wilts
Printed in Great Britain by Information Press, Ltd, Eynsham, Oxon.

Preface

The rapid growth in biotechnology over the last 15 years has led to an upsurge in interest in microbial technology by scientists who were trained initially in other fields. Many biochemists, molecular biologists, geneticists, virologists, endocrinologists, and clinicians are interested in developing their work using microbial culture. The objectives of these workers may be very diverse, ranging from the isolation of a stable enzyme from a hyperthermophile to the expression of a human protein by a recombinant yeast or bacterium. Once the product of interest has been obtained in pure form there is a need to generate enough material for more detailed study. This objective may be achieved by optimizing culture conditions and directing the activities of the producing microorganism. This book has been written to help such scientists progress their project to the point of scale-up.

Optimization of product yield can be achieved by medium design and control of the chemical and physical environment of the microorganism. However, to effect such control strategies by purely empirical techniques is often too laborious to be practical. Advances in microbial physiology have made possible a rational approach to optimization based on analysis of cultures, growth kinetics, and biochemical pathways. The application of statistical optimization methods, widely used in other fields, has also much to offer microbiology and biotechnology. The choice of material for this text has been influenced by both the need for practical information to enable the isolation, handling, and culture of organisms and the necessity to generate and analyse data enabling the development of a process. We have therefore included chapters covering the 'husbandry' of microbiology (culture storage, medium design, and the use of laboratory fermenters), the generation of data by chemical and physical analysis, and the interpretation of such data. Data interpretation is considered from two points of view. Kinetic analyses of growth and product formation, pioneered by Pirt and colleagues, have frequently illuminated the development of fermentation processes. More recently, the analysis of the flux of metabolites through intermediate biochemical pathways has helped to elucidate the important factors in metabolic engineering which has become possible through the application of molecular biology techniques in microbial physiology.

The data obtained by the fundamental analysis approach can also be valuable later on in scaling-up a process, where problems are often due to a poor understanding of the physiology of the industrial microorganism. Thus, we envisage that this volume will also be of use to biochemical engineers who are involved in fermentation process development. Last, but by no means least, we trust that this volume will also be a useful source to research students and undergraduate project students.

Edinburgh and Hatfield P. M. R.
May 1997 P. F. S.

Contents

List of contributors   xvii

Abbreviations   xix

1. Sources of microorganisms and their preservation   1

David Smith

1. Introduction   1
  Microorganism stability   1
  Reasons for maintaining collections   2
  Characterization of microorganisms   2
  Data storage and retrieval   3
  Guidelines for the establishment and operation of collections   3

2. Sources of microorganisms and microbial databases   4
  Organizations   4
  Databases   6
  Microbial resource collections   7

3. Preservation and maintenance   8
  Preservation techniques available   8
  Adaptations to continuous growth used for preservation   9
  Dehydration techniques   11
  Cryopreservation   18
  Summary   21

References   21

2. Isolation and growth of hyperthermophiles   23

Richard J. Sharp and Neil D. H. Raven

1. Introduction   23

2. The isolation of hyperthermophiles   23
  Geothermal environments   23
  Sampling geothermal environments   24

3. Media for the growth of hyperthermophiles   26
  Liquid media   26
  Preparation of solidified media   28

4. Growth and bioreactors for hyperthermophiles   31
  Introduction   31
  Continuous culture of *Pyrococcus furiosus*   32

Gas-lift reactors   32
Biomass yields   35

5. Development of vessels for the study of barophilic
hyperthermophiles   41

6. Cryopreservation of hyperthermophiles   42
Introduction   42

7. Culture procedures for hyperthermophiles   45

References   50

3. Design and optimization of growth media   53

Randolph L. Greasham and Wayne K. Herber

1. Introduction   53

2. Medium design   53
Complex media   54
Chemically defined media   55

3. Nutritional requirements   57
Carbon source   57
Nitrogen source   59
Oxygen   60
Inorganic ions   60
Growth factors   61

4. Inducers   61

5. Non-nutritional components   62
Selective agents   62
Solidifying agents   62

6. Environmental factors   62

7. Medium optimization   64
Full factorial search   65
Statistical search   65
Pattern search   69

Acknowledgement   72

References   73

4. Working with laboratory fermenters   75

Stephen Collins

1. Introduction   75

2. Laboratory requirements   76

3. Choice of vessel   76

4. Sterilization   78

5. Aeration and agitation   81

6. Aseptic connections   81
     Septum ports   82
     Line connections   82
     Steam sterilizable connectors   83

7. Inoculation   83

8. Sampling   84
     Syringe   84
     Hoods   84
     Sample valves   85

9. Media   86
     Sterilization of large volumes   86
     Microbial growth in media supply lines   86
     Salt balance   87

10. Process measurement and control   87
     pH   87
     Dissolved oxygen tension   90
     Temperature   92
     Foam   93
     Dissolved CO_2 93
     Redox   93
     Vent-gas analysis   94
     Biomass   94

11. Continuous culture   94
     Sterilization and the storage of media   94
     Control and measurement of flow   95
     Measurement and control of volume   95
     Interruption of steady state   96

12. Computer data logging and control   96
     Typical functions of fermentation software   97
     Remote access   97
     Alarms   97
     What to monitor   98
     What to control   98
     Example: control of a fed-batch process   98

References   101

Further Reading   101

5. Measurement of biomass   103

Andrew P. Ison and Gavin B. Matthew

1. Introduction   103

General remarks 103
What is biomass? 103
Specific and volumetric rates 104
Off-line and on-line measurement 104

2. Chemical methods 104
Bioluminescence and chemiluminescence 104
DNA analysis 107
Fluorescence 108
Near infrared spectroscopy 109

3. Microscopic methods 110
Direct count microscopy 110
Viable cell counts 111
Epifluorescence 113
Image analysis 113

4. Physical methods 114
Dry weight methods 114
Packed cell volume 117
Turbidimetry 118
Nephelometry 120
Electrical counting and sizing 120
Flow cytometry 121
Dielectric permittivity 121
Other techniques 125

5. Mathematical modelling methods 125
Mass balance analysis 125
Mass spectrometry 125

6. Conclusions 126

References 127

Further reading 128
General biomass measurement 128
Chemical methods 129
Microscopical methods 129
Physical methods 129
Mathematical methods 129

6. Fermenter vent-gas analysis 131

Peter M. Salmon and Barry C. Buckland

1. Introduction 131

2. Methods for vent-gas analysis 131
Thermal conductivity 131
Flame ionization 132
Gas chromatography 132

Electrochemical sensors 133
Infrared (IR) absorbtion 134
Paramagnetism 136
Mass spectrometry 139

3. Installation and operation 145
Sample probes 145
Sample transport 146
Knock-out pots, coolers, filters, dryers, and absorbers 147
Multistream sample manifolds 148
Pressure, temperature, and flow control 149
Monitoring an analyser system 150
Fermenter pressure, volume, air flow, and dissolved oxygen 151
Data collection 151

4. Calculated variables 152
Well-mixed liquid and gas phases 152
Alternative mixing models 156
Estimation of aqueous concentrations of volatile organic compounds 157
The respiratory quotient 160

References 162

7. The analytical chemistry of microbial cultures 165

David M. Mousdale

1. Introduction 165
The analytical approach to microbial fermentations 165
General aspects of methodology 166
Sampling and sample monitoring 166

2. The utilization of inputs 166
Carbohydrates 166
Oils 170
Nitrogen sources 170
Phosphate and other inorganic anions 175

3. The accumulation of fermentation metabolites 178
Product and side-products 178
Products of carbohydrate metabolism 178
Amino compounds 180
Ammonia 180
Peptides, proteins, and enzymes 181
Thiol compounds 183
Other common metabolites 184
Carbon dioxide 185
Pigments 185

4. The insoluble phase (biomass and pelletable material) 185
Biomass measurement in complex media 185

Biomass (pellet) composition	188
Biomass compositions and elemental analyses	189
5. Carbon and nitrogen mass balances	189
References	191

8. Analysis of microbial growth data — 193

Michael J. Bazin, Ann P. Wood, and David Paget-Brown

1. Introduction	193
Definitions	193
Kinetic functions	195
Culture systems	197
2. Parameter estimation	197
Estimation of Monod growth constants from steady-state chemostat data	198
The 'washout' method	199
Growth yields	201
3. Simulation	202
Numerical solution of differential equations	204
Dynamic parameter estimation	205
4. Analytical methods	208
References	211

9. Metabolic flux analysis — 213

William H. Holms

1. Introduction	213
Basic principles	213
Definitions and units	214
The central metabolic pathways (CMPs)	214
Components of the CMPs	216
2. Flux analysis of *E. coli* ML308 growing on glucose, pyruvate, or fumarate as sole sources of carbon	219
The data	219
Construction of a flux or throughput diagram	222
3. Interpretation of flux analysis	231
Fluxes in CMPs must balance one another	231
What does acetate excretion tell us?	231
4. Intervention to modulate acetate excretion	232
Intervention by restriction of feedstock uptake	232
Intervention by enzyme inhibition	234

Contents

Intervention by deletion of acetate excretion mechanism 234
Intervention to improve position of precursors 234
Other means of diminishing acetate excretion 239
Conclusions 239

5. What controls flux? 239
Theories 239
Determination of flux—a statement of the obvious 241

6. Applications of flux analysis in the real world 245

7. Conclusions 246
General 246
E. coli ML308 246
Control of CMPs 246

References 247

A1. List of suppliers 249

A2. Addresses of culture collections, microbial databases, and national and international culture collection organizations 253

Index 263

Contributors

MICHAEL J. BAZIN
Division of Life Sciences, King's College London, Campden Hill Road, London W8 7AH, UK.

BARRY C. BUCKLAND
Merck Research Laboratories, PO Box 2000, Rahway, NJ 07065, USA.

STEPHEN COLLINS
Chiron Vaccines SPA, Via Fiorentina 1, Siena, Italy.

RANDOLPH L. GREASHAM
Merck Research Laboratories, PO Box 2000, Rahway, NJ 07065, USA.

WAYNE K. HERBER
Merck & Co. Inc., PO Box 4, West Point, PA 19486, USA.

WILLIAM H. HOLMS
Bioflux Ltd, Robertson Institute of Biotechnology, 54 Dumbarton Road, Glasgow G11 6AQ, Scotland, UK.

ANDREW P. ISON
Department of Chemical and Biochemical Engineering, University College London, Torrington Place, London WC1E 7JE, UK.

GAVIN B. MATTHEW
Department of Chemical and Biochemical Engineering, University College London, Torrington Place, London WC1E 7JE, UK.

DAVID M. MOUSEDALE
Bioflux Ltd, Robertson Institute of Biotechnology, 54 Dumbarton Road, Glasgow G11 6AQ, Scotland, UK.

DAVID PAGET-BROWN
Division of Life Sciences, King's College London, Campden Hill Road, London W8 7AH, UK.

NEIL D. H. RAVEN
CAMR, Porton Down, Salisbury, Wiltshire SP4 0JG, UK.

P. MALCOLM RHODES
Bioscot Ltd, King's Buildings, West Mains Road, Edinbrugh EH9 3JF, Scotland, UK.

PETER M. SALMON
Merck Research Laboratories, PO Box 2000, Rahway, NJ 07065, USA.

Contributors

RICHARD J. SHARP
CAMR, Porton Down, Salisbury, Wiltshire SP4 0JG, UK.

DAVID SMITH
International Mycological Institute, Bakenham Lane, Egham, Surrey TW20 9TY, UK.

PETER F. STANBURY
Division of Biochemistry and Microbiology, University of Hertfordshire, Hatfield, Herts AL10 9AB, UK.

ANN P. WOOD
Division of Life Sciences, King's College London, Campden Hill Road, London W8 7AH, UK.

Abbreviations

a.m.u.	atomic mass unit
ADP	adenosine diphosphate
Arg	arginine
ATCC	American Type Culture Collection
ATP	adenosine triphosphate
BAP	Biotechnology Action Programme
BRIDGE	Biotechnology Research for Innovation, Development, and Growth in Europe
CAMR	Centre for Applied Microbiology and Research
CBS	Centraalbureau voor Schimmelcultures
CEC	Commission of the European Community
CER	carbon dioxide evolution rate
CMPs	central metabolic pathways
DCW	dry cell weight
DIMDI	Deutches Institut für Medizinsche Dokumentation und Information
DSM	Deutsche Sammlung von Mikroorganismen und Zelkulturen
e.m.f.	electromotive force
ECCO	European Culture Collection Organization
EDTA	ethylenediaminetetraacetic acid
ETS	electron transport system
FEMS	Federation of the European Microbiological Societies
GC	gas chromatography
Glu	glutamine
Gly	glycine
HPLC	high-performance liquid chromatography
IC	ion chromatography
ICDH	*iso*citrate dehydrogenase
ICECC	Information Centre for European Culture Collections
ICL	*iso*citrate lyase
ICRO	International Cell Research Organisation
IMI	International Mycological Institute
IPA	propanol-2-ol
IPTG	isopropylthio-β-D-galactoside
JFCC	Japan Federation for Culture Collections
LMG	Laboratorium voor Microbiologie Universiteit Ghent
MESH	2-mercaptoethanol
MINE	Microbial Information Network Europe
MIRCENs	Microbial Resource Centres
MPN	most probable number

MSDN	Microbial Strain Data Network
m/z	mass-to-charge ratio
NADP	nicotinamide–adenine dinucleotide phosphate
NAG	Numerical Algorithm Group
NCIMB	National Collection of Industrial and Marine Bacteria
NCYC	National Collection of Yeast Cultures
NDIR	non-dispersive infrared (analyser)
NIR	near-infrared (spectroscopy)
NMR	nuclear magnetic resonance
OGA	oxoglutarate
OPA	*o*-phthaldialdehyde
Orn	ornithine
OUR	oxygen uptake rate
PCA	perchloric acid
PEP	phosphoenolpyruvate
PID	proportional integral differential
PPG	propylene glycol
PPP	pentose phosphate pathway
Pro	proline
PTFE	poly(tetrafluoroethylene)
PTS	phosphoenolpyruvate-dependent phosphotransferase system
RF	radio frequency
RIKEN	The Institute of Physical and Chemical Research
THF	tetrahydrofuran
TLC	thin-layer chromatography
UKCC	United Kingdom Culture Collection
UKFCC	United Kingdom Federation for Culture Collections
UNEP	United Nations Environment Programme
UNESCO	United Nations Educational, Scientific, and Cultural Organization
USFCO	United States Federation of Culture Collections
WDCM	World Data Center on Microorganisms
WFCC	World Federation for Culture Collections

1

Sources of microorganisms and their preservation

DAVID SMITH

1. Introduction

1.1 Microorganism stability

It is essential when working with microorganisms that the strains employed are representative of the species and possess the full range of properties typical of the organism. These properties must not be allowed to deteriorate or change throughout the duration of the study or use of the microorganism. It is therefore imperative that the source of the strain is reputable. If the strain is collected specifically for the study, it must be fully characterized and described so that variance from the original characteristics can be noticed. The organism must also be stored in such a way that it remains both viable and stable. Studies using a wrongly named or atypical strain may generate invalid data and be a waste of time and resources. When isolating an organism from its natural environment, and growing on a synthetic growth medium under laboratory conditions in isolation from its co-habitors, the first step in the process of selecting and generating a 'laboratory culture' has been taken. In a mixed population the cell-line most suited to the growth conditions provided will dominate. Therefore the medium, temperature, pH, and water activity of the growth medium must be carefully selected to be as close to the substrates utilized in the organism's natural environment as possible, to minimize selection. Once suitable conditions have been chosen, the most appropriate method of preservation must be employed to prevent change that would normally result from continuous growth and subculture. In order to prevent variation resulting from mistakes in replication, recombination, or segregation of polyploids, growth and metabolism must be minimized. This can be achieved by dehydration or lowering the temperature below a level where both chemical and physical changes can occur. The loss of expression of a single gene could result in the failure of the microorganism to behave as expected.

1.2 Reasons for maintaining collections

Many types of work require readily available microorganisms. The delays incurred in acquiring them from other sources or trying to re-isolate them from their natural habitat can be unacceptable. Indeed, it may be impossible to obtain the same isolate again. It is quite common that an organism has only been isolated once and repeated attempts to re-isolate from the same location have failed.

The cost in time and resources to update, purify, characterize, and name organisms for use are generally prohibitive. Rarely is the expertise available in one centre, outside microbial resource collections, to enable laboratories to collect their own named organisms for their work.

Many studies require the use of identical replicates and sufficient stocks must be laid down to provide them. If these are not prepared and stored correctly then long-term work may be jeopardized. In-house collections can be established to make strains available as required. However, this may be impracticable where investment in preservation facilities is not justified by the number or value of the organisms being stored. Service collections have been established to provide cultures for use by the scientific community. Generally they preserve several replicates over and above a reserve seed stock which is used to provide cultures for subsequent batches. If large numbers of replicates are required suitable arrangements for the preparation of such large stocks can be made with service collections to ensure a customer's needs are met.

1.3 Characterization of microorganisms

It is essential that organisms are characterized sufficiently, so that subsequent samples or subcultures can be compared and proven unchanged. The accepted variation of a strain within a species makes the description of the species insufficient as a record of that strain. It is important to record the extent to which the strain differs from the species description. The measurement and recording of properties is a highly satisfactory means of characterizing strains. Several approaches have been used such as enzyme and metabolite production, isoenzyme patterns, molecular structure, genetic markers, and gene probes.

The measurement of properties can give an indication of the strain's potential uses as well as being a means of identifying it and checking stability during storage and use. Having knowledge of such properties can reduce unnecessary prescreening of strains every time an organism is required for a different process or product.

There are several methodologies which can be used to help characterize a strain sufficiently so that a record can be kept for future reference to confirm strain stability. A review of these techniques used in the biosystematics of filamentous fungi carried out by Bridge and Hawksworth (1) discusses the study and recording of biochemical and physiological activities. Methods, including thin-layer chromatography (TLC), high-performance liquid chromatography (HPLC), electrophoresis to determine isoenzyme patterns, and DNA hybridization are described as aids for characterizing filamentous fungi. Other characters which are quite simple to record such as growth in the presence of inhibitors at different temperatures and pH values, assimilation of carbon and nitrogen sources, and enzyme activities are all utilized. The use of the APIZYM testing system (API) is one of the more common rapid methods used to characterize bacteria and fungi.

The determination and recording of such characteristics are essential to enable proper and adequate quality control of strains in use.

1.4 Data storage and retrieval

The proper recording and storage of strain data is as important as the correct maintenance and preservation of the organism. Documentation describing the organism, including information on the name, source, growth conditions, preservation, and properties (see Section 1.3) must be maintained. Computer software and hardware is becoming commonplace in the microbiology laboratory and this provides the ideal means of storing strain data. The format for storage is a matter of choice, but it may be advisable to adopt that which many European collections have developed for common use. A project sponsored, in part, by the European Commission through its Biotechnology Action Programme (BAP) and subsequently their Biotechnology Research for Innovation, Development and Growth in Europe (BRIDGE) programme has developed the Microbial Information Network Europe (MINE) database (2, 3). Although such a format would undoubtedly enable the storage of information on most properties of organisms it may be too complex for non-service collections.

Whatever means of storage of data is chosen the need for, and the use of, the information recorded, must be considered so that it can be retrieved and utilized easily.

1.5 Guidelines for the establishment and operation of collections

The World Federation of Culture Collections (WFCC) have outlined requirements and procedures for the maintenance of culture collections in *Guidelines for the establishment and operation of collections of cultures of microorganisms* (4). In order that the user of strains is confident the organism will perform in the same way each time it is retrieved or supplied from a collection, controlled procedures to give a reproducible product must be established. The essence of a well-organized collection is careful quality control. The WFCC guidelines help to set the basic framework, but these must be extended to ensure optimum results. Following the guidelines can offer a degree of procedural control, but in the future it may be necessary for collections to obtain a more formal accreditation (5).

The aims and objectives of a collection must be carefully considered and laid down with a detailed programme for collecting and preserving strains. The long-term security of the collection must be a priority and there must be a schedule for the re-stocking and re-preservation of strains, depending on the frequency of use and longevity in the preservation method. All methods must be carefully defined and monitored to maintain reproducibility, an all too important requirement when studying microbial physiology.

Recommendations are made to ensure long-term funding for the long-term aims of the collection (4). It is emphasized that due attention be made to safety, quarantine, and other regulations. This is particularly important when supplying strains off-site. It is imperative that relevant information is provided with the strain to ensure that appropriate precautions and containment can be employed in handling the organism on receipt. One of the requirements that is quite often overlooked is the need to provide adequate staffing to access, preserve, maintain, and check the stability of strains. The curation of a collection is quite often given low priority and considered to be of secondary importance. The most appropriate preservation method to serve the needs of the collection should be chosen and adequate records must be kept.

Information is available from several sources on collection management maintenance and preservation of strains and, if needed, where and how to obtain suitable and authentic strains of microorganisms.

2. Sources of microorganisms and microbial databases

Full address details of the sources and organizations listed in this section are given in Appendix 2.

2.1 Organizations

Several organizations have been founded to support the activities of microbial resource collections. They operate on a national, regional, or international level. Country-based federations for culture collections function at the national level, the European Culture Collection Organization (ECCO) at the regional level, and the World Federation for Culture Collections (WFCC) at the world level. Microbial Resource Centres (MIRCENs) are a network of institutions which operate at national level providing international benefit.

2.1.1 National organizations

The United Kingdom Federation for Culture Collections (UKFCC) has the objectives to promote the use of collections, to facilitate communication between them and their users, to save endangered collections, to encourage the establishment of specialized collections, to promote research in systematics and preservation, to encourage the distribution of culture data using information technology, and to represent culture collections and their users in national and international forums. Their activities include holding scientific meetings on subjects related to collection activities and liaison with organizations at regional and international level.

Other national organizations with similar objectives and activities operate in other countries, for example the Japan Federation for Culture Collections (JFCC) and the United States Federation of Culture Collections (USFCC).

2.1.2 United Kingdom Culture Collection (UKCC)

The UKCC was established following the Government response to an Office of Science and Technology review of the UK based culture collections. A single point of contact was recommended and the Culture Collection Advisory Group (CCAG) was established within the Biotechnology and Biological Sciences Research Council (BBSRC) to advise UK collections on a united strategy for marketing, cataloguing, database provision, and collaborative activities.

Additionally, a new virus collection will be set up at the European Collection of Animal Cell Cultures, Porton Down. The UKCC will be accessible through an electronic enquiry point on the INTERNET which will provide information on services and access to information on *ca.* 50 000 strains of organisms held. The UKCC is a consortium of ten collections with expertise covering identification, preservation, patent strain storage and applied microbiology covering algae, animal cells, bacteria, fungi (including yeasts), protozoa, and viruses of importance to industry, agriculture, health, and academia.

2.1.3 European Culture Collections Organization (ECCO)

ECCO was established to offer a forum for European culture collection curators to discuss collaboration and to exchange ideas and information about all aspects of culture collection activities. Annual meetings are held to discuss various issues including rapid identification techniques, patent deposits, databases, and systematics. Currently there are 43 member collections and membership is open to representatives of any microbial resource centre that provides a professional service on demand without restriction, that accepts cultures for deposit, that produces catalogues and is housed in a country with microbiological societies affiliated to the Federation of the European Microbiological Societies (FEMS). Member collections must also be affiliated to the World Federation for Culture Collections (WFCC). Currently, ECCO is discussing the expansion of its activities and membership beyond culture collection representatives.

2.1.4 World Federation for Culture Collections (WFCC)

The WFCC seeks to promote and foster activities that support the interest of culture collections and their users. Their activities include keeping members informed on matters relevant to culture collections in its newsletter, organization of a congress every four years, and standing committees reporting on patent depositions, postal, quarantine and safety regulations, safeguard of endangered collections, education, publicity, standards and biodiversity. The standards committee produced guidelines (see Section 1.5) which were agreed by the board and have proven to be a useful guide for the establishment and operation of culture collections. The WFCC has overseen the activities of the World Data Center on Microorganisms, (WDCM see Section 2.2.3) with which all WFCC member collections must register.

2.1.5 Microbial Resource Centres (MIRCENs)

The MIRCEN network was started by United Nations Environment Programme (UNEP), UNESCO, and International Cell Research Organization (ICRO) to preserve and exploit microbial gene pools, make them readily accessible to developing countries, and to carry out research and development in environmental microbiology and biotechnology. The MIRCEN network activities are published in the reports on MIRCEN research in the *World Journal of Microbiology and Biotechnology* (6). There are 22 MIRCENs in 18 countries (6) covering a variety of specialization from *Rhizobium* collections, through fermentation, food and waste recycling, culture collections, to biotechnology. They provide training and information to meet the objectives of the MIRCEN network outlined above.

2.2 Databases

2.2.1 Microbial Strain Data Network (MSDN)

The MSDN is an information and communication network for microbiologists and biotechnologists providing electronic mail, bulletin boards, computer conferences, and databases. It is distributed on several hosts and links databases through electronic gateways in several countries including Germany, France, The Netherlands, Canada, and Japan. Several microbial resource collections make their strain lists available on-line through MSDN, these include the American Type Culture Collections (ATCC), Centraalbureau voor Schimmelcultures (CBS) and the International Mycological Institute (IMI). Information is accessible on microbiological laboratories and their specialization, as well as databases holding strain data. The use of the network is facilitated by regional offices: the Tropical Database, Brazil; the Distributed Information Center, Pune, India; Australian Collection of Microorganisms, Queensland, Australia; Germany, and a North American helpdesk is provided by the ATCC, USA. The MSDN is available through INTERNET: MSDN@CGNET.COM.

2.2.2 Microbial Information Network Europe (MINE)

The MINE project was initiated under the Commission of the European Community (CEC) Biotechnology Action Programme and continued under the CEC BRIDGE Programme. It is an integrated catalogue project, incorporating a European network of microbial collection databanks. Specially designed data formats were created for fungi (2) and bacteria (3). The data from 42 collections on approximately 80 000 strains have been integrated into the database. Further information on this database is available from the coordinator at the Centraalbureau voor Schimmelcultures (see below). The data in-put was co-ordinated by 11 national nodes and integrated by two data integrating nodes, one for bacteria at Laboratorium voor Microbiologie Universiteit (LMG) Ghent, Belgium, and for fungi the Centraalbureau voor Schimmelcultures (CBS), The Netherlands. The data was standardized by committees of scientists for each group of organisms. Further details can be found in the booklet *European laboratory without walls: in the field of MINE, The Microbial Information Network Europe* (7).

2.2.3 World Data Center on Microorganisms (WDCM)

The WDC is sponsored by UNEP, UNESCO, and The Institute of Physical and Chemical Research (RIKEN); the database holds information on collections, the species they hold, and details on their specialization. Data is held on 481 collections from 60 countries and lists the names of 786 328 strains. Currently, strain data is not held. The data mainly covers fungi (44%) and bacteria (43%), giving the source of species thus enabling the user to find suppliers for the organisms they require. The data is also available in the *World directory of collections of cultures of microorganisms* (8). This catalogue of collections and their holdings presents indexes by country, main subjects studied, organisms held, culture availability, staff, and services offered.

Data can be accessed on the Internet through gopher software such as WDC BioGopher by entering "Gopher fragans.riken.go.jp70".

2.3 Microbial resource collections

Microorganisms are maintained by many laboratories and institutions for many different reasons. Many collections make their strains available to the scientific community and offer many different services. Collections are not just sources of cultures, they provide information on collection methodology, systematics, and organism characterization. They accept strain deposits either in their open collections or they may keep them confidentially as safe deposits. Many act as International Depository Authorities for organisms cited in patents under the Budapest Treaty rules (1977). The data on the strains of several of these collections are available on databases described in Section 2.2 above. They can also be contacted directly. Appendix 2 lists the larger collections listed in the *World directory of collections of cultures of microorganisms* (8). The WDCM has 303 collections registered supplying bacteria, 231 supplying fungi, 165 supplying yeasts, 87 supplying viruses, 65 supplying algae, 34 supplying animal cell lines, 23 supplying plasmids, and 8 supplying plant cell lines, therefore only a small representative list can be included here.

3. Preservation and maintenance

3.1 Preservation techniques available

Many preservation techniques have been used to preserve microorganisms. Many workers are beginning to realize the consequences of simply placing cultures of their research and working strains in the refrigerator until they are required again. This procedure and other methods that allow the continuous growth of organisms is an unsatisfactory method for maintaining strains for the long-term, for example during a study, project, or process. Organisms adapt to the artificial growth conditions provided and may lose valuable properties. The techniques that have been developed and used fall into three basic categories:

- continuous growth
- dehydration
- frozen storage

These categories can be further subdivided. Continuous growth includes all techniques that allow the organism to grow and metabolize during storage. There are several procedures available that increase the time period between subcultures, i.e. transfer to fresh media. These include manipulation of growth conditions by limiting carbon, nitrogen, and energy sources, lowering the temperature, or preventing dehydration. Alternatively, dehydration or drying can be used to preserve organisms: techniques include air-drying, desiccation in or above a desiccant, or drying in a vacuum either from the liquid or frozen state. Frozen storage or cryopreservation is storage at a temperature where the organism is frozen to reduce or completely prevent metabolism and physical change. Selection of the most appropriate technique is quite crucial. Careful consideration is needed to ensure that the organism is maintained in such a way that the properties required for its use are retained. Not all the techniques described above are suitable. The continuing growth of cultures on agar, often done to provide instant access to working strains, is unsuitable if you wish to ensure that the strain does not deteriorate and change or become replaced with a contaminant. On each occasion the strain is transferred to fresh medium there is a risk of selecting an atypical portion of growth as inoculum or, indeed, of contaminating the strain. The medium and the incubation conditions for growth can be different from organism to organism and it is important that these are optimal for the strain. It is not appropriate to discuss such conditions here. The techniques required, to retain replicate strains which will give reproducible results, must go some way to reduce or prevent variation and the possibility of contamination or replacement. Information on culture media and conditions can be found in Smith and Onions (9) for fungi and Kirsop and Doyle (10) for fungi, bacteria, and other microorganisms.

3.2 Adapations to continuous growth used for preservation

3.2.1 Storage under a layer of paraffin

This method has been used successfully for both bacteria (11) and fungi (9). It reduces the growth rate of organisms by reducing oxygen availability and reduces dehydration by preventing evaporation from the medium and organism. The details of this method are given in *Protocol 1*, which requires that the cultures are grown on any suitable non-selective medium and that bacterial strains should be in late logarithmic growth phase or have sporulated.

Protocol 1. Storage on agar under a layer of oil

Equipment and reagents

- Medicinal quality liquid paraffin, specific gravity 0.830–0.890 (autoclaved twice at 121°C for 20 min on consecutive days)
- Metal segmented trays (375 mm × 175 mm divided into 25 mm × 25 mm squares to take 60 × 30 ml Universal bottles (Denley))
- Sterile solid growth medium in 30 ml Universal bottles: set at 30° slope. Select the most appropriate growth medium for the organism.
- Sterile inoculating needle or loop

A. *Inoculation and storage*

1. Inoculate at least two Universal bottles for each strain to be maintained.

2. Label one culture as reserve stock, the other(s) as working stock.

3. Incubate at optimum growth temperature until the organism has reached maturity.

4. Add 8–10 ml of liquid paraffin to cover the slope to a maximum depth of 10 mm over its highest point.

5. Store the oiled cultures, with the screw cap loose, in metal divided racks at 15–20°C.

B. *Recovery of sample*

1. Remove a portion of the working stock culture using a sterile needle or loop.

2. Drain as much oil as possible from the inoculum.

3. Inoculate fresh growth medium (it is often best to inoculate a slope so that the adhering oil can drain and the organism can grow up the slope away from the oil at the point of inoculation).

Protocol 1. *Continued*

4. The reserve stock culture is used only when re-preservation becomes necessary when all the inoculum has been removed when it is contaminated or when the shelf-life expiry date[a] set for the organism has been reached.

[a] Although many fungi have survived for 44 years at the International Mycological Institute, it is advisable to set a re-preservation programme of between 2 and 10 years (see ref. 9).

Bacteria are expected to survive 2–4 years if preserved according to *Protocol 1* (11, 12). Many fungi survive much longer periods; several have been found to retain viability following 40 years in storage (9). However, if this is the sole method of long-term preservation a shorter time between transfer is recommended. Some more sensitive organisms should be subcultured on a two-yearly basis (9) and it would be wise to transfer all others before ten years.

This method of preservation allows growth under very special conditions and therefore any variant cell present that grows best under these conditions will dominate and outgrow the rest of the population. This may result in a culture which no longer has the same properties as the original. Therefore long-term storage by this method is not recommended. This technique is discussed in this chapter as it provides a useful back-up for delicate cells that may not survive some of the following techniques.

As stated in *Protocol 1*, when preserving cultures by this method, it is advisable to prepare at least two bottles. One to provide a working culture, the other as a reserve stock for use as inoculum and re-preservation if the working culture fails to recover, becomes contaminated, or deteriorates.

3.2.2 Water storage

This is a technique that again allows some growth, but it is one which can be modified to reduce growth almost to a standstill. Metabolism is still possible and therefore the cell will deteriorate and eventually die if not transferred. The method described here (*Protocol 2*) requires the organisms to be grown on agar and blocks of this agar with a covering of the organism are removed from the plates for storage in water. Alternatively, cells can be harvested and transferred from the growth vessel to water in another sterile screw-cap tube or bottle for storage (12). This latter technique will minimize the amount of nutrients in the storage container and therefore minimize growth and metabolism. For both methods, cultures are grown on suitable growth media until sporulation occurs. Non-sporulating bacteria should be grown until they reach late logarithmic phase; mycelial fungi can be transferred to storage when growth is reasonably prolific.

Protocol 2 is recommended for fungi, in particular phytopathogenic fungi, for storage periods of between 2 and 7 years (9, 13). The modified method, harvested spores and cells in water, is recommended for fungi, yeasts, plant pathogenic bacteria, and actinomycetes (12,14).

Protocol 2.   Storage of fungi in water

Equipment and reagents

- Sterile distilled water (10 ml in 30 ml Universal bottles, at least two per culture)
- Mature cultures on agar media in Petri dishes
- Metal segmented racks (375 mm × 175 mm divided into 25 mm × 25 mm sections to take 60 × 30 ml Universal bottles (Denley))

A. *Storage*

1. Cut agar blocks 6 mm^3 through the colony of the organism,^{a} generally from the growing edge.

2. Transfer 20–30 agar blocks to 10 ml of sterile distilled water in two or more 30 ml Universal bottles.

3. Label one bottle as reserve stock and the other(s) as working stock.

4. Screw the caps of the Universal bottles tightly and store at a temperature between 20°C and 25°C.

B. *Recovery*

1. Remove an agar block from the working stock and place the organism face down on a suitable growth medium, incubate under optimum growth conditions. Use the reserve stock when re-preservation is necessary (see *Protocol 1*).

^{a}Sporulating or non-filamentous organisms can be harvested without the agar and simply suspended in water. Recover the organism by placing a small amount of the suspension on to suitable growth medium.

3.3 Dehydration techniques

The methods discussed in this section involve drying in various desiccants or support media and drying under vacuum by L-drying or freeze-drying.

3.3.1 Drying in a desiccator or support medium

The removal of water from a biological system will reduce the possibility of chemical or biochemical reactions and therefore reduce the chance of variation or deterioration. Many support or desiccant media have been used to achieve this method of preservation. Soil, sand, or silica gel for fungi (9), silica gel or porcelain beads for fungi and bacteria (12), paper replicates or silica gel for yeasts (15). The method covered here is one adapted from a method by Perkins (16) for storage in non-indicator silica gel (*Protocol 3*).

11

Protocol 3. Storage in silica gel

Equipment and reagents

- Coarse non-indicator silica gel
- 30 ml glass Universal bottles (a minimum of 2 per culture)
- 100 mm deep waterproof tray filled to a depth of 30 mm with water
- −20°C freezer
- Sterile 5% (w/v) solution of non-fat skimmed milk cooled to 5°C
- Refrigerator
- Sterile Pasteur pipettes
- Airtight storage boxes
- Indicator silica gel

A. *Storage*

1. One-third fill the 30 ml Universal bottles with the coarse non-indicator silica gel and sterilize in an oven at 180°C for 2–3 hours.

2. Place the bottles into a tray of water up to the level of the silica gel and place the tray in a − 20°C freezer, leave overnight to freeze.

3. Prepare a suspension of the sporulating microorganisms in the cooled 5% (w/v) skimmed milk (at 5°C).

4. Add approximately 1 ml of the suspension, using a Pasteur pipette, to at least two bottles of silica gel for each strain whilst they remain in the frozen water.

5. After 20 min or longer when the bottles can be easily moved, remove the Universal bottles from the ice and agitate them to disperse the suspension.

6. Label one bottle as reserve stock and the other(s) as working stock.

7. Incubate the bottles at 25°C until the crystals readily separate when shaken, this may take one to two weeks.

8. Screw the bottle caps down tightly and store at 4°C in an airtight container, include an open Universal containing indicator silica gel to absorb water.

B. *Recovery*

1. Sprinkle a few crystals from the working stock on to a suitable growth medium and incubate under appropriate growth conditions.

2. If the organism fails to grow, attempt again, this time streaking a silica gel crystal over the agar to dislodge the cells and discarding the silica gel crystal before incubation.

Modifications of this technique usually involve the suspending medium where 10% (w/v) skimmed milk and 3% (w/v) inositol or 5% (w/v) honey is used for protecting bacteria during storage (12). Another variation is to use different or smaller storage vessels, capped vials or tubes, or McCartney bottles.

Recommended storage times for organisms protected by this method vary. Success with yeasts appears to be limited. Only 50% of strains preserved by this method at the National Collection of Yeast Cultures (NCYC) survived the method (15). However, sporulating fungi can be maintained for periods of 20 years or more, but it is recommended, following experience at IMI, that the majority of cultures should be re-preserved before 8 years as a large proportion of strains only survive for 8–11 years (9).

3.3.2 L-drying

This method of drying under vacuum without freezing has been used successfully for bacteria that are particularly sensitive to the initial freezing stage of freeze-drying (17). It has also been used for vesicular arbuscular mycorrhizal fungi (18). *Protocol 4* describes the method used at the National Collection of Industrial and Marine Bacteria (NCIMB Ltd) (17).

Protocol 4. L-drying after the method of Dando and Bousfield, 1991 (17)

Equipment and reagents

- 0.5 ml neutral glass ampoules containing numbered (with the strain number of the organisms being preserved) and dated strips of filter paper, plugged with sterile cotton wool and sterilized by autoclaving at 121°C for 15 min (19)
- 'Mist desiccans': 100 ml horse serum + 33 ml nutrient broth (Unipath Ltd, CM1) are mixed and 10 g glucose dissolved slowly while shaking. Sterilize by pressure filtration and dispense in 5 ml aliquots (17)
- Ram rod: metal needle/loop handle with a collar fixed at 60 mm from tip

- Manifold with connections for 0.5 ml glass ampoules
- Water bath at 20°C
- Vacuum tubing and valve for connecting to vacuum pump with an incorporated phosphorus pentoxide trap
- Vacuum rotary pump
- Freeze-dryer with secondary drying manifold (Modulyo 4K)
- Air/gas glass-blower's torch
- Twin jet air/gas sealing torch
- Glass cutter

A. *L-drying*

1. Prepare a dense suspension of the cells in 'mist desiccans' and add approximately 0.1 ml to each replicate ampoule to be dried. Avoid leaving the suspension on the sides of the ampoules.

2. Replace the cotton wool plug and trim to 10 mm and push it down, aseptically, to just above the strip of filter paper (approximately 60 mm down the ampoule) with a ram rod.

3. Attach the ampoule vertically to the manifold and fix in place so that the ampoules are immersed to a depth of 40–50 mm in the + 20°C water-bath.

4. Attach the manifold to the rotary vacuum pump via a closed valve and the phosphorus pentoxide desiccant trap.

5. Switch on the vacuum pump with the valve closed. Quickly open the valve for approximately 0.5 sec and then quickly close it.

Protocol 4. *Continued*

6. Open the valve very gradually until the ampoule contents begin to degas. Manipulate the valve to avoid violent bubbling in the ampoule. Close the valve if violent bubbling occurs. Degassing will be complete in about 5 min.

7. Open the valve fully to allow drying to take place.

8. Remove the ampoules and constrict, using an air/gas glass-blower's torch, 10 mm above the cotton plug and transfer to the secondary drying manifold of the freeze-dryer.

9. Dry overnight, seal at the constriction with the twin flame air/gas torch.

10. Store in racked drawers at a convenient temperature.[a]

B. *Recovery*

1. Scratch the ampoule at the centre of the cotton wool plug using a glass cutter.

2. Snap open the ampoule, remove the cotton plug, and add 0.1 ml sterile distilled water.

3. Replace the plug and allow 15–30 min for absorption of water.

4. Streak the contents on to a suitable growth medium and incubate under optimum conditions

[a] Ampoules can be stored at room temperature, but storage at a lower temperature will reduce the rate of deterioration thus increasing the shelf-life of the dried cells.

At NCIMB bacteria have been preserved by this procedure successfully for 15 years. It has been very useful for preserving spirilla and *Azomonas insignis*, cells which are normally sensitive to freeze-drying (17).

3.3.3 Freeze-drying

Freeze-drying is dehydration by the sublimation of ice at reduced pressure. The method used to achieve this normally depends upon the equipment used. The centrifugal or spin-freezer methods depend upon evaporative cooling and rely upon atmospheric heat, and that conducted through the equipment, to drive the freeze-drying process. The vacuum pump on the freeze-dryer removes the air and facilitates the diffusion of water vapour from the freeze-drying material to the water trap. The latter can be a desiccant such as phosphorus pentoxide or a refrigeration system. Freeze-drying will not occur if there is no significant difference in the water vapour pressure above the freeze-drying material and the water trap. Effectively the condenser (water trap) should be around 20 °C lower than the sample, or if a desiccant is used there must be sufficient available to absorb all the water to be removed from the samples. Although the spin-freeze method is perhaps the most common (*Protocol 5*), methods that enable controlled cooling to freeze the material are more successful. Equipment that has a pre-freezing stage such as a shelf freeze-drier is extremely useful.

Protocol 5. Spin or centrifugal freeze-drying

Equipment and reagents

- Sterile 10% (w/v) skimmed milk + 5% (w/v) inositol[a]
- Freeze-drier (Edwards High Vacuum International) with spin-freeze and manifold accessories (Modulyo 4K)
- 0.5 ml (normal capacity) neutral glass ampoules (Anchor Glass Co. Ltd) heat sterilized and labelled with the strain number of the organism to be freeze-dried
- Sterile lint caps fitted to the 0.5 ml ampoules individually

- Sterile non-absorbent cotton wool formed into plugs pushing into the neck of 0.5 ml glass ampoules and trimmed to 10 mm in depth
- Air/gas glass-blower's torch (Vacuum Industrial Products Ltd)
- Phosphorus pentoxide
- Twin flame air/gas sealing torch (Vacuum Industrial Products Ltd)
- Glass cutter in support handle
- Sterile distilled water

A. *Freeze-drying*

1. Prepare a suspension of spores or cells in sterile 10% (w/v) skimmed milk and 5% (w/v) inositol

2. Add approximately 0.2 ml of the spore or cell suspension to each sterile ampoule using a Pasteur pipette and cover each with a sterile lint cap.

3. Load the filled ampoule into the spin-freeze racks of the Modulyo 4K freeze-drier.

4. Place the loaded racks into the spin-freeze accessory and spin the ampoules.

5. Evacuate the chamber and continue to spin the ampoules for 30 min.

6. Leave the ampoules in the chamber while evacuating for a further 3 h (at this point the moisture content by dry weight of the material would be approximately 5%).

7. Admit air into the freeze-drier chamber and remove the ampoules.

8. Remove the lint caps and plug the ampoules with sterile cotton wool compressed to 10 mm in depth approximately 10 mm above the top of the freeze-dried material.

9. Constrict the plugged ampoule 10 mm above the cotton plug using the air/gas torch. The bore of the constriction should remain greater than 1 mm, the outer diameter approximately 2.5 mm.

10. Place the ampoules on the manifold, which replaces the spin-freeze accessory, evacuate and dry over phosphorus pentoxide.

Protocol 5. *Continued*

11. Heat-seal the ampoules at the point of constriction using the twin flame air/gas torch (at this point the moisture content should be 1–2% by dry weight).

B. *Recovery*

1. Scratch the ampoule at the centre of the cotton wool plug using the glass cutter.

2. Snap open the ampoule, remove the cotton plug, add about 0.3 ml sterile distilled water, replace the plug and allow 30 min for absorption of water.

3. Streak the contents on to a suitable growth medium and incubate under optimum conditions.

[a] There are many suspending media used to protect cells (20).

The retention of viability of many fungi also depends upon ensuring that the suspension and cells remain frozen during drying until the water content is reduced significantly ($< 5\%$).

Fungal cells must be dried below $-15\,°C$ until this level of moisture content is reached (20). Residual moisture content at the end of the process is also quite critical; this should be about 2% to retain cell viability. If the water content is too high approximately 10% shorter survival periods will result. For example, the viability of *Aspergillus niger* and *Penicillium ochrochloron* decreased by 50% during the first year of storage at IMI (20). If the water content is below 1% it is possible that the removal of structural water could cause permanent damage to the cells. Storage at temperatures of $15-20\,°C$ proved successful at IMI, but others recommend lower storage temperatures, for example $+4\,°C$ (21).

The method can be controlled much more efficiently on a shelf freeze-drier to achieve the above parameters. Protocols can be developed to preserve individual organisms. *Protocol 6* outlines a method which can be modified to suit more susceptible cells.

Protocol 6. Shelf-freeze drying at IMI

Equipment and reagents

- Sterile 10% (w/v) skimmed milk + 5% (w/v) inositol
- Shelf freeze-drier Minifast 3400 (Edwards High Vacuum International)
- Sterile 2 ml preconstricted long-necked vials with butyl rubber bungs (vampoules)
- Glass cutter in support handle
- Air/gas glass-blower's torch (Vacuum Industrial Products Ltd)

For recovery:
- Sterile distilled water
- Sterile cotton plugs to fit the neck of the vampoules

A. *Shelf-freezing*

1. Pre-cool the shelf of the Minifast 3400 freeze-drier to $-35\,°C$.

2. Prepare a suspension of spores or cells in sterile 10% (w/v) skimmed milk and 5% (w/v) inositol

3. Remove the bung from each vampoule and add approximately 0.5 ml of suspension using a Pasteur pipette.

4. Replace the rubber bung to the marked, partially closed level and load on to the pre-cooled shelf of the freeze-drier.

5. Place the sample probe into a vampoule with sterile 0.5% (w/v) skimmed milk and 5% inositol as a control.

6. Close the chamber door.

7. When the control sample temperature reaches $-20\,°C$ evacuate the chamber.

8. Using the T-matic temperature controller hold the shelf temperature at $-35\,°C$ for 3 h and then raise the shelf temperature 0.08 °C min to $+10\,°C$.

9. When the pressure in the chamber is close or equal to the pressure measured just above the vacuum pump, seal the ampoules by lowering the shelf stoppering device to push in the bungs.

10. Bring the chamber to atmospheric pressure and unload the vampoules.

11. Heat-seal the vampoules at the neck below the bung with the air/gas glass-blower's torch.

12. Store the vampoules at approximately 18 °C.

B. *Recovery*

1. Scratch the glass vampoule at the pre-constriction with a glass cutter and snap open.

2. Add 0.5 ml of distilled water and place a sterile cotton wool plug into the neck of the open vampoule.

3. After 30 min, streak the contents of the vampoule on to a suitable growth medium and incubate at an appropriate temperature.

[a] Storage temperature can be in the range $-70\,°C$ to room temperature; the lower the temperature the slower will be the deterioration.

Freeze-drying should be optimized for different cell types and if this is done it is successful for bacteria, sporulating fungi, and yeasts. It is generally unsatisfactory for eukaryotic microalgae. More development is required to achieve successful methods for algae and protozoa, although cyanobacteria are more likely to survive.

3.4 Cryopreservation

Frozen storage of cells at temperatures where no chemical or physical change can occur is the ideal method of preservation. To determine the optimum conditions for a particular cell could be time-consuming. It requires optimum growth conditions for the organism to prepare the cells for removal of water during cooling, the most suitable cryoprotectant must be found, and then the optimum cooling and subsequent thawing protocols must be employed. Generally, a routine method is chosen for the cells and only when difficulties are encountered is an optimum protocol devised. Slow cooling in 10% (v/v) glycerol followed by rapid warming (*Protocol 7*) is quite often selected. Optimum conditions can be determined by the use of a cryogenic light microscope (23) where the effects of different protocols on the cell can be observed and the least stressful conditions used. A method for the cryopreservation of hyperthermophiles is given in Chapter 2, *Protocol 5*.

Protocol 7. Cryopreservation

Equipment and reagents

- Sterile 10% (v/v) glycerol[a]
- 2.0 ml sterile graduated cryotubes[b] labelled with strain number (LabM)
- Sterile Pasteur pipettes
- Liquid nitrogen
- Controlled rate freezer (Planer Products Ltd)
- Liquid nitrogen storage freezer with metal drawer rack inventory control system (Statebourne Cryogenics)

A. *Cryopreservation*

1. Prepare the spore or cell suspensions in 10% (v/v) glycerol.

2. Pipette 0.5 ml of the cell suspension into the 2.0 ml sterile cryotubes.

3. Cool in a controlled rate freezer to −50°C.[c]

4. Transfer to a metal drawer rack in the liquid nitrogen storage freezer to complete cooling to the storage temperature.

B. *Recovery*

1. Thaw the cryotube rapidly by placing it in a water-bath at +37°C or in the chamber of the controlled cooler on a warming cycle until the sample ampoule, monitored with a temperature probe, thaws.

---

[a] There are many suspending media (cryoprotectants) that can be used for different cells (9).
[b] The Prolab microbank system can be used where the cryotubes are filled with cryoprotectant and glass beads. Recovery of the strain can be achieved by chipping off a bead and placing it in growth medium (22).
[c] The optimum cooling rate for the cell type should be employed. Cooling at −10°C/min may be applied as a routine.

3.4.1 Cryoprotection

Cell cryoprotection is normally obtained by placing the cells in a cryoprotective additive and allowing them to equilibrate in it, between 1 and 2 h is normally sufficient. The most commonly used are glycerol or dimethylsufoxide. However, there are extensive lists of chemicals that have been used (9). It is quite common to find naturally occurring osmoregulatory chemicals in cells which protect against the stresses of cooling. The stresses are primarily concentration effects and mechanical damage caused by the presence of ice. The presence of such chemicals can be induced by growing the cells to be preserved under osmotic stress, and, in a few cases, this has been successful at IMI. In other instances, suspending cells in an aqueous solution can be damaging in itself and slightly air-dried spores can be frozen dry with greater success (24).

3.4.2. Cooling rate

Although different cooling rates can have dramatic effects on cells it is normally a combination of cryoprotectant and suitable cooling rate that allows the successful freezing of cells. Normally, slow cooling causes cell shrinkage as the cell loses water when ice is formed outside the cell thus concentrating the extracelluar solution. As the cell membrane is not normally elastic, membrane deletions can occur as it folds in on itself. If on warming, this material cannot be re-incorporated into the cell membrane, the cell may rupture. Some fungal cells have been seen to survive this by losing cytoplasm and on thawing remaining at only 70–80% of their original size, eventually resynthesizing membrane and growing normally. This has been observed in *Lentinus edodes* the Shiitake mushroom (25). Addition of a cryoprotective agent, one that mimics water and can replace it, prevents shrinkage and the cell survives well.

Fast cooling normally induces intracellular ice, an event which is lethal to many vegetative cells. Although many fungi and a few algae can withstand ice formation within the cell it is best avoided as it can cause sublethal damage causing, at the very least, delays in recovery (9).

3.4.3 Storage temperature

Organisms are stored at many subzero temperatures, from $-10\,°C$ in the icebox of a refrigerator to $-196\,°C$ immersed in liquid nitrogen. However, it is only when the cell cytoplasm is frozen that the organism is considered to be in frozen storage. In some fungi the cytoplasm does not freeze until $-25\,°C$ to $-30\,°C$ (26). Therefore, in the freezer at $-10\,°C$ to $-25\,°C$ metabolism can still occur and in some cells can occur down to $-70\,°C$. It is not until $-130\,°C$ is reached that the structure of frozen water is stable. Organisms should be stored in freezers that maintain temperatures of $-135\,°C$ or below or in liquid nitrogen ($-196\,°C$) to achieve stability.

Table 1. Response of microorganisms to preservation techniques

Organism	Protocol 1 Oil storage	Protocol 2 Water storage	Protocol 3 Silica gel storage	Protocol 4 L-drying	Protocol 5 Spin freeze-drying	Protocol 6 Shelf freeze-drying	Protocol 7 Cryopreservation in liquid nitrogen
Algae	Not applicable in most cases	Used in regular subculture; successful for some species	Not applicable	Not used for these organisms	Not applicable to most cells; only Cyanobacteria survive well	See *Protocol 5*	Most appropriate method
Animal cell lines	Not applicable	Not applicable	Not applicable	Not applicable	Not applicable	Not applicable	Protocols developed for all cell lines
Bacteria	Useful but only for short-term	A useful method for short-term storage; Enterobacteriaceae do not recover well	A great number of species fail, but several survive	A good long-term method particularly those sensitive to freeze-drying	Good, but some bacteria are sensitive	Controlled cooling will allow more cells to survive	Successful for most species
Fungi (filamentous)	Good long-term method; some sensitive species	Good short-term method for most species	Only useful for sporulating fungi but not Oomycota well	Many fungi are sensitive usually low survival	Most sporulating fungi survive; some sensitive	All sporulating species except some Oomycota	Successful for nearly all species
Plant cell lines	Not applicable	Not applicable	Not applicable	Not applicable	Not applicable	Not applicable	Best technique available, some cells are sensitive and some fail to survive
Plasmids	Not applicable	Not applicable	Little used	Not normally used	Useful method although poor technique may cause failure	Limited information, should be better than *Protocol 5*	Most useful method
Viruses	Not applicable	Not applicable	Little used	Not normally used	Plant viruses survive better than animal viruses	Useful method used extensively in vaccine preparations	Most useful method
Yeasts	Not an ideal method but has been used	A useful method for 5 years storage for most species	Poor recoveries are quite normal, useful for some species	Little information available	Strain specific, but quite often low recoveries result	Little information on use of improved techniques	Most appropriate method. Most cells survive with high recoveries

3.4.4 Warming rate for recovery of the cell

Having successfully frozen the cell, all the good work can be undone if the cell is damaged during thawing. Normally, rapid thawing is required to avoid recrystallization of ice and other deleterious effects (27). This is usually achieved by placing ampoules in a water-bath at 37 °C until the last ice crystal melts or in a controlled rate cooler on a thaw cycle.

3.5 Summary

Cryopreservation, particularly in liquid nitrogen or in freezers at −135 °C or below, is the best preservation method for all cell types. The handling techniques, freezing protocol, cryopreservation, and thawing rates can be optimized for the particular cell. Once the cell is successfully frozen and stored, the shelf-life is considered to be infinite. Freeze-drying is probably considered a more useful technique if the cells are to be distributed from the collection. However, fewer organisms survive this technique and recovery of cells is lower than from cryopreservation. Other methods discussed here are useful but have their limitations. The applicability of the seven protocols discussed in this chapter is summarized in *Table 1*.

References

1. Bridge, P. D. and Hawksworth, D. L. (1990). *Genet. Eng. Biotechnol.*, **10**, 9–11.
2. Gams, W., Hennebert, G. L., Stalpers, J. A., Jansens, D., Schipper, M. A. A., Smith, J. *et al.* (1988). *J. Gen. Microbiol.*, **134**, 1667–89.
3. Stalpers, J. A., Kracht, M., Jansens, D., De Ley, J., Van der Toorn, J., Smith, J., *et al.* (1990). *Systemat. Appl. Microbiol.*, **13**, 92–103.
4. Hawksworth, D. L., Sastramihardja, I., Kokke, R. and Stevenson, R. (1990). Guidelines for the establishment and operation of collections of cultures of microorganisms. World Federation for Culture Collections, WFCC Secretariat, Brazil.
5. Stevenson, R. E. and Jong, S. C. (1992). *World J. Microbiol. Biotechnol.*, **8**, 229–35.
6. Ratledge, C. and Da Silva, E. (1990). *World J. Microbiol. Biotechnol.*, **6**, 3–5.
7. Aguilar, A. (ed.) (1990). *European laboratory without walls: In the field of MINE, the microbial information network Europe*. Commission of the European Communities, Brussels.
8. Sugawara, H., Ma, J., Miyazaki, S., Shimura, J. and Takishima, Y. (ed.) (1993). *World directory of collections of cultures of microorganisms: bacteria, fungi and yeasts* (4th edn). World Federation for Culture Collections World Data Center on Microorganisms, Saitama, Japan.
9. Smith, D. and Onions, A. H. S. (1994). *The preservation and maintenance of living fungi* (2nd edn). IMI Technical Handbooks, no. 2, International Mycological Institute, Egham, UK.
10. Kirsop, B. E. and Doyle, A. (ed.) (1991). *Maintenance of microorganisms and cultured cells: a manual of laboratory methods* (2nd edn). Academic Press, London.

11. Lapage, S. P. and Redway, K. F. (1974). *Preservation of bacteria with notes on other microorganisms.* Public Health Laboratory Service Monograph Series No. 7 (ed. A. T. Willis and C. H. Collins). HMSO, London.
12. Malik, K. A. (1991). In *Maintenance of microorganisms and cultured cells: a manual of laboratory methods* (2nd edn), (ed. B. E. Kirsop and A. Doyle), pp. 121–132. Academic Press, London.
13. Boeswinkel, H. J. (1976). *Trans. Br. Mycol. Soc.*, **66**, 183–5.
14. McGinnis, M. R., Padhye, A. A., and Ajello, L. (1974). *Appl. Microbiol.*, **28**, 218–22.
15. Kirsop, B. E. (1991). In *Maintenance of microorganisms and cultured cells: a manual of laboratory methods* (2nd ed.), (ed. B. E. Kirsop and A. Doyle), pp. 161–82. Academic Press, London.
16. Perkins, D. D. (1962). *Can. J. Microbiol.*, **8**, 591–4.
17. Dando, T. R. and Bousfield, I. J. (1991). In *Maintenance of microorganisms and cultured cells: a manual of laboratory methods* (2nd edn), (ed. B. E. Kirsop and A. Doyle), pp. 57–63. Academic Press, London.
18. Tommerup, I. C. (1988). *Trans. Br. Mycol. Soc.*, **90**, 585–91.
19. Rudge, R. H. (1991). In *Maintenance of microorganisms and cultured cells: a manual of laboratory methods* (2nd edn), (ed. B. E. Kirsop and A. Doyle), pp. 31–43. Academic Press, London.
20. Smith, D. (1986). *The evaluation and development of techniques for the preservation of fungi.* A thesis submitted to London University for the degree of Doctor of Philosophy.
21. Heckly, R. J. (1978). *Adv. Appl. Microbiol.*, **24**, 1–53.
22. Chandler, D. (1994). *Mycol. Res.*, **98**, 525–6.
23. Smith, D. (1992). *Lab. Pract.*, **41**, 25–28,
24. Holden, A. and Smith, D. (1992). *Mycol. Res.*, **96**, 473–6.
25. Roquebert, M. F. and Bury, E. (1993). *World J. Microbiol. Biotechnol.*, **9**, 641–7.
26. Morris, G. J., Smith, D., and Coulson, G. E. (1988). *J. Gen. Microbiol.*, **134**, 2987–906.
27. Smith, D. (1993). In *Stress tolerance of fungi* (ed. D. H. Jennings), pp. 145–171. Marcel Dekker, Inc., NY.

2

Isolation and growth of hyperthermophiles

RICHARD J. SHARP and NEIL D. H. RAVEN

1. Introduction

This chapter discusses the problems encountered in the isolation and cultivation of hyperthermophilic microorganisms and presents procedures and guidance for working with the more common hyperthermophiles. We define hyperthermophiles as organisms with growth optima of $> 75\,°C$. This excludes thermophilic *Bacillus* and *Thermus* species which have recently been discussed in other reviews (1, 2). The chapter will describe procedures which have been applied to the growth of both hyperthermophilic Archaea and Bacteria.

2. The isolation of hyperthermophiles

2.1 Geothermal environments

Many environments are extremely inhospitable to man and most micro-organisms, but provide unique ecological niches which are colonized by specialized groups of microorganisms. These environments encompass extremes of temperature, pH, salinity, pressure, and radiation. The majority of the organisms colonizing these environments have only been isolated within the past 10–20 years as techniques for their growth and study have developed. Many are members of the Archaea, first described from the work of Woese and Fox (3) as a third primary kingdom, the Archaebacteria, and now designated the Archaea (4). The Archaea include the methanogens, extreme halophiles, and the majority of hyperthermophiles. The hyperthermophiles have received considerable attention, both as a potential source of highly thermostable biocatalysts and for their apparent evolutionary antiquity. There are a number of recent reviews covering aspects of the ecology, biology, molecular biology, and biotechnology of extremophiles and the Archaea (5–17).

Geothermal environments are distributed across the earth and are primarily associated with areas of tectonic activity. Major geothermal areas studied as a source of hyperthermophilic microorganisms include New Zealand, Iceland, Yellowstone USA, Italy, The Azores, and Japan. Ground water percolates into the earth where, at depths of 500–3000 m, it is heated by magma. Under hydrostatic pressure the water does not initially boil, but as the temperature increases thermal expansion forces the water back up to the surface. As the pressure decreases, the water boils, forcing more water to the surface resulting in the eruption of geysers and hot springs.

The pH of terrestrial thermal environments generally falls within the ranges 1–2.5 or 6.0–8.5. These reflect the chemical composition of the two main components, sulfuric acid with a pK_a of 1.8 and sodium carbonate and sodium bicarbonate with a pK_a of 6.3 and 10.2. The origin of the buffering agents and the dissolved minerals carried to the surface by hot water have a profound effect on the surface environment and colonizing microbial population.

Solfatara fields, associated with acid soils, the presence of sulfur, acidic hot springs, and boiling mud pots are generally located within active volcanic regions where the heat source is at a depth of up to 5 km. The water temperature is 150–300 °C at depths of 500–3000 m. Steam and volcanic gases comprising principally CO_2, N_2, H_2S, and H_2 are emitted at the surface, where H_2S is oxidized chemically and biologically to sulfur and sulfuric acid. The low pH results in the corrosion of rocks and the formation of acidic muds. Geothermal areas away from volcanic activity are heated by deep lava flows or dead magma chambers where at 500–3000 m the water is generally below 150 °C. These, typified by the upper geyser basin in Yellowstone National Park, are associated with freshwater hot springs and geysers, at neutral to alkaline pH. The ground water returns to the surface and contains dissolved minerals such as silica and dissolved gases such as CO_2 and H_2S. The concentration of H_2S is relatively low and with the larger volumes of water, surface oxidation has little effect on the pH. The CO_2 is dissipated and silica is precipitated, resulting in an increase in the pH. The pH in these environments often stabilizes at pH 8–9 and these areas are frequently heavily encrusted with silicates. Similar marine environments are found at great depths in ocean rifts such as the East Pacific Rise (2500–2600 m) or the Guaymas basin (2000 m), where temperatures of 350–400 °C have been recorded in the vents. The surrounding sea water at 4 °C results in a very steep temperature gradient.

2.2 Sampling geothermal environments

Most of the hyperthermophilic microorganisms isolated and characterized from geothermal environments have been derived from samples collected and transported to the laboratory at ambient temperature. The need to maintain samples at the original source temperature during transfer is not normally a problem. Samples collected, stored at 2–6 °C and subsequently examined 4–5 years later have enabled the isolation of a number of organisms.

Studies using most probable number (MPN) techniques, demonstrated little decrease in the numbers of thermophilic methanogens in samples stored in a cold room for 3 years. *Methanobacterium thermoautotrophicum*, for example, was isolated from samples stored for 5 years (18).

Samples should be stored at 4–6°C since, although the hyperthermophiles are unable to grow at mesophilic temperatures, the growth of mesophiles can result in deterioration of the samples. Where gas-tight sample bottles are used, cooling the sample will cause the development of a negative pressure resulting in an influx of air when the sample tube is opened. To avoid pressure changes the sample tube should be completely filled with liquid during sampling. The exclusion of air will also aid the survival of obligate anaerobes.

Sampling of hot springs, geysers, and solfataric pools should be treated with extreme caution. The ground may be unstable and the eruption of geysers cannot always be predicted. The measurement of pH, temperature, dissolved oxygen, conductivity, and other physical parameters are best done directly at the site being sampled. Where direct measurement is impossible large samples should be collected to enable indirect measurements to be made. A range of appropriate portable equipment is now available. It is vital to ensure that spare probes and appropriate pH buffers are also available. For sampling terrestrial sites it is useful to have an extension rod fitted with appropriate clamps to carry probes or sample bottles.

Sampling containers commonly used include 2–5 ml cryotubes (Nalgene), 25 ml Universal bottles (Sterilin) or, for the isolation of thermophilic anaerobes, glass serum bottles fitted with butyl rubber stoppers which can be sealed with aluminium crimp caps. The addition of a drop of 1% sodium dithionite will ensure reducing conditions are maintained. As a redox indicator a drop of 1% resazurin indicates oxidizing conditions by the formation of a red colour. (This reaction becomes unreliable below 4.5 since it also acts as a pH indicator.)

Thermoacidophiles maintain a pH gradient across their membrane during active metabolism, ensuring a near neutral internal cytoplasm. When the temperature is reduced and metabolism ceases the maintenance of this gradient is disrupted and may result in death of the cells. To avoid this, samples should be neutralized by the addition of $CaCO_3$ immediately after collection.

Protocol 1. Collection of samples from marine geothermal environments

This procedure has been used for the isolation of marine hyperthermophiles from vents in shallow waters off the coast of Vulcano, Italy (19), at depths of 2–10 m and vent and sediment temperatures of 103°C. *Pyrodictum occultum, Pyrodictum brockii* (20), *Pyrococcus furiosus* (21), and *Pyrococcus woesei* (22), for example, have been isolated using this procedure.

Protocol 1. *Continued*

Equipment and reagents

- Syringes fitted with enlarged inlet ports
- Glass serum bottles
- Butyl rubber septa and aluminium crimp caps
- Crimper for aluminium cap
- Resazurin solution 1 g/litre
- Anaerobic gas—H_2/CO_2 (80:20) or oxygen-free nitrogen
- Sulfur
- Sodium dithionite solution, 1%
- Trace element solution: Nitrilotriacetic acid 1.5 g, $MgSO_4 \times 7 H_2O$ 3.0 g, $MnSO_4 \times 2 H_2O$ 0.5 g, NaCl 1.0 g, $FeSO_4 \times 7 H_2O$ 0.1 g, $CoSO_4 \times 7 H_2O$ 0.18 g, $CaCl_2 \times 2 H_2O$ 0.1 g, $ZnSO_4 \times 7 H_2O$ 0.18 g, $CuSO_4 \times 5 H_2O$

0.01 g, $KAl(SO_4)_2 \times 12 H_2$) 0.02 g, H_3BO_3 0.01 g, $Na_2MoO_4 \times 2 H_2O$ 0.01 g, $NiCl_2 \times 6 H_2O$ 0.025 g, $Na_2SeO_3 \times 5 H_2O$ 0.3 mg, Distilled water 1000.0 ml. First dissolve nitrilotriacetic acid and adjust pH to 6.5 with KOH, then add minerals. Final pH 7.0 (with KOH).
- SME medium (20): NaBr 0.05 g, H_3BO_3 0.015 g, $SrCl_2 \times 6 H_2O$ 7.5 mg, $(NH_4)_2SO_4$ 10.0 mg, Citric acid 5.0 mg, KI 0.05 mg, $CaCl_2 \times 2 H_2O$ 0.75 g, KH_2PO_4 0.5 g, $NiCl_2 \times 6 H_2O$ 2.0 mg, Trace minerals 10.0 ml, Resazurin 1.0 mg, Yeast extract 2.0 g, Sulfur, powdered 30.0 mg, $Na_2S \times 9 H_2O$ 0.5 g, Distilled water 1000.0 ml. Adjust pH to 5.5 with 10 N sulfuric acid.

Method

1. Agitate the sediment as deeply as possible and draw into a syringe fitted with an enlarged inlet.

2. At the surface, transfer the hot samples to serum bottles filled with H_2/CO_2 (80:20) or N_2 containing 3 g sulfur and 10 µl of resazurin solution (1 g/litre) and immediately seal with rubber stoppers.

3. Remove residual oxygen by injecting a drop of sodium dithionite solution (1%).

4. To enrich for microorganisms such as *Pyrococcus*, for example, add 1 ml of the sample to 10 ml of sulfur-containing culture medium (e.g. SME) and maintain under N_2 or H_2/CO_2 (80:20) with 1 bar overpressure.

5. After one day's incubation at 100°C coccoid cells become visible in successful enrichments.

6. Transfer the cultures to fresh medium and purify by three series of serial dilutions.

3. Media for the growth of hyperthermophiles

3.1 Liquid media

The media used for the cultivation of hyperthermophiles are varied, but all contain a basic mineral salts and trace element component often derived from media developed originally for the cultivation of more moderate thermophiles (e.g. 23, 24). Many organic media components, particularly sugars, will be degraded when held for prolonged periods above 60°C.

Since hyperthermophilic microorganisms are exposed to high temperatures for prolonged periods of time it is valuable to avoid any unnecessary prior exposure of the media to heat. This minimizes both inorganic precipitate formation and organic thermal decomposition. For this reason, all hyperthermo-phile media used in our laboratories are routinely sterilized by filtration (where a component is present which is not readily solubilized and filter-sterilized, e.g. starch, it is autoclaved separately as a concentrated stock solution).

Elemental sulfur is essential for the growth of many hyperthermophiles in closed bottles. Even where it does not appear to be essential, for example, for *Pyrococcus furiosus*, it may give increased cell densities and longer storage times as viable cultures. One problem with the use of sulfur is that it is virtu-ally insoluble in water and melts at less than 120°C thus losing its micro-crystalline form. This means that its sterilization is problematical for normal laboratory use since neither filter sterilization nor autoclaving at 121°C is suitable. Three procedures are routinely used to produce sterilized sulfur, (a) tyndallization, where wetted sulfur is heated at 100°C for 1 hour on three consecutive days, (b) autoclaving at 112–115°C in the presence of air for 30–60 minutes, and (c) dissolving the sulfur in concentrated sulfide solutions and autoclaving conventionally at 121°C for 15 minutes. Although all three procedures have been used successfully, procedure (b) may be preferable since procedure (a) theoretically does not kill all microorganisms (with the discovery of microaerophilic/aerotolerant hyperthermophiles, e.g. *Pyrobacu-lum aerophilum*) and procedure (c) can only provide a limited quantity of elemental sulfur upon dissociation of the polysulfides formed, because of the requirement for at least equimolar sulfide to be also supplied.

Protocol 2. Liquid medium for the growth of *Pyrococcus furiosus* (see ref. 25, modified from ref. 20)

Equipment and reagents

- Static incubator set at 90–100°C
- Oxygen-free nitrogen cylinder
- Filters, 0.2 μm (presterilized, disposable), e.g. Ministart NML (Sartorius)
- Glass serum bottles, e.g. 50 ml or 125 ml
- Butyl rubber septa, 20 mm diameter
- Aluminium crimp caps, for the above
- Crimper
- Needles (presterilized, disposable), 25 gauge, 25 mm long
- Autoclave tape
- Magnesium salts solution (per litre): 180 g $MgSO_4 \cdot 7H_2O$, 140 g $MgCl_2 \cdot 6H_2O$
- Solution A (per litre): 9 g $MnSO_4 \cdot 4H_2O$, 2.5 g $ZnSO_4 \cdot 7H_2O$, 2.5 g $NiCl_2 \cdot 6H_2O$, 0.3 g $KAl(SO_4)_2 \cdot 12H_2O$, 0.3 g $CoCl_2 \cdot 6H_2O$, 0.15 g $CuSO_4 \cdot 5H_2O$
- Solution B (per litre): 56 g $CaCl_2 \cdot 2H_2O$, 25 g NaBr, 10 g KI, 4 g $SrCl_2 \cdot 6H_2O$
- Solution C (per litre): 500 g K_2HPO_4, 7.5 g H_3BO_3, 3.3 g $Na_2WO_4 \cdot 2H_2O$, 0.15 g $Na_2MoO_4 \cdot 2H_2O$, 0.005 g $NaSeO_3$
- Solution D (per litre): 10 g $FeCl_2 \cdot 4H_2O$. Make up in 1 M HCl
- Vitamin solution (per litre): 200 mg pyri-doxine hydrochloride 100 mg thiamine hydrochloride, 100 mg riboflavin, 100 mg nicotinic acid, 100 mg DL-calcium pan-tothenate, 100 mg lipoic acid, 40 mg biotin, 40 mg folic acid, 2 mg cyanocobalamin. Make up in 50% v/v ethanol
- Resazurin solution, 1 g/litre
- Peptone (Difco)
- Yeast extract (Difco)
- L-cysteine
- Medium (per litre): Add the following, in order and with mixing, to 900 ml H_2O. 10 ml magnesium salts solution, 1 ml Solution A, 1 ml Solution B, 1 ml Solution C, 1 ml Solution D, 1 ml vitamin solution, 1 ml resazurin solution, 28 g sodium chloride, 5 g peptone, 1 g yeast extract, 0.5 g L-cys-teine. Adjust the pH to 7.0 at room temper-ature with 2 M NaOH and the volume to 1 litre with distilled water

Protocol 2. *Continued*

Method

1. Weigh out 0.2 g of elemental sulfur (from a stock ground to a fine powder using a pestle and mortar) and pour into a 50 ml serum bottle (or 0.5 g for 125 ml bottle).

2. Cap the serum bottle with a butyl rubber septum and cover the top with aluminium foil. Hold foil loosely in place with a strip of autoclave tape.

3. Autoclave the covered bottle at 112–115°C for 30 min.

4. Prepare the growth medium as described above.

5. Remove the autoclave tape from the bottle, lift the septum, and introduce 20 ml of medium via a 0.2 μm sterile filter.

6. Replace the septum and seal the top with an aluminium crimp cap; flush the headspace at room temperature for 5 min with oxygen-free nitrogen via 25-gauge needles, with a sterile filter on the inlet side.

7. Place the bottle in a 100°C incubator for 1 h, take out, and allow to cool. A pale straw colour indicates that the medium is reduced.

8. Inoculate bottle with a 1% inoculum from a previous stock culture of *Pyrococcus furiosus*, again aseptically and without introducing air, via a 25-gauge needle.

9. Incubate at 90–100°C for 8–16 hours depending upon the age of the stock culture.

10. Examine a sample of the culture by phase-contrast microscopy at 400 × magnification using a Helber counting chamber with Thoma ruling (Weber Scientific). The cell count should be in the region of $1–3 \times 10^8$/ml. Continue incubation if it is below this level.

11. Remove from the incubator and allow to cool. Flush the headspace again with filter-sterilized, oxygen-free nitrogen for 5 min and leave a slight overpressure.

12. Store the bottle at 4°C. Cultures prepared in this manner routinely remain viable for at least 6 months.

3.2 Preparation of solidified media

A number of gelling agents have been used for the preparation of plating media. The inability to grow discrete single colonies for the characterization, enumeration, and purification of cultures has been a considerable impediment to the study of hyperthermophiles.

3.2.1 Agar

Agar is used as the gelling agent in most bacteriological media. Agar melts at temperatures between 85 and 100°C and resolidifies between 35 and 45°C depending upon the grade of agar and degree of polymerization. It is suitable for the culture of most thermophilic bacteria up to 65–70°C, above which the agar becomes rapidly dehydrated. Increasing the agar concentration up to 4% w/v enables its use up to 75°C for limited incubation periods. Incubating plates in plastic bags can help to reduce water loss particularly in incubators with fan-assisted air circulation, however, the build up of condensate can result in very wet conditions on the plates. Plastic Petri dishes start to buckle at temperatures above 65°C, therefore the use of glass dishes is necessary. Agar is hydrolysed when autoclaved at low pH and fails to gel when cool. Where agar is used as the gelling agent for acidophiles the salts and nutrients should be adjusted to the correct pH and added after sterilization to molten concentrated agar.

3.2.2 Polyacrylamide

Thermoproteus tenax has been cultured on plates containing 5% polyacrylamide (containing 1.3 g/L *N,N'*-methylene bisacrylamide polymerized with sodium persulfate and *N,N,N',N'*-tetramethylethylenediamine) in a desiccator under N_2 equilibrated with an anaerobic modification of *Sulfolobus* medium (23, 26).

3.2.3 Silica gel

Media solidified with silica gel has been applied to the isolation and study of bacteria under hydrostatic pressure (27) and some thermophilic and hyperthermophilic microorganisms. Silica gel must be dissolved in alkali (7% w/v KOH) and is solidified by the addition of a strong mineral acid (2% phosphoric acid). It must then be equilibrated with other medium components (18). It is generally considered to be relatively laborious to prepare. Polysilicate or water glass has also been used as a solid support for enrichments of marine isolates (22).

3.2.4 Gelrite

Gelrite was first described by Lin and Casida (28) for the cultivation of thermophilic bacteria. Their initial studies examined the growth of *Bacillus stearothermophilus*, *Alicyclobacillus acidocaldarius*, *Thermus thermophilus*, and *Thermus aquaticus* at incubation temperatures up to 70°C. Gelrite (deacylated gellan gum PS-60) is derived from a polysaccharide produced by a species of *Sphingomonas* and marketed by Kelco (a division of Merck). Gelrite has been shown to remain solid under elevated pressure at temperatures up to 120°C. In contrast to agar, gelrite requires the presence of cations for gelation (30). Divalent cations (e.g. Ca^{2+} and Mg^{2+}) appear to give greater gel strengths at much lower concentrations than monovalent cations (e.g. Na^+ and K^+). For marine hyperthermophiles this does not present a problem since the concentrations of both divalent and monovalent cations in sea water based media are already sufficiently high to give firm gels. For terrestrial hyperthermophiles, however, the concentrations of the cations required are frequently higher than the organisms would be exposed to in their natural environment, therefore, care has to be taken to provide a combination of cation and Gelrite concentrations which is not inhibitory to growth but gives a firm gel at the required temperature. Since this varies from organism to organism, along with a much wider pH range for growth, it is impossible to give generalized conditions for the plating of terrestrial hyperthermophiles. By contrast, marine-based formulations should generally be easily interchangeable, providing that the nutritional requirements of the organism are met. Examples of the application of Gelrite for the cultivation of hyperthermophiles include *Sulfolobus* species (31), *Pyrococcus abyssi* (32), *Pyrococcus woesei* (22), and *Hyperthermus butylicus* (33). A procedure which has successfully been used in our laboratories for the recovery of single colonies of the most frequently grown hyperthermophile, the heterotrophic marine archaeon *Pyrococcus furiosus*, is described in *Protocol 3*.

Protocol 3. Plating of *Pyrococcus furiosus* on Gelrite medium

Equipment and reagents

- Glass Petri dishes (90 mm diameter)
- Glass beads (2 mm diameter)
- Glass Universal bottles (25 ml capacity)
- Serum bottles (50 ml capacity)
- Sterile disposable filters (0.2 μm), e.g. Ministart
- Anaerobic chamber
- Incubator
- Gelrite
- Growth medium: 2 × concentration given in *Protocol 2*—see step 2 in method below.
- Oxygen-free nitrogen

Method

1. Autoclave the Petri dishes, glass beads, and a 2% solution of gelrite in water at 121°C for 15 min (20 ml aliquots in 25 ml glass bottles). Place the hot molten gelrite solution (>80°C) in an incubator at 80°C.[a]

2. Prepare *Pyrococcus furiosus* growth medium at 2 × concentration (ref. 25, *Protocol 2*), with 1 g/L sodium sulfide•$9H_2O$[b] added as the last component but directly before the adjustment of the pH to 7.0. Filter-sterilize immediately in 20 ml aliquots into 50 ml capacity serum bottles.[c] Place in the incubator at 80°C for 10 min.

3. Prepare serial dilutions of the culture in aliquots of anaerobic growth medium (e.g. 1 ml transfers via syringe and needle into 9 ml of medium) and label the glass plates with the range required.

4. Add bottles of Gelrite solution individually to bottles of 2 × medium, mix by repeated inversion, and pour the contents (40 ml) into a glass Petri dish (plates set almost immediately). Repeat for the required number of plates.

5. Pour 5–10 glass beads on to the surface of each plate and dispense 100 μl aliquots of the serially diluted culture. Replace the lids and swirl the plates to distribute the culture uniformly. Invert the plate allowing the beads to drop on to the plate lid.[c]

---

6. Place the plates in the anaerobic chamber, seal and purge with sterile oxygen-free nitrogen for 5 minutes at room temperature.

7. Place in the incubator and continue purging with nitrogen for 15 min whilst the anaerobic chamber and contents are warming (this removes any residual oxygen from the medium and also condensate from the glass lids caused by pouring the plates at high temperature).

8. Seal the anaerobic chamber with a positive pressure of nitrogen (0.5–1 bar) and increase the incubator temperature to 90°C. Incubate for approximately 3 days at this temperature, allow to cool, and open the anaerobic chamber.[c]

[a] The molten Gelrite solution can be actively deoxygenated by gassing with filter-sterilized nitrogen. This has not been found to be necessary for *Pyrococcus furiosus*.
[b] For organisms with an obligate sulfur requirement, the sodium sulfide solution can be replaced by a saturated polysulfide solution (approximately 20% by weight S^0 suspended in a freshly prepared 50% solution of $Na_2S \cdot 9H_2O$ and autoclaved at 121°C for 15 minutes).
[c] These steps are carried out on the laboratory bench; media preparation for more fastidious anaerobes may require the use of an anaerobic cabinet.

3.2.5 Starch

Starch has been used as a solidifying agent for the cultivation of several thermophiles and hyperthermophiles including *Pyrobaculum islandicum* (34), *Thermoplasma acidophilum* and *Thermoplasma volcanium* (35), and thermo-acidophiles from solfataras in Naples (36).

4. Growth and bioreactors for hyperthermophiles

4.1 Introduction

The growth of microorganisms at temperatures up to 113°C, under pressures up to 300 bar, in medium which can contain up to at least 7% salt, and actively producing H_2S presents a considerable challenge to the design of laboratory equipment and fermentation systems. Similarly, microbes growing at temperatures up to 96°C and at pHs as low as 1 present a different set of challenges.

With a few exceptions most small-scale and large-scale fermentation equipment are constructed from stainless steel or glass, or a combination of the two. Stainless steel combines robustness, good machinability, and resistance to corrosion through the addition of chromium. The leaching of heavy metal ions from stainless steel reactors has, however, been reported to seriously inhibit the growth of some microorganisms (37). To provide enhanced resistance to corrosion in specific chemical environments other elements are added, giving a range of stainless steels each with particular characteristics (38).

The addition of nickel improves the ability of stainless steel to form a protective oxide film (passive film) over the surface, especially in the presence of strong oxidizing acids such as HNO_3. This process is known as passivation. When exposed to strong hydrochloric acid, acidity dominates the mildly oxidizing capacity of dissolved oxygen and corrosion is rapid. In dilute phosphoric acid, stainless steels are generally passive, particularly in the presence of dissolved oxygen or oxidizing ions such as the ferric ion. Organic acids are considerably less corrosive than inorganic acids. Acetic acid solutions are on the boundary of being passive or active. Austenitic stainless steels become active as the temperature is increased.

The addition of molybdenum to stainless steel improves resistance to pitting corrosion, particularly in the presence of liquids with high chloride contents. Halide ions are particularly effective in penetrating passive films and causing pitting (39, 40)

Various protective layers have been applied to protect the surface including halar, enamel, and Teflon. On a small scale, where culture vessels are not operated for extended periods under pressure, glass vessels provide an ideal, versatile, and relatively economic system for cultivation. Where stainless steel vessels or components are to be used they should be selected with regard to the grade of steel either AISI 316 or Carpenter 20 (US grades) (38).

4.2 Continuous culture of *Pyrococcus furiosus*

A glass continuous culture vessel was described by Brown and Kelly (41) for the culture of *Pyrococcus furiosus*. The reactor comprised a 2 litre, glass round-bottomed flask maintained at 98°C by a heating mantle controlled through a proportional controller. The vessel was fitted with a gas inlet sparger and the exit gas was passed through sodium hydroxide to remove H_2S. The medium was supplied from a polycarbonate reservoir via a peristaltic pump and anaerobicity maintained by sparging with nitrogen. Teflon perfluoro-alkyl tubing was used for the medium feed lines with silicone tubing in the pump head. The reactor was operated at a volume of 750 ml using an artificial sea water medium supplemented with 0.1% yeast extract and 0.5% tryptone. After each change in dilution rate 2 g of sulfur was added to ensure it remained in excess. A constant volume was maintained using a dip tube connected in parallel to the medium feed pump. At dilution rates of 0.8/h, cell densities reached a maximum of 1.6×10^8 cells/ml.

4.3 Gas-lift reactors

A glass, gas-lift reactor has been described (25) for the growth of *Pyrococcus furiosus* under continuous culture in the absence of sulfur. The 2 litre gas-lift reactor provided relatively high-mass transfer rates at low shear forces. Steady-state cell densities were found to increase with higher gas-flow rates up to 0.5 vol/vol/min of nitrogen yielding 3×10^9 cells/ml at a dilution rate of 0.2/h. The reactor (*Figure 1*) has been used to develop defined and minimal medium for *Pyrococcus furiosus* (42) and improved conditions for the

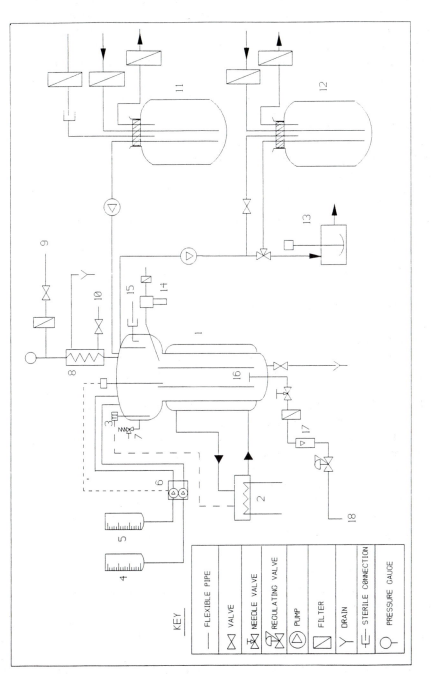

Figure 1. Gas-lift reactor for the culture of *Pyrococcus furiosus* and other hyperthermophiles: 1, vessel; 2, oil bath; 3, temperature controller; 4, acid reservoir; 5, alkali reservoir; 6, pH controller; 7, safety valve; 8, condenser; 9 exhaust; 10, cold water supply; 11, medium reservoir; 12, product reservoir; 13, centrifuge; 14, sample port; 15, inoculation port; 16, sparger; 17, gas flow meter; 18, gas supply.

Table 1. Growth of *Pyrococcus furiosus*

Reference	Carbon source	Presence of sulfur	Sparging	Temp °C	Vessel	Culture	Doubling time	Yields (g/L)	Cell count (Cells/ml)
21	Starch Maltose Peptone YE	Prevents H$_2$ inhibition	N$_2$	100	300 litre enamelled vessel	Batch	37 min	0.22	3×10^8
21	tryptone YE	30 g/L	—	98	125 ml vials 750 ml	Batch	1–2 h, D of	—	3×10^8
41	tryptone YE Maltose	10 g/L	N$_2$	98	fermenter 400 litre	Continuous	0.2–0.7 h	—	1×10^8
43	—	—	Ar	85–88	fermenter 1.5 litre	Batch	—	1–2.7	—
44	YE	10 g/L	N$_2$	98	fermenter	Continuous	D of 0.5 h^{-1}	0.47	1×10^8
45	YE	10 g/L	N$_2$	98	fermenter	Batch	—	—	—
46	tryptone YE	10 g/L	N$_2$	98	4–8 litre fermenter	Batch	—	0.3–0.5	—
47	peptone starch YE	10 g/L	H$_2$CO$_2$	98	—	Batch	—	—	6.2×10^9
25	Peptone Pyruvate YE	—	N$_2$	95	500 ml fermenter	Batch	1 h	—	2×10^8
25	Peptone	—	N$_2$	95	2 litre gas lift	Continuous	—	4	3×10^9

YE, yeast extract.

cultivation of, for example, *Pyrococcus woesei*, *Pyrobaculum islandicum*, and *Thermococcus litoralis* and is described in *Protocol 4*.

4.4 Biomass yields

While the number of different species of hyperthermophiles identified has increased dramatically over the past 10 years, *Pyrococcus furiosus* (21) has received much of the attention, primarily in studies of its enzymology and metabolism, since it is relatively easy to grow and gives cell yields in excess of 10^8/ml, which is high compared with hyperthermophiles in general. A number of groups have grown the organism in a variety of fermentation systems and on widely different scales of operation (*Table 1*). Cultivation in a 300-litre enamelled vessel (21) yielded some 0.22 g of cell paste per litre. Bryant and Adams (43) reported variable yields of 1–2.7 g wet weight per litre without sulfur but sparging the medium with argon.

Pyrococcus produces hydrogen which, unless removed, appears to inhibit growth of the organism. The addition of sulfur to the medium results in hydrogen removal by the formation of H_2S. Alternatively, sparging of the culture with gases such as nitrogen or argon removes hydrogen from the medium. Similarly, the growth of *Pyrococcus woesei* was significantly enhanced using a dialysis membrane reactor (Bioengineering, Switzerland) at 90 °C where cell densities of 2×10^9/ml were reached (48).

Protocol 4. Construction and operation of a high-temperature anaerobic gas-lift reactor for the growth of *Pyrococcus furiosus* (modified from ref. 25)

Equipment and reagents

- All-glass, concentric tube bioreactor—comprising:

(a) A central column section (80 mm o.d. × 500 mm) with a rounded base. The base has a 45 mm diameter port with a glass, Duran-type screw thread. The top 10 cm of the column section widens to 100 mm and a glass rim with a ground-glass surface is fitted. A standard, stainless steel fermenter top plate (e.g. LH Fermentation/Inceltech) can then be clamped on top with a silicone gasket in between to ensure a gas-tight seal. At least 10 ports are required in the top plate (condenser, media in, media out, acid in, alkali in, inoculation port, temperature probe, pH electrode, safety valve).

(b) An external glass jacket (100 mm o.d. × 400 mm) is installed to envelop the lower 400 mm of the column section and two small flanged glass ports are fitted on opposite sides, one at the bottom and the other at the top. Silicone tubing can be pushed over the glass flanges and held in place by

Jubilee clips. This allows the circulation of a heated fluid through the outer jacket.

(c) A glass draft tube (60 mm o.d. × 400 mm) is inserted within the central column section. The draft tube has two sets of three glass lugs (~8 mm long) near the top and bottom, respectively. Silicone tubing (~20 mm long) is stretched over each lug and used to position the draft tube within the vessel. A bottom clearance of 5–10 mm is generally suitable.

(d) A glass condenser which consists of a tightly spiralled inner coil of glass tubing (5 mm o.d.) and an outer glass jacket (40 mm o.d. × 200 mm) through which cold water can be passed.

(e) The entire assembly can be fabricated readily by a competent glassblower and sterilized (with the ports closed or covered as appropriate) by placing in an autoclave. As an alternative, a chemically resistant version of a commercially available air-lift bioreactor is now being manufactured (FT Applikon).

Protocol 4. *Continued*

- Temperature-controlling circulating bath (Haake F3M, Fisher)
- Resistance thermometer (PT100, class A, three-wire ThermoElectric)
- Combined pH electrode (Ingold 465-35-K9, Mettler Toledo)
- pH controller (Model 500 series III, LH Fermentation/Inceltech)
- Acid and alkali reservoirs
- Gas distribution tube, porosity 2 (Fisher)
- Polypropylene closure with bulkhead fitting (Nalgene)
- Duran-type bottle cap (with 30 mm diameter, centred, drilled hole)
- Gas flow meters
- PTFE filters, autoclavable (ACRO50 0.2 μm, Gelman Sciences)
- Needle valve
- Oxygen-free nitrogen
- Silicone tubing (various diameters as appropriate)
- Synth 260 synthetic oil, silicone tubing compatible (Fisher)
- Jubilee clips
- Glass reservoir bottles, 20 litres
- Silicone bungs
- Steel rods (hollow, $\sim$ 5 mm I.D. $\times$ 100 mm and 500 mm)
- Steel discs ($\sim$ 50 mm diameter)
- Clamps (various)
- Sterile 1 ml glass pipettes
- Cable ties
- PTFE tape
- Aluminium foil
- Autoclave tape
- Peristaltic pumps (Watson Marlow)
- Cartridge filters, autoclavable (Sartobran, Sartorius)
- Stainless steel push-fit tubing connectors (manufactured in-house)
- Safety valve (Inceltech)
- Sampler (Inceltech)

A. *Bioreactor assembly—bioreactor vessel and gas distributor assembly—see Figure 1*

1. Pass a polypropylene bulkhead fitting through the holed Duran cap and tighten on both sides to give a watertight seal.

2. Push some silicone rubber tubing over the stem of the outside of the bulkhead fitting and insert a gas distribution tube, stem first, on the opposite side, again forming a watertight seal.

3. Push a length of silicone tubing over the end of the gas distribution tube and connect a PTFE membrane filter to the other end.

4. Insert a butyl rubber washer into the base of the Duran cap and screw the cap into the bottom of the vessel.

5. Sterilize the whole assembly by autoclaving, and mount in a suitable frame giving support at the base and the sides.

6. Connect the exposed side of the filter with silicone tubing to a flow meter, needle valve and oxygen-free nitrogen cylinder, all in series. Reinforce all connections with cable ties.

B. *Condenser assembly*

1. Push one end of the shell and coil condenser through a silicone rubber disc or bung housed within a top plate port fitting to form a gas-tight seal. Cover both ends of the condenser in aluminium foil and sterilize by autoclaving.

2. Remove a blank port fitting from the top plate and replace aseptically with the condenser assembly.

3. Attach a cold water supply to the lower port of the condenser jacket with silicone tubing and similarly connect the upper port either to a drain or to a chiller unit for recirculation. Reinforce all tubing connections with cable ties.

C. *Temperature control*

1. Fill the temperature-controlled, heated circulating bath with a synthetic oil compatible with the silicone tubing.

2. Connect the silicone tubing from the bath outlet to the lower port of the vessel jacket. Connect the jacket outlet similarly to the bath inlet to allow circulation of the heated oil. Secure the silicone tubing with Jubilee clips.

3. Connect the resistance thermometer lead to the external control socket of the bath and insert the probe (sterilize by immersion in 70% ethanol) through a top plate port. Form a gas-tight seal by wrapping the stem with PTFE tape.

   Note: The bath now controls the temperature of the medium in the bioreactor directly.

D. *pH control*

1. Clamp the acid and alkali reservoirs to a stand and connect via a length of silicone tubing to a 1 ml glass pipette.

2. Clamp the reservoirs temporarily at their bases and fill with 2 M HCl and 2 M NaOH, respectively. Cap both with a holed silicone bung, pass a short steel rod through the centre, and join via a short length of silicone tubing to PTFE filters.

3. Cover the glass pipettes in aluminium foil and hold in place with autoclave tape and autoclave the assemblies.

4. Feed the silicone tubing through the acid and alkali pumps of the pH controller, respectively.

5. Insert the 1 ml pipettes through two further top plate ports and again form gas-tight seals with PTFE tape. Remove the clamps on the two lines

E. *Media supply and product collection*

1. Select large silicone bungs to fit the necks of 20 litre glass bottles. Make four evenly spaced holes in each bung and insert two short and two long tightly fitting steel rods. Adjust the depth of each rod so that equal lengths of steel tube are present on the top of the bung.

2. For each bung, drill four holes in two steel discs so that the rods can pass through them. Drill a fifth central hole in both discs and through

Protocol 4. *Continued*

the centre of the bung. Position one disc on each side of the bung and insert a tight fitting bolt from the bottom through both discs and the centre of the bung. Locate a nut over the exposed end of the bolt.

3. Attach short lengths of silicone tubing to the lower ends of the two long rods and point in opposite directions (so that the very bottom edge of the reservoir is reached). Insert the bung into the neck of the bottle and tighten the nut down (this compresses the bung in the neck so forming a gas-tight seal).

4. *For use as a medium reservoir* connect one of the two long rods to a PTFE vent filter and the other via a length of silicone tubing to a 1 ml glass pipette wrapped in aluminium foil and taped in place with autoclave tape. Connect one of the short steel rods to a further PTFE filter and the second to a tubing connector and blank.

5. *For product reservoirs* connect one of the short steel rods to a PTFE filter, as for the medium reservoir, but join the other via a length of silicone tubing to a 1 ml glass pipette wrapped in aluminium foil. Similarly, connect one of the long rods to a further PTFE filter, but connect the other to a tubing connector and blank.

6. Sterilize both assemblies by autoclaving.

7. Feed the medium reservoir line through a peristaltic pump and insert the 1 ml pipette through a top plate port. Hold in position and seal by wrapping with PTFE tape.

8. Feed the product recovery line through a second peristaltic pump, operating at a higher speed in the opposite direction, and insert its 1 ml pipette through a further top plate port. Insert the pipette deeper to fix the product take-off height from the bioreactor and, therefore, regulate its working volume. Again form a gas-tight seal by wrapping in PTFE tape.

F. *Sampling and inoculation*

1. Insert a close fitting silicone bung or disc in one of the top plate ports and compress with the screw closure. This can be installed prior to autoclaving the vessel assembly for use as an inoculation port.

2. Attach a length of silicone rubber to the outlet side of the sampler and join to a PTFE filter. Screw a glass Bijou bottle into the culture trap and connect via a length of silicone tubing to a 1 ml glass pipette. Wrap the 1 ml pipette in aluminium foil and sterilize the whole assembly by autoclaving.

3. Clamp the sampling assembly to the side of the top plate and insert the 1 ml pipette through a top plate port to below the level of the product take-off tube. Again form a gas-tight seal by wrapping with PTFE tape.

4. Connect a syringe to the PTFE filter with a short length of silicone tubing so that drawing on the rubber plunger pulls the culture into the trap by vacuum

5. Once in use, disposable, plastic Bijou bottles can be used in place of glass bottles for collecting samples.

G. *Medium preparation*

1. Link a cartridge filter via its OUT side with a short length of silicone tubing to a tubing connector and blank closure. Autoclave the assembly, then connect to the media inlet port. To ensure that the two closures are joined aseptically, spray 70% ethanol over the connectors as a precaution.

2. Connect the IN side of the cartridge filter to a length of silicone tubing and pass through a peristaltic pump.

3. Prepare 20 litres of growth medium and weight the open end of the silicone tubing, with a hollow steel rod, at the bottom of the holding bottle.

4. Switch the pump on and bleed the air from the filter. Reinforce the tubing connections to the cartridge filter with cable ties.

5. Continue pumping until all the medium has passed through the filter into the sterile medium reservoir.

6. Remove the filter and connector from the bottle and refit the blank closures.

7. Back-flush the filter with distilled water prior to reassembly (as in Step G1) and re-sterilization.

H. *Set-up*

1. During the initial set-up fill the bioreactor by switching on the pump from the medium reservoir. Switch on the product pump when the required level is reached.

2. Connect the nitrogen (or alternative inert gas) supply and regulate the flow with the needle valve and gas flow meter.

3. Establish pH control by setting the pH controller to the required pH and the acid and alkali feeds to switch on at 0.1 pH units above and below this set point, respectively. Standardize the pH values obtained from the electrode by measuring the pH of small samples obtained from the sample port using a standard bench pH meter. Once in operation, the pH measured at 20°C is normally 0.3–0.5 pH units higher (dependent upon the medium employed) than the reading at 90°C providing the electrode is still functioning properly.

4. Lower the medium feed rate and switch the heating bath on. Switch the bath to regulate on its own internal temperature reading and set at 5°C above that required for the bioreactor.

Protocol 4. *Continued*

5. Allow the bath temperature and the bioreactor temperatures to reach equilibrium (the differential between the bioreactor and bath temperatures is routinely 2–3 °C at low dilution rates) then switch the bath back to external control via the temperature probe immersed in the bioreactor. Adjust the temperature setting accordingly.

6. Introduce a supply of coolant to the condenser.

7. Once the bioreactor is in full operation leave it running at a low dilution rate (~ 0.05/h) for 2–3 days to confirm the sterility of the entire system.

8. After this period inoculate the bioreactor with a seed culture (1% or more) via the inoculation port. Allow the culture a further 2–3 days to reach a steady state before beginning experimentation/biomass production.

I. *Operation*

1. Once the culture has become established in the bioreactor, take readings at least daily for the following parameters: temperature, pH (*in situ*), pH (at room temperature), gas flow rate, dilution rate, cell density, and optical density using standard procedures.

2. Record both cell density and optical density to provide a more reliable indicator of cell growth. Direct cell counts can vary independently of the optical density (at 600 nm) by several-fold. Optical density generally correlates well with true biomass production using L-cysteine as the reducing agent, but it can give distorted readings with other reductants (e.g. titanium citrate and sodium sulfide) due to the formation of inorganic precipitates.

3. For routine experimentation dilution rates of 0.125/h and above are convenient, since three volume changes occur in the bioreactor in a 24-hour period. This allows a parameter to be altered sequentially each day with results approximating to equilibrium values being obtained.

4. For biomass production a dilution rate of 0.4/h is convenient (since 19.2 litres of product is generated in a 24-hour period). Fresh medium and a fresh product receiver can then be supplied for the following day's production.

5. The product can be harvested directly from the fermenter, but this requires either constant centrifugation or concentration by cross-flow filtration. Neither are convenient due to the wear and tear on the centrifuge (potentially being left in operation unmonitored) and the autolytic nature of *Pyrococcus* at high concentrations. Routinely, therefore, biomass is collected for a 24-hour period with the product receiver immersed in a bath cooled at 4°C.

6. Media and product reservoirs can be kept anaerobic if necessary by sparging at a slow rate with nitrogen. Biomass can similarly be harvested anaerobically using a closed continuous centrifuge system, e.g. a Sorvall SS34 rotor with a KSB continuous centrifuge attachment, purged with nitrogen before use. The assembly can be transferred to an anaerobic cabinet for anaerobic recovery of the biomass.

5. Development of vessels for the study of barophilic hyperthermophiles

The development of bioreactors for the growth and study of hyperthermophiles, under both high temperature and pressure, has progressed with the isolation of marine hyperthermophiles under high hydrostatic pressure from thermal vents on the ocean floor.

Some of the simpler systems developed to study the effects of temperature and pressure growth have involved the use of modified autoclaves. To study the growth of *Methanococcus thermolithotrophicus* on hydrogen 10 ml nickel tubes with a liquid:gas ratio of 1:2 were used in a set of autoclaves connected in series. With the application of an hydraulic pump and a 2.5 kW heating device, changes in temperature (up to 400°C) and pressure (up to 4000 bar) could be obtained within 10 minutes (49).

Other relatively simple systems include the use of pressurized syringes. Yayanos *et al.* used a cylindrical sample chamber fitted with a piston which separated the sample from the pressurizing fluid and transferred pressure to the sample during pressurization and sampling. Sampling was achieved by pumping preheated hydraulic fluid into the pressure vessel at the same rate as the liquid was removed from the syringe thus ensuring that constant temperature and pressure was maintained during sampling (50).

A relatively simple, pressurized, temperature-gradient instrument consisting of eight pressure vessels in parallel with each other in an aluminium block enabled the study of temperature and pressure effects on the growth of microorganisms. A linear temperature gradient was maintained across the block by circulating thermostatted fluids at two different temperatures. A temperature gradient from −20°C to 100°C could be maintained. Capped glass or polyethylene tubes containing either liquid or solid medium in short (20 mm) culture tubes or in long glass capillaries (762 mm) were placed in pressure vessels made from type 316 high-pressure stainless steel. Each vessel was pressurized to between 1 and 1100 bar. The equipment was used to study the boundaries of temperature and pressure for the growth of deep-sea isolate CNPT-3 (51).

A continuous culture system to study isolates from crude oil reservoirs was developed, consisting of a 1 litre stainless steel reaction vessel with walls 20 mm thick. The reaction vessel was supplied with media hydraulically pumped from a sealed reservoir. The effluent was removed through an overflow port provided with a plug valve controlled micrometering valve. Mixing was achieved through fluid recycling via a bypass loop using a magnetically coupled gear pump. There was no gas phase present in the system. The apparatus was used to culture an anaerobic, rod-shaped sewage isolate at 65°C. The organism was initially cultured in the reaction vessel at atmospheric pressure in batch phase to a density of 3.5×10^5 cells/ml. The feed was initiated at 50 ml/h and reached a cell density of 4×10^7/ml at 102 h. The pressure was then increased over a period to 200 bar when the population increased to 2.5×10^8/ml and was maintained for 3 days. The rod-shaped cells were observed to take up a coccoidal shape (52).

A bioreactor designed for the study of growth at temperatures up to 260°C and pressures up to 350 bar comprised a transparent sapphire cell permitting observation of the growth medium. The cell comprised a single crystal sapphire tube (Union Carbide) of approximately 30 ml capacity. A gas compressor introduced gases at pressures above those normally supplied from cylinders, and a magnetically driven pump recirculated vapour through the liquid phase to promote vapour–liquid equilibrium. Vapour recirculation accomplished the stirring of the liquid phase and the proportion of a thermodynamic equilibrium between the vapour and liquid phase. The vessel and pump were maintained in an oven. Studies with *Methanococcus jannaschii*, an extremely thermophilic methanogen isolated from a deep-sea hydrothermal vent, indicated that at 90°C increasing pressures from 7.8 to 100 bar accelerated the production of methane and cellular protein and increased the maximum growth temperature of the organism from 90 to 92°C (53). A similar reactor was used for the spectrophotometric assay of hydrogenase activity in cell-free extracts of *Methanococcus jannaschii*. The system was adapted to enable the rapid high-pressure gas injection of substrate into an equilibrated enzyme solution (54). Subsequently, the system was further modified with a large stainless steel vessel and more powerful pump enabling pressures up to 1000 bar. The system was used to study the growth and methane production of *Methanococcus jannaschii* (55). A version of this system using a stainless steel and glass lined reactor was used to study the growth of a deep-sea archaeon, ES4 (56). Growth and metabolism as a function of temperature and pressure was found to be very sensitive to the experimental conditions (stainless steel or glass lined vessels) used.

6. Cryopreservation of hyperthermophiles

6.1 Introduction

The most extensive publicly available collection of hyperthermophilic archaea and bacteria is held by the Deutsche Sammlung von Mikroorganismen und Zellkulturen (DSM) at Braunschweig in Germany (see Appendix 2). Although lyophilization has been shown to be an effective method for the long-term storage of some hyperthermophiles, cryopreservation in glass capillaries has been shown by the DSM to be the most generally applicable procedure (57). At CAMR, hyperthermophiles such as *Pyrococcus furiosus* have been successfully maintained in this manner for at least 6 years in the vapour phase of liquid nitrogen (58). Recently, a modification of this procedure has been introduced which has been shown, to date, to be effective for the storage of more than 20 species of hyperthermophiles for periods of at least a year (Raven and Sharp, unpublished observations). This method takes advantage of the phenomenon that anaerobic hyperthermophiles are generally less sensitive to oxygen at room temperature, and is also applicable to aerobic hyperthermophiles. Concentration of cell suspensions has been found to be counter-productive for some of the organisms. If cultures are found not to survive the original deposition using this procedure then the more rigorous method employed by Hippe (57) to eliminate oxygen combined with the use of cryoprotectants (e.g. 10% v/v glycerol or 5% v/v dimethyl sulfoxide) and lower storage temperatures may be required.

Protocol 5. Cryopreservation of hyperthermophiles in glass capillaries

Equipment and reagents

- −70°C freezer
- Glass capillaries, 50 μl, 100 mm long (Sigma)
- Cryovials, 5.0 ml, 92 mm long (Nalgene)
- Cryomarkers (Nalgene)
- Polycarbonate cryoboxes, 9 × 9 array, 133 mm × 133 mm × 95 mm (Nalgene)
- Glass test tubes, rimless, 100 mm × 12 mm (Fisher)
- Aluminium caps
- Forceps, straight, fine point, 150 mm long (Fisher)
- Sterile syringes, 1 ml
- Sterile needles, 25 gauge, 0.5 mm × 25 mm (Becton Dickinson)

- Vacuum flask, stainless steel, i.d. > 100 mm
- Liquid nitrogen
- Solid carbon dioxide (dry ice)
- Ethanol

For recovery
- Scissors or nail clippers
- Sterile syringes, 1 ml
- Sterile needles, 25 gauge, 0.5 mm × 25 mm (Becton Dickinson)
- Serum vials (50 ml or less) containing sterile culture medium (20 ml or less) and sealed with a rubber septum plus aluminium crimp cap
- Ethanol

A. *Deposition*

1. Place the number of glass capillaries required into a glass test tube and cover with an aluminium cap; autoclave (121°C for 15 minutes).

2. Label a 5.0 ml cryovial with the strain designation using a cryomarker.

3. Take a freshly grown culture of the organism to be preserved and allow to cool at room temperature on the bench.

3a. *For thermoacidophiles*, withdraw a sample of known volume aseptically via a sterile syringe and needle (a pipette tip may be used for

43

Protocol 5. *Continued*

aerobes). Read the pH and add measured aliquots of a filter-sterilized 1 M sodium bicarbonate solution until the pH reaches 6.0. Add
a proportional volume of the sodium bicarbonate solution to the
stock culture to similarly adjust the pH.

4. Where concentrated samples are to be preserved, transfer the contents of the bottle aseptically to an appropriately sized sterile centrifuge tube and pellet the cells by centrifugation (5000–10 000 *g* for
   10 min). Decant the supernatant and resuspend the cells in fresh
   medium (prepared anaerobically where appropriate and adjusted to
   pH 6.0 for thermoacidophiles) taking care to minimize mixing with
   the overlying air.

5. Assemble two sterile 1 ml syringes and 25-gauge needles and withdraw a sample of the culture or culture concentrate. Replace the
   protective sterile needle cover.

5a. *For anaerobic cultures* fill the syringe with the headspace gas of the
    culture and discharge prior to withdrawing a sample.

6. Dislodge any air/gas bubbles within the syringe by flicking the barrel
   with the needle pointing vertically upwards. Discharge the air/gas
   from the syringe by pushing in the syringe plunger as required (still
   within the needle cover).

7. Remove a single glass capillary from the test tube with a pair of
   forceps and pass swiftly through a hot Bunsen flame. Take off the
   needle housing and inject the culture through the needle into one
   end of the horizontal glass capillary until it reaches approximately
   10 mm from the opposite end. Pass the needle through the flame
   and replace the housing.

8. Place one end of the glass capillary into a flame and carefully heat-
   seal it without causing the contents to discharge.

9. With the second syringe and needle, withdraw some culture from the
   open end of the capillary up to the full length of the inserted needle.
   If the capillary is not properly sealed at the other end this will cause
   the entire contents of the capillary tube to be extracted; in this event
   the injection and sealing steps should be repeated. Once completed,
   pass the needle through the flame and replace in the needle housing.

10. Hold the open end of the capillary with a second pair of forceps (still
    holding the closed end with a pair of forceps) and position the capil-
    lary in the flame at the junction of the air/liquid interface. Heat until
    the glass softens then briskly pull the ends in opposite directions to
    seal the capillary tube.

11. Break off and discard the unwanted portion of the extended capillary

tube. Trim the new end and seal neatly by placing it carefully in the flame for a few seconds. The sealed capillary should be no more than 90 mm long.

12. Place the sealed capillary in the vapour phase of liquid nitrogen (the contents freeze almost instantaneously), then place in the labelled cryovial embedded in a dry ice/ethanol bath before transferring to a cryobox in a −70°C freezer.

B. *Recovery from glass capillaries*

1. Open the cryobox, still within the −70°C freezer, and withdraw a single capillary from the cryovial.

2. Place the capillary at room temperature and allow to thaw (occurs within a few seconds).

3. Dip one end of the capillary tube into ethanol and pass it briefly through a flame.

4. Dip the blades of a pair of scissors or jaws of a pair of nail clippers into ethanol and also pass through a flame.

5. Snip the now sterile end of the capillary off behind a screen and, keeping the capillary tube horizontal, repeat the sterilization and tip removal procedure with the other end.

6. Using a syringe, insert the needle into one end of the capillary and withdraw the contents.

7. Insert this same needle (with syringe still attached) through the septum of an appropriately labelled medium bottle and withdraw a sample. (This ensures that the small aliquot of culture is mixed in a larger volume so guaranteeing its subsequent injection into the growth medium.)

8. Replace the needle housing (with the syringe attached) and hold the syringe with the needle pointing vertically up.

9. Mix the contents of the syringe, then dislodge any air/gas bubbles by flicking the syringe barrel and expel any air/gas from the syringe.

10. Inject the contents of the syringe into the culture bottle and incubate under appropriate conditions.

7. Culture procedures for hyperthermophiles

Procedures for the cultivation of hyperthermophiles vary according to the different groups (marine, terrestrial, acidophilic, etc.), but many of the general operations discussed and outlined for the cultivation of the marine isolate *Pyrococcus furiosus* may be applied. The three examples which follow summarize the media and techniques used for the cultivation of (a) thermo-acidophiles of the genus *Sulfolobus*, (b) the terrestrial hyperthermophilic archaeon, *Pyrobaculum islandicum*, and (c) the hyperthermophilic marine bacterium *Thermotoga maritima*.

Protocol 6. Cultivation of *Sulfolobus* species

Equipment and reagents

For A
- Trace elements' solution (per litre): 20 g $FeCl_3 \cdot 6H_2O$, 1.8 g $MnCl_2 \cdot 4H_2O$, 4.5 g $Na_2B_4O_7 \cdot 10H_2O$, 0.22 g $CuCl_2 \cdot 2H_2O$, 0.03 g $NaMoO_4 \cdot 2H_2O$, 0.03 g $VOSO_4 \cdot 2H_2O$, 0.01 g $CoSO_4$. Dissolve in 950 ml double-distilled water. To achieve complete dissolution, adjust the pH to < 1.5 with 9 M H_2SO_4, and adjust the final volume to 1 litre
- Medium (according to Brock *et al.*, ref. 23) (per litre): 1.3 g $(NH_4)_2SO_4$, 0.28 g KH_2PO_4, 0.25 g $MgSO_4 \cdot 7H_2O$, 0.07 g $CaCl_2 \cdot 2H_2O$, 1 ml trace elements' solution, 1 g yeast extract. Adjust the pH to 2.0 with H_2SO_4

For B
- Gelrite
- 20 mM $MgCl_2$
- 6 mM $CaCl_2$
- Petri dishes

For C
- Gelrite
- 9K medium with iron (per litre): 3 g $(NH_4)_2SO_4$, 0.66 g $K_2HPO_4 \cdot 3H_2O$, 0.5 g $MgSO_4 \cdot 7H_2O$, 0.1 g KCl, 0.02 g $FeCl_3 \cdot 6H_2O$, 14 mg $Ca(NO_3)_2 \cdot 4H_2O$. Make up to 1 litre with double-distilled water and adjust the pH to 3.0 with H_2SO_4
- 20 mM tetrathionate
- 2 mM NaCl
- 0.2% (w/v) casamino acids[a]
- 16 mM $MgCl_2$

A. *Liquid medium*

Media for the growth of *Sulfolobus* species have generally been derived from mineral solutions developed for the growth of autotrophic acidophiles (e.g. refs 24, 60). An example is the medium of Brock *et al.* (23) used in the original report of *Sulfolobus*.

1. Autoclave the medium at 121°C for 15 min.

2. Inoculate the medium.

3. Incubate at 70°C with moderate aeration.

Note: In a survey of commonly grown *Sulfolobus* isolates, Grogan (60) examined a wide range of phenotypic characteristics. Several of these properties were present in all the strains examined. We have observed improved growth of all these *Sulfolobus* strains by adopting the conditions shown by Grogan to give improved growth. These are:

(a) increasing the growth temperature to 75–80°C;

(b) increasing the medium pH to 3.5, where the medium pH is controlled;

(c) including starch (2 g/litre) and/or a polypeptide (e.g. tryptone, 2 g/litre) in the culture medium.

B. *Solidified medium*

This medium was modified by Grogan (60) to provide a convenient solidi-fied medium for the growth of *Sulfolobus*. Again Gelrite was found to be a suitable gelling agent and colonies could be produced at high effi-ciency in as little as 4 days.

Method

1. Dissolve 12–14 g of Gelrite in 1 litre of distilled water by boiling and stirring.
2. Add an equal volume of (presterilized) double concentrated growth medium of Brock *et al.* (23), supplemented with 20 mM $MgCl_2$ and 6 mM $CaCl_2$. Heat to 60°C and add to the gel solution.
3. Adjust the pH of the medium as necessary and pour the gel into Petri dishes.
4. Inoculate either by streaking or spreading as appropriate, and incu-bate at 75°C in a closed container.

Note: The gel is stable for incubations up to 75–80°C giving high plating efficiencies. Colonies are 1 mm in diameter. For heterotrophic growth, basal media can be supplemented with organic substrates such as 0.2% tryptone and 0.1% yeast extract or 0.1% yeast extract and 0.2% glucose (60).

For lithotrophic growth, media can be supplemented with 5–10 mg/litre sulfur, although most strains appear to show enhanced growth with the addition of low levels (0.05–0.2 g/litre) of yeast extract or meat extract (36).

C. *Alternative solidified medium (derived from ref. 31)*

An alternative solidified medium has been reported by Lindstrom and Sehlin (31) for *Sulfolobus* isolates, able to augment growth by the oxidation of solu-ble sulfur compounds (e.g. tetrathionate). This medium was derived from an iron-free variant of the 9K mineral medium of Silverman and Lundgren (59).

1. Dissolve 16 g of gelrite in 1 litre of distilled water.
2. Autoclave the suspension at 121°C for 20 min and then maintain the gel at >70°C.
3. Add an equal volume of double-strength 9K basal medium supple-mented with 20 mM tetrathionate, 2 mM NaCl, 0.2% (w/v) casamino acids[a] and 16 mM $MgCl_2$, to the molten gel.[b]
4. Mix the solution and pour into Petri dishes and allow to solidify.

[a] Other *Sulfolobus* strains prefer alternative carbon sources to casamino acids and carbohydrates (e.g. starch); polypeptides (e.g. tryptone) and yeast extract may be substituted as required.
[b] An overlay technique may be used for strains growing by the oxidation of elemental sulfur. Colloidal sulfur is prepared by combining a concentrated polysulfide solution with acidified double-strength medium (both preheated to 70°C) to give a final pH of 3. Cell dilutions are immediately added to this suspension and combined with an equal volume of half-strength gelrite (8 g/litre), mixed vigorously, and poured directly on to the supporting gel.

Protocol 7. Cultivation of *Pyrobaculum islandicum* strain GEO3 (DSM 4184)

The mineral salts solution of Allen (24) has also been used as the basal medium for the growth of anaerobic hyperthermophiles such as *Pyrobaculum islandicum* (34).

Equipment and reagents

- Basal medium of Allen (24)
- Peptone (Difco Bacto)
- Yeast extract (Difco Bacto)
- Resazurin, 1 g/litre
- Sulfur

- Sodium sulfide ·9H$_2$O
- Stoppered, crimped serum bottles (*Protocol 2*)
- Nitrogen gas cylinder

A. *Liquid medium*

1. Make up the following medium:

   - Basal medium of Allen (24)   for 1 litre
   - Peptone (Difco Bacto)   0.5 g/litre
   - Yeast extract (Difco Bacto)   0.2 g/litre
   - Resazurin solution (1 g/l)   1 ml
   - Sulfur[a]   20 g/litre
   - Sodium sulfide ·9H$_2$O[b]   0.5 g/litre

   Make up to 1 litre and adjust the pH to 6.0 with H$_2$SO$_4$.

2. Grow cultures in stoppered, crimped serum bottles (see *Protocol 2*).

3. Pressurize with N$_2$ (300 kPa) and incubate statically at 100°C.

Notes:
[a] Sodium thiosulfate·5H$_2$O (2 g/litre) can be substituted for elemental sulfur for growth in bioreactors or on solid medium.
[b] L-cysteine (0.5 g/litre) can be substituted for sodium sulfide to produce a medium which is readily filter-sterilized.

B. *Solidified medium*

Huber *et al.* (34) obtained growth on culture medium solidified with 20% starch. After 7 days anaerobic growth at 85°C small greenish-black colonies developed.

Note: under equivalent conditions, gelrite plates (1%) are only semi-solid due to the low levels of monovalent and divalent cations.

C. *Culture storage (34)*

After incubation at 100°C for 2–3 days, small (10 ml) liquid cultures maintained at 4°C can serve as inocula for up to 3 months. Long-term stocks can be maintained by cryopreservation in glass capillaries.

Protocol 8. Cultivation of *Thermotoga maritima* strain MSB8 (DSM 3109)

The heterotrophic marine bacterium *Thermotoga maritima* has been grown on both MMS medium and SME medium (61). Good growth has also been observed on *Pyrococcus furiosus* medium (25) modified as follows.

Equipment and reagents

- Modified SME mineral salts (*Protocol 2*)
- Starch, soluble
- Peptone
- Yeast extract
- 1 g/litre Resazurin
- L-cysteine
- 0.22 μm filter,
- Stoppered, crimped serum bottles or reservoir
- Oxygen-free nitrogen

A. *Liquid medium*

1. Make up the following medium:

   - Modified SME mineral salts (see *Protocol 2*)
   - Starch   0.5 g/litre
   - Peptone   0.2 g/litre
   - Yeast extract   1 g/litre
   - Resazurin solution (1 g/litre)   1 ml
   - L-cysteine   0.5 g/litre

1. Autoclave soluble starch in a bottle or reservoir at 5 × concentration (12.5 g/litre).

2. Dissolve the remaining medium components at 1.25 × concentration, adding the L-cysteine last.

3. Adjust pH to 6.5 at room temperature.

4. Filter-sterilize through a 0.2 μm filter into the starch solution.

5. Stopper and crimp the bottle.

6. Displace oxygen from the bottle by purging with filter-sterilized, oxygen-free nitrogen.

7. Inoculate and place the bottle in a static incubator at 80°C.

8. Incubate for up to 24 hours.

B. *Solidified medium*

Huber *et al.* (61) observed round white colonies of *Thermotoga maritima* after 3 days growth on MMS medium solidified with agar (0.8%) at the sub-optimal temperature of 65°C. More rapid colony formation is observed on the liquid medium above solidified with gelrite (0.8%), where an optimal incubation temperature of 80°C can be maintained.

C. *Culture storage*

Huber *et al.* (61) showed that cultures stored at both 4°C and unusually −20 °C could serve as inocula for at least a year, even when oxygen had penetrated the bottle as indicated by the colour of the resazurin. Long-term stocks can be maintained by cryopreservation in glass capillaries.

References

1. Sharp, R. J. and Williams, R. A. D. (1995). In Thermus *species. Biotechnology handbooks*, Volume 9, Plenum Press, New York.
2. Sharp, R. J., Riley, P., and White, D. (1992). In *Thermophilic bacteria* (ed. J. K. Kristjansson), pp. 19–50, CRC Press., Boca Raton, Florida.
3. Woese, C. R. and Fox, G. E. (1977). *Proc. Natl. Acad. Sci. USA*, **74**, 5088.
4. Woese, C. R., Kandler, O., and Wheelis, M. L. (1990). *Proc. Natl, Acad. Sci. USA*, **87**, 4576.
5. Brock, T. D. (ed.) (1986). *Thermophiles, general molecular and applied microbiology.* John Wiley and Sons, New York
6. Kandler, D. and Zillig, W. (1986). In *Archaebacteria 85.* Gustav Fischer, Stuttgart.
7. Herbert, R. A. and Codd, G. A. (1986). *Microbes in extreme environments.* Academic Press, London.
8. Da Costa, M. S., Duarte, J., and Williams, R. A. D. (1989). In *Microbiology of extreme environments and its potential for biotechnology*, FEMS Symposium No. 49. Elsevier, London and New York.
9. Edwards, C. (ed.) (1990). *Microbiology of extreme environments.* Open University Press, Milton Keynes.
10. Herbert, R. A. and Sharp, R. J. (1992). In *Molecular biology and biotechnology of extremophiles*, pp. 1–331.. Blackie and Son, Glasgow
11. Kristjansson, J. K. (1992). In *Thermophilic bacteria*, pp. 1–228. CRC Press, Boca Raton.
12. Danson, M. J., Hough, D. W., and Lunt, G. G. (1992). Editors *The archaebacteria: biochemistry and biotechnology.* Portland Press, London and Chapel Hill.
13. Cowan, D. A. (1992). *Tibtech*, **10**, 315.
14. Herbert, R. A. (1992). *Tibtech*, **10**, 395.
15. Horikoshi, K. (1995). *Curr. Opin. Biotech.*, **6**, 292.
16. Blöchl, E., Burggraf, S., Fiala, G., Lauerer, G., Huber, G., Huber, R., *et al.* (1995). *World J. Microbiol.*, **11**, 9.
17. Yayanos, A. A. (1995). *Annu. Rev. Microbiol.*, **49**, 777.
18. Wiegel, J. (1986). In *Thermophiles, general, molecular and applied microbiology* (ed. T. D. Brock), pp. 17–37. John Wiley, New York.
19. Stetter, K. O. (1982). *Nature*, **300**, 258.
20. Stetter, K. O., König, H., and Sackebrandt, E. (1983). *System. Appl. Microbiol.*, **4**, 535.
21. Fiala, G. and Stetter, K. O. (1986). *Arch. Microbiol.*, **145**, 56.
22. Zillig, W., Holz, I., Klenk, H.-P., Trent, J., Wunderl, S., Janekovic, D., *et al.* (1987). *System. Appl. Microbiol.*, **9**, 62.

23. Brock, T. D., Brock, K. M., Belly, R. T., and Weiss, R. L. (1972). *Arch. Mikrobiol.*, **84**, 54.
24. Allen, M. B. (1959). *Arch. Mikrobiol.*, **32**, 270.
25. Raven, N., Ladwa, N., Cossar, D., and Sharp, R. J. (1992). *Appl. Microbiol. Biotechnol.*, **38**, 263.
26. Zillig, W., Stetter, K. O., Schäfer, W., Janekovic, D., Wunderl, S., Holz, I. *et al.* (1981). *Zbl. Bakt. Hyg., I. Abt. Orig.*, **C2**, 205.
27. Dietz, A. S. and Yayanos, A. A. (1978). *Appl. Environ. Microbiol.*, **36**, 966.
28. Lin, C. C. and Casida, Jr, L. E. (1984). *Appl. Environ. Microbiol.*, **47**, 427.
29. Deming, J. W. and Baross, J. A. (1986). *Appl. Environ. Microbiol.*, **51**, 238.
30. Kang, K. S., Veeder, G. T., Mirrasoul, P. J., Kaneko, T., and Cottrell, I. W. (1982). *Appl. Environ. Microbiol.*, **43**, 1086.
31. Lindstrom, E. B. and Sehlin, H. M. (1989). *Appl. Environ. Microbiol.*, **55**, 3020.
32. Erauso, G., Reysenbach, A.-L., Godfroy, A., Meunier, J.-R., Crump, B., Partensky, F., *et al.* (1993). *Arch. Microbiol.*, **160**, 338.
33. Zillig, W., Holz, I., Janekovic, D., Klenk, H.-P., Imsel, E., Trent, J., Wunderl, S., Forjaz, V., Coutinho, R., Ferreira, T. *et al.* (1990). *J. Bacteriol.*, **3959**, 172.
34. Huber. R., Kristjansson, J. K., and Stetter, K. O. (1987). *Arch. Microbiol.*, **149**, 95.
35. Segerer, A., Langworthy, T. A., and Stetter, K. O. (1988). *System. Appl. Microbiol.*, **10**, 161.
36. Segerer, A. and Stetter, K. O. (1992). In *The Prokaryotes* (2nd edn) (ed. A. Balows., H. G. Trüper, M. Dworkin, W. Harder, and K. H. Schleifer), pp. 684–701. Springer-Verlag, New York.
37. Sonnleitner, B. (1984). In *Adv. Biochem. Eng.*, **30**, 70.
38. Sharp, R. J. and Munster, M. (1986). In *Microbes in extreme environments* (ed. R. A. Herbert and G. A. Codd), pp. 215–96. Academic Press., London
39. Tiller, A. K. (1982). In *Corrosion processes* (ed. R. N. Parkins), pp. 104–7. Applied Science, London.
40. Wakerley, D. S. (1979). *Chem. Industry*, **656**, 979.
41. Brown, S. H. and Kelly, R. M. (1989). *Appl. Environ. Microbiol.*, **55**, 2086.
42. Raven, N. and Sharp, R. J. (Submitted).
43. Bryant, F. O. and Adams, M. W. W. (1989). *J. Biol. Chem.*, **264**, 5070.
44. Costantino, H., Brown, S., and Kelly, R. (1990). *J. Bacteriol.*, **172**, 3654.
45. Blumentals, I. I., Robinson, A., and Kelly, R. M. (1990). *Appl. Environ. Microbiol.*, **56**, 1992.
46. Koch, R., Zablowski, P., Spreinat, A., and Antranikian, G. (1990). *FEMS Microbiol. Lett.*, **71**, 21.
47. Schafer, T. and Schönheit, P. (1991). *Arch. Microbiol.*, **155**, 366.
48. Rödger, A., Ogbonna, J. C., Märkl, H., and Antranikian, G. (1992). *Appl. Microbiol. Biotechnol.*, **37**, 501.
49. Bernhardt, G., Jaenicke, R., and Lüdemann, H.-D. (1987). *Appl. Environ. Microbiol.*, **53**, 1876.
50. Yayanos, A. A., van Boxtel, R., and Dietz, A. S. (1983). *Appl. Environ. Microbiol.*, **46**, 1357.
51. Yayanos, A. A., van Boxtel, R., and Dietz, A. S. (1984). *Appl. Environ. Microbiol.*, **48**, 771.
52. Bubela, B., Labone, C. L., and Dawson, C. H. (1987). *Biotech. Bioeng.*, **29**, 289.

53. Miller, J. F., Almond, E. L., Shah, N. N., Ludlow, J. M., Zollweg, J. A., Streett, W. B., Zinder, S. H., and Clark, D. S. (1988). *Biotech. Bioeng.*, **31**, 407.
54. Miller, J. F., Nelson, C. M., Ludlow, J. M., Shah, N. N., and Clark, D. S. (1989). *Biotech. Bioeng.*, **34**, 1015.
55. Miller, J. F., Shah, N. N., Nelson, C. M., Ludlow, J. M., and Clark, D. S. (1988). *Appl. Environ. Microbiol.*, **54**, 3039.
56. Nelson, C. M., Schuppenhauer, M. R., and Clark, D. S. (1991). *Appl. Environ. Microbiol.*, **57**, 3576.
57. Hippe, H. (1991). In *Maintenance of microorganisms and cultured cells* (ed. B. E. Kirsop and A. Doyle), p. 101. Academic Press.
58. Connaris, H., Cowan, D., Ruffett, M., and Sharp, R. J. (1991). *Lett. Appl. Microbiol.*, **13**, 25.
59. Silverman, M. P. and Lundgren, D. G. (1959). *J. Bacteriol.*, **77**, 642.
60. Grogan, D. W. (1989). *J. Bacteriol.*, **171**, 6710.
61. Huber, R., Langworthy, T. A., König, H., Thomm, M., Woese, C. R., Sleytr, U. B *et al.* (1986). *Arch. Microbiol.*, **144**, 324.

3

Design and optimization of growth media

RANDOLPH L. GREASHAM and WAYNE K. HERBER

1. Introduction

The primary objective in developing a microbial culture medium is to ensure that the required nutrients are present in appropriate forms and at non-inhibitory concentrations. This objective can be quite challenging when considering the tremendous diversity of microorganisms present in nature, exhibiting diverse nutritional requirements ranging from simple chemicals, such as atmospheric carbon dioxide and a few inorganic salts, to complex chemicals, such as lipids, vitamins and nucleotides. Microbes that gain their energy from the photooxidation of inorganic electron donors and use carbon dioxide as their sole carbon source are referred to as photolithotrophs. Microbes that gain their energy from the chemical oxidation of inorganic electron donors and use carbon dioxide as their sole carbon source are referred to as chemolithotrophs. Microbes that photooxidize organic electron donors and use both carbon dioxide and organic carbon are called photoorganotrophs. The remaining microbes that oxidize organic electron donors which are also used as carbon sources are called chemoorganotrophs. This chapter will focus on the design and preparation of media that support the cultivation of chemoorganotrophs, many of which are economically important, especially in the food and pharmaceutical industries. The approach and optimization strategies that will be presented may be applied, in principle, towards the design and preparation of media for the other three nutritional types of microbes.

2. Medium design

Microbes, like other living organisms, require sources of carbon, nitrogen, oxygen, hydrogen, and inorganic ions as well as an exogenous source of energy for growth. Some microbes may also require specific nutrients; that is, those which they are unable to synthesize such as essential amino acids and vitamins. There are basically two types of medium formulations used to provide microbes with their required nutrients, namely chemically defined (or synthetic) and complex. As implied, the former usually consists of both organic and inorganic ingredients that are chemically defined. The complex formulations are composed of one or more nutritional components that can not be easily defined. When a complex medium contains several chemically defined nutrients and only one complex component it may be referred to as a semi-defined (or semi-synthetic) medium.

The initial approach in designing a cultivation medium is greatly influenced by how much is known about the microbe. If the identity of the microbe is known, a literature search will frequently yield one or more chemically defined or complex formulations that will support cell growth. Catalogues from various culture depository centres such as the American Type Culture Collection (ATCC) and from various suppliers of dehydrated media (Difco Laboratories, BBL Microbiology Systems, and Oxoid Unipath) are excellent resources. There are also several comprehensive books on this subject, including the *Handbook of microbiological media* (1), the *Manual of industrial microbiology and biotechnology* (2), and the 8th edition of *Bergey's manual of determinative bacteriology* (47). If the identity of the microbe is unknown, the cultivation medium, especially for a chemoorganotroph, is commonly formulated with complex ingredients to supply not only the basic nutrients but also any required growth factors. This practice is commonly employed in the pharmaceutical industry where many unidentified natural isolates are cultivated in search of new bioactive metabolites such as antifungals, antibacterials, and antiparasitics.

2.1 Complex media

Many of the complex media ingredients employed to cultivate microorganisms which support the production of bioactive metabolites are by-products and waste materials from the agriculture and food industries or extracts of biological materials. These materials are attractive not only for their nutritional value but also their relatively low cost. However, in selecting one or more of these materials for both laboratory culture and industrial fermentations, special attention must be given to consistency of quality. Since complete chemical characterization of a complex medium ingredient is usually very difficult (if at all possible), consistency may be determined by measuring the level of one or more key constituents, such as carbohydrate and amino nitrogen, as well as subjecting the ingredient to a 'use' test. The 'use' test is usually performed at the shake-flask scale under established growth conditions to measure the level of microbial activity (growth, metabolite production, enzyme production, etc.) that is supported by a particular lot of the complex nutrient. Several lots procured from two or more suppliers over at least a 12 month period are usually sufficient to establish consistency of quality.

Complex media employed for the initial cultivation of a wide variety of microbes are typically formulated with one or more carbon (0.5–7%) and

Table 1. Media for the production of commercially important secondary metabolites[a]

MSD803 (Mevinolin)	(%)	Avermectin	(%)	Efrotomycin	(%)
Corn steep liquor	1.5	Cerelose	4.5	Primary yeast	1
CPC starch	2.0	Peptonized milk	2.4	Distiller's solubles	3
Corn meal	0.1	Autolysed yeast	0.25	Glycine	0.05
Soybean meal	0.4	Polyglycol P2000	0.25 (by vol.)	L-phenylalaine	0.3
Glucose	0.5			Cornstarch	2
Soybean oil	0.25 (by vol.)			Dimethylformamide	1 (by vol.)
$(NH_4)_2SO_4$	0.4			Sodium thiosulfate	0.31
KH_2PO_4	0.03			Mobil par-*S*-defoamer	0.25 (by vol.)
$CaCO_3$	0.6				
pH 6.7		pH 7.0		pH 7.0	

[a] Components given as %.

nitrogen (0.5–4%) sources. The required inorganic nutrients are usually added as constituents of tap water and complex medium components. As will be discussed later (Section 3.4) trace elements may also be added directly or as an aliquot of a trace element solution to ensure their presence. This practice, or an abbreviated form, is quite attractive in laboratories and production facilities where deionized water (or its equivalent) is used instead of tap water to dissolve the medium components. In some locations, the quality of tap water can contribute significantly to inconsistent fermentation performance. Examples of complex medium formulations that have been used to support initial cell growth and production of economically important, bioactive metabolites are presented in *Table 1*. Mevinolin is a potent cholesterol-lowering agent (3), avermectin is a highly effective antiparasitic agent (4), and efrotomycin is an antibiotic agent that exhibits growth promoting activity in animals (5). Frequently, more than one complex medium formulation is employed during initial growth studies, especially when screening for new microbial metabolites.

2.2 Chemically defined media

Chemically defined media are used routinely at laboratory scale to develop a fundamental understanding of the nutritional requirements of the microbe that is impossible with complex media (6). Traditionally, chemically defined media have been unattractive at commercial scales for the production of secondary metabolites because of their relatively high cost and support of low productivities. However, these media are gaining popularity for the production of recombinant proteins (7), especially when optimized to achieve production

Table 2. Typical elemental composition of microorganisms

Element	Bacteria	Yeast	Fungi
	(average % dry cell weight)		
Carbon	48	48	48
Nitrogen	12.5	7.5	6
	(average g/100 g dry cell weight)		
Phosphorus	2.5	1.7	2.5
Sulfur	0.6	0.13	0.3
Potassium	2.8	2.5	1.4
Magnesium	0.3	0.3	0.2
Sodium	0.8	0.06	0.26
Calcium	0.56	0.2	0.75
Iron	0.11	0.26	0.15
Copper	0.02	0.006	—
Manganese	0.006	0.004	—
Molybdenum	—	0.0002	—

[a] Modified from Zabriskie *et al.* (9)

levels equal to or greater than those achieved with complex media. Also, chemically defined media have the inherent characteristic of supporting consistent fermentation performance, an important characteristic for any fermentation process. Fermentation processes developed with chemically defined media often yield to rapid scale-up. They appear to be less sensitive to large-scale sterilization conditions than complex medium formulations.

Although complex medium formulations continue to dominate the fermentation industry, there are occasions when encouraging levels of a secondary metabolite are achieved employing relatively inexpensive chemically defined media (8). The use of these and semi-defined media have the potential of not only enhancing fermentation process consistency but also product isolation and purification.

The initial formulation of a chemically defined medium may be rationally developed based on the chemical composition of the microbe (*Table 2*). For example, the amount of carbon and nitrogen required to support the growth of yeast to a dry cell weight (DCW) of 60 g/L is calculated as follows:

Carbon source: glucose, estimate 51% cell yield (10)

$$\left(\frac{60 \text{ g DCW}}{L}\right)\left(\frac{\text{g glucose}}{0.51 \text{ g DCW}}\right) = 117.6 \text{ g glucose/L;}$$

Nitrogen source: ammonium sulfate

$$\left(\frac{60 \text{ g DCW}}{L}\right)\left(\frac{0.075 \text{ g N}}{\text{g DCW}}\right)\left(\frac{132 \text{ g (NH}_4)_2\text{SO}_4/\text{mol(NH}_4)_2\text{SO}_4}{28 \text{ g N/mol (NH}_4)_2\text{SO}_4}\right)$$
$$= 21.2 \text{ g (NH}_4)_2\text{SO}_4/L.$$

Similar calculations are employed in determining the amount of the remaining nutrients. Since most yeasts are known to require biotin, this growth factor must also be added to the medium. Frequently, a small amount of yeast extract (0.001–0.05%) may be added initially to the formulation in an effort to meet any unknown growth factor requirements of the microbe.

As well as the relative concentrations of nutrients in a medium reflecting the composition of the cells it is also extremely important to design a medium such that growth in batch culture is limited by the exhaustion of a medium component and not by the accumulation of toxic microbial products. Thus, the biomass in the stationary phase of a batch culture may be starved of a selected nutrient but should not be poisoned. Furthermore, the identity of the growth limiting substrate is critical, especially for the production of secondary metabolites where the exhaustion of a particular nutrient initiates product formation. Depending on the secondary metabolite, the limiting nutrient may be the carbon, nitrogen, or phosphate source.

3. Nutritional requirements

As discussed in Section 2, microorganisms require sources of carbon, nitrogen, oxygen, hydrogen, inorganic ions, specific nutrients, and an exogenous source of energy. Having a fundamental knowledge of the role(s) these nutrients play in cell growth, as well as biosynthesis of primary and secondary metabolites, can be of great value in developing cultivation media. This section considers the provision of the various nutritional requirements.

3.1 Carbon source

Microbes utilize reduced carbon compounds (*Table 3*) for the production of cell mass and metabolites (primary and secondary) as well as for an energy source. During carbon metabolism high-energy phosphate compounds such as ATP are produced either by substrate level phosphorylation or oxidative phosphorylation (aerobic respiration). These compounds are utilized for cellular biosynthesis and cell maintenance. Also, some of the energy captured by these compounds is lost as heat, and the more reduced the carbon source the more heat will be generated. Thus, growth is an exothermic reaction. The balance between the amount of heat produced by the culture system and that lost from it will depend on the scale of the process. Laboratory cultures will lose more heat than they produce and, thus, will need to be heated, whereas industrial scale fermentations may produce more heat than is lost and therefore need to be cooled.

Caution must be exercised in establishing the initial carbon concentration since too high a level can reduce cell growth. Reduction in bacterial growth performance is commonly observed when the level of the primary carbon source is excessive, for example glucose exceeding 50 g/L. At these levels, the

Table 3. Carbon and nitrogen sources used in the development of fermentation media

Carbon sources:

Cerelose (commercial glucose•H_2O)	Oils (soybean, corn, and cottonseed)
Maltose	Corn starch, dextrins, and hydrolysates
Fructose	Methanol
Glycerol	Whey (65% lactose)
Molasses (Black strap or cane)	

Nitrogen sources:

Meals (soybean, corn gluten, linseed, peanut and fish)	
Flours (cottonseed and soybean)	
Yeast extract or hydrolysates	Inorganic ammonium salts
Dried yeast	Ammonia gas
Peptone	Sodium nitrate
Corn steep liquor	Urea
Distiller's solubles	

bacteria experience dehydration (plasmolysis). However, yeast and moulds have a low dependency on water, allowing them to tolerate glucose concentrations in excess of 200 g/L. The level of carbon source is also important in medium designed to support the production of a secondary metabolite. At certain concentrations, a carbon source may repress one or more enzymes employed for the synthesis of a secondary metabolite, referred to as carbon catabolite repression or carbon source repression (11). This type of repression is clearly observed when glucose is present in cephalosporin C production medium at a concentration of 165 mM. Two enzymes required for the biosynthesis of cephamycin C in *Nocardia lactamdurans* (δ(α-aminoadipyl)-cysteinyl-valine synthetase and deacetoxycephalosporin C synthase) are repressed by glucose (12).

One approach commonly employed in maintaining glucose below the growth inhibitory level (either for growth or product formation) is to start with a lower initial concentration and then add glucose, as a high concentration syrup, intermittently or continuously during the fermentation cycle. Glucose feeding is rather straightforward when conducted in highly instrumented stirred-tank bioreactors, but rather tedious when conducted in shake flasks. Also, as glucose is added to these flasks, higher cell masses are usually experienced, frequently resulting in oxygen limitation. To a certain extent, this situation may be addressed by using baffled flasks and/or reducing the medium volume in the flask, such as reducing the volume in a 250 ml shake flask from 50 ml to 25 ml or even 12 ml. The evaporation problems frequently experienced at lower volumes can usually be addressed by maintaining a high relative humidity (approximately 90%) in the incubation chamber.

If catabolite repression is encountered an alternative to the adoption of feed strategies is to explore alternative carbon sources such as other mono-saccharides, polysaccharides, oligosaccharides, or oils.

3.2 Nitrogen source

Microbes require nitrogen to support the biosynthesis of nitrogenous metabolites, both primary and secondary. The primary metabolites include purines, pyrimidines, and amino acids. Penicillin, chloramphenicol, and tetra-cycline are only a few of the well-known, nitrogen-containing secondary metabolites. Both organic and inorganic sources of nitrogen may be used in microbiological media and some examples of commonly found constituents of economically important media are presented in *Table 3*. The choice of nitrogen source can have a major effect on the pH drift occurring during microbial growth. Ammonium salts, such as ammonium sulfate, will usually produce acid conditions as the ammonium ion is utilized and free acid liber-ated. On the other hand, nitrates will normally cause an alkaline drift as they are metabolized. Ammonium nitrate will first cause an acid drift as the ammonium ion is utilized and nitrate assimilation is repressed. When the ammonium ion has been exhausted there is an alkaline drift as the nitrate is used as an alternative nitrogen source. Thus, such nitrogen sources require the incorporation of effective buffers into the medium (usually in the form of phosphates or organic buffers) or the use of electronic pH control systems. An alternative approach to limit pH drift is the use of the ammonium salt of a weak acid—for example, ammonium succinate. In this case, as the ammo-nium ion is consumed the organic acid accumulates which, due to its poor ionization, only affects the pH marginally. This solution is observed occasion-ally in the design of antibiotic production media for shake-flask culture where high phosphate buffer concentrations may inhibit product formation. It is also worth remembering that if nitrate is used as a nitrogen source then ammonium molybdate must be incorporated as a trace element because it is a cofactor of nitrate reductase.

Organic nitrogen sources can also cause pH drift in a culture. If the pri-mary carbon source (such as glucose) becomes limited then amino acids in the medium (providing the primary nitrogen source) may be utilized as car-bon. During amino acid metabolism deamination occurs, often resulting in the accumulation of ammonia. This situation may be addressed by buffering or re-designing the medium composition. Also, the level of ammonium ion in the medium may be reduced by adding an ammonium ion-trapping agent to the medium such as natural zeolite (13).

The concentration of nitrogen in the medium may not inhibit growth but still repress the biosynthesis of secondary metabolites. For example, Young *et al.* (14) demonstrated that ammonium chloride at 200 mM repressed the synthesis of lincomycin but did not repress cell growth. A stringent feeding strategy must be employed during the penicillin fermentation to ensure that the nitrogen level is optimal for high penicillin production (15).

3.3 Oxygen

Oxygen is also a key element of microbial cells, frequently found as a constituent of macromolecules (nucleic acids, proteins, lipopolysaccharides, etc.) as well as primary and secondary metabolites. This 'oxygen demand' is usually met with medium ingredients such as water and organic compounds, especially carbohydrates. Molcular oxygen plays a key role in generating energy for the cell by serving as a final hydrogen or electron acceptor during aerobic respiration. This source of molecular oxygen is supplied as gaseous oxygen during aeration of the culture. Continuous air sparging is required due to the low solubility of gaseous oxygen in water, 6.99 p.p.m. at 35 °C (16). Meeting the molecular oxygen demand can become a major concern when high cell densities and high broth viscosities are reached.

3.4 Inorganic ions

Cultivation media routinely include phosphate, sulfate, potassium, calcium, magnesium, manganese, zinc, and ferric ions to meet the mineral requirements of most microbial cells. Of these eight ions, the first two are usually required at higher concentrations. Organic phosphate plays an active role in intermediary metabolism, especially as a constituent of 'high energy' compounds such as adenosine triphosphate, adenosine diphosphate, and arginine phosphate. Phosphate is also a constituent of phospholipids and nucleic acids and a regulator of certain enzymes of both primary and secondary metabolism (17). Sulfate is required for the biosynthesis of sulfur-containing amino acids and certain secondary metabolites, most notably the β-lactam antibiotics. This sulfate was found to be an excellent sulfur source for the biosynthesis of the cephamycin C molecule (18). The remaining ions (potassium, calcium, magnesium, manganese, zinc, and iron) plus copper, cobalt, and molybdenum are commonly referred to as the inorganic micronutrients or trace elements. As implied by this terminology, these ions are only required in trace amounts as cofactors or activators for many enzymic systems and as biosynthetic regulators of several secondary metabolites (19). Often, inorganic micronutrients are added to the growth medium as contaminants in other medium components, as shown in *Table 4*, and/or as contaminants in tap water. However, to ensure that all these mineral elements are present, an aliquot of a trace element solution is frequently added to the cultivation medium. An example of a trace element solution used in the inoculum medium for the mevinolin fermentation (21) is composed of (per litre): 1 g of $FeSO_4 \cdot 7H_2O$, 1 g of $MnSO_4 \cdot 4H_2O$, 25 mg of $CuCl_2 \cdot 2H_2O$, 100 mg of $CaCl_2 \cdot 2H_2O$, 56 mg of H_3BO_3, 19 mg of $(NH_4)_6Mo_7O_{24} \cdot H_2O$, and 200 mg of $ZnSO_4 \cdot 7H_2O$. Ten millilitres of this trace element solution are added to one litre of inoculum medium. Metal hydroxides may precipitate at a pH higher than 8 and, thus, trace elements are often dissolved in acids to ensure

Table 4. Contamination levels of trace metals found in medium components[a]

Component	g/L	Mg	Mn	Zn	Fe	Ca	Cu	Co	Mo
		Concentration contributed by component (μM)							
Glucose	40.0	<1.6	<0.36	<0.03	<0.36	<0.5	<0.32	<0.34	<0.77
Yeast extract	5.0	108	<0.18	11.0	5.9	39.0	0.32	0.17	0.58
Potassium phosphate	13.6	<0.8	<0.18	0.11	0.53	<0.5	<0.16	<0.17	<0.38
Sodium citrate	9.8	<1.6	<0.36	0.08	<0.35	16.0	<0.31	<0.33	<0.76
Sodium sulfate	1.0	<0.16	0.07	<0.04	<0.04	<0.5	<0.03	<0.03	<0.08

[a] Modified from Scott *et al.* (20).

solubility. Alternatively, chelating agents such as EDTA may be incorporated into trace element solutions. Although these mineral elements are minor constituents of a cultivation medium, their level is important. The stimulatory and inhibitory levels of these elements on yeast growth were thoroughly reviewed by Jones and Greenfield (22).

3.5 Growth factors

Those compounds that microbes require for growth but are unable to synthesize are referred to as growth factors (23). For example, several vitamins (biotin, thiamine, inositol, and pantothenic acid) are required for the cultivation of certain strains of *Saccharomyces cerevisiae*. Amino acids are also considered to be growth factors when required for the cultivation of microorganisms auxotrophic for one or more amino acids. The fastidious bacterium *Leuconostoc paramesenteroides* requires, in addition to several vitamins and amino acids, both purines and the pyrimidine, uracil (24). These growth factors may be added to the cultivation medium separately or as constituents of complex nutrients.

4. Inducers

Compounds added to the cultivation medium to initiate the biosynthesis of a desired product are usually called inducers. One of the most commonly used inducers in molecular biology is isopropylthio-β-D-galactoside (IPTG). By adding this inducer to the cultivation medium, recombinant *Escherichia coli* cells (containing the *lac* promoter) are encouraged to produce large amounts of the desired protein product. The microbe does not metabolize the IPTG added to the medium (25). However, when galactose is used (in the absence of glucose) to induce foreign protein expression in yeast cells carrying the GAL10 promoter (26), this inducer may be metabolized during protein expression. Inducers are also requried in making other microbial products, especially enzymes. The presence of the inducer D-xylose in the cultivation medium is required for the production of D-glucose isomerase by *Streptomyces* (27).

5. Non-nutritional components

5.1 Selective agents

Medium formulations which include a compound that inhibits or suppresses the growth of microbes other than the one desired are referred to as selective. The selective agents may be toxic chemicals (tetrathionate, phenylethanol, etc.), dyes (methylene blue, eosin, etc.), or antimicrobials (ampicillin, kanamycin, nystatin, etc.). Selective media are usually employed to isolate a particular microbe from a mixed population such as isolation from clinical or environmental sources; however, they have also proved useful in keeping selective pressure on a recombinant microbe during cultivation. For example, the *kan* gene may be cloned on the same *E. coli* plasmid that carries a foreign protein gene. When this microbe is cultivated in a selective medium containing kanamycin, only the recombinant cells carrying the antibiotic resistance gene will be propagated. Cells that lose the plasmid would be inhibited by kanamycin (28).

5.2 Solidifying agents

Many of the medium formulations that support submerged growth will also support surface growth when a solidifying agent is included. The most widely used solidifier is agar, a polysaccharide extract from marine algae. It has the unique physicochemical property of melting at 84 °C and solidifying at 38 °C. A solid medium is achieved with an agar concentration of 15 g/L. Lower agar concentrations (approximately 7.5 g/L) will produce semi-solid media, which may be desirable for cultivating microbes that can grow only under low oxygen tension (such as motile, microaerophilic species).

6. Environmental factors

During medium development and optimization, several environmental factors are important, including the hydrogen ion concentration, temperature, formation of foam, and medium sterilization. The pH of the cultivation medium frequently affects the growth of the microbe and in some cases affects the biosynthesis of primary and secondary metabolites. The optimum pH range for growing bacteria, yeasts, and fungi is 6.5–7.5, 4.5–5.5, and 4.5–5.5, respectively (29). Control of pH in shake-flask cultivations is usually achieved with buffers, including organic buffers (Tris and MOPS), whereas the control of pH in bioreactors is routinely accomplished by the automatic addition of acid or base.

The temperature at which microorganisms are cultivated is also important. Those that grow best at 5–15 °C, 20–40 °C, and 45–60 °C are referred to as psychrophilic, mesophilic, and thermophilic, respectively (29). Although most cultivations are performed at the optimum temperature for growth, some may be performed at lower-than-optimum temperatures to slow down cell growth. This latter approach may be useful during the growth phase of a fermentation cycle where meeting the dissolved oxygen demand can be quite difficult, especially if a nutritionally rich medium is employed. Foam formation during microbial cultivation is undesirable but sometimes unavoidable. Although foam formation is usually not a serious problem at the shake-flask scale, it is indeed an important concern in bioreactors. A number of antifoams are effective in controlling foam formation, including the silicones and polyalkylglycols (polyethylene glycol and polypropylene glycol), and partially oxidized animal and vegetable oils (lard oil, and soybean oil, respectively). The silicones and polyalkylglycols are highly active at low concentrations, minimizing any influence they may have on product recovery. In some fermentations, the vegetable oil serves not only as an antifoam but also as a carbon source, greatly reducing its level prior to product recovery. During medium development, several antifoams at various concentrations are usually evaluated initially at the shake-flask scale with the best candidates evaluated in bioreactors.

Medium sterilization is a crucial part of medium design playing a pivotal role in a properly formulated culture medium. Sterilization is routinely accomplished by a batch process employing heat and pressure, although continuous sterilizers are favoured in large-scale industrial processes. The primary goal of the sterilization operation is to eliminate all viable microbes from the medium. A side-effect that must be considered is the possibility of chemical alteration of the medium components. One obvious deleterious effect is the destruction of heat-labile components such as vitamins (pyridoxine, riboflavin, thiamine). Another damaging reaction is the property exhibited by certain amino acids (arginine, glutamine, tryptophan) which undergo chemical rearrangement reactions upon exposure to excessive temperatures. Another harmful reaction which may occur during sterilization is the complexing of certain components, resulting in precipitation reactions and the net reduction in the bioavailability of nutrients which are otherwise present chemically. For instance, many di- and trivalent metal cations react with phosphates to form an insoluble precipitate. This problem can be overcome by the incorporation of a chelating agent in the medium.

Another approach to avoid these unfavourable reactions is to sterilize certain medium components separately and supplement the culture medium with post-sterile additions. For instance, glucose is commonly heat-sterilized as a concentrated stock solution to avoid Maillard reactions which occur between reducing sugars and primary amines. Heat-labile components are usually sterilized by filtration and again added to the medium as a post-sterile addition. It is common practice to examine the sensitivity of the culture medium to heat sterilization and to reformulate as the process matures to larger scales of operation.

7. Medium optimization

Once initial cultivation of the desired microbe is achieved, the medium is frequently subjected to optimization studies. Medium optimization generally refers to finding the conditions (appropriate nutrients, nutrient concentrations, temperature, aeration, etc.) that will support the best cell growth and/or synthesis of a particular microbial product. However, this endeavour should be performed within the context of the overall process objectives. For example, a medium optimized for supporting high levels of a particular secondary metabolite may also enhance the levels of its analogues, greatly reducing downstream isolation/purification yields. Thus, an improved medium formulation that minimizes the synthesis of the analogue but falls short in supporting maximum titres may still be considered optimized if the final production target is reached. As indicated in this example, having a good sense of the overall process objective is very important when conducting a successful optimization study.

A critical part of the medium optimization process is the ability to accurately measure the dependent variable, such as a recombinant protein, a secondary metabolite, or an enzyme activity for bioconversion. A robust assay is especially important to obtain a quantitative determination of the product of interest in fermentation medium or cell lysates. Fortunately, there have been great advances in the analytical technology available to the investigator (see Chapters 5, 6, and 7).

An optimization strategy that has been commonly used in the laboratory is the one-variable-at-a-time method in which one independent variable is optimized while the others are held constant. The optima for the remaining variables are determined using the same approach, provided the variables do not interact with one another. However, variables frequently do interact, preventing the use of this optimization approach from always yielding an optimum set of conditions (30). This approach can also be quite time consuming especially if several medium components are being examined. An alternative optimization strategy which has become popular for medium optimization especially in industry, is the use of statistically designed experiments that allow the investigator to evaluate more than one independent variable at a time. Two of these search methods that have proven to be effective are discussed in this chapter. In addition, a non-statistical optimization strategy (Simplex optimization) proven to be quite successful in rapidly identifying the experimental optimum is also presented. As expected, the success of these optimization methods can be greatly influenced by what is known about the physiology, metabolism, and stability of the microbe, including plasmid stability in recombinant microbes. Also, because of the relatively large number of experiments required to optimize a medium, these experiments are usually performed in shake-flask culture. The performance achieved in shake flasks is frequently achieved in batch-operated fermenters (31); however, there are exceptions.

7.1 Full factorial search

As discussed earlier, there are many nutritional factors (independent variables) that can affect microbial growth and product synthesis. Employing a full factorial search can be successful but time consuming. An evaluation of only six nutrients at three concentrations would require a total of 3^6 or 729 separate experimental trials. This large number of trials, combined with relatively long fermentation cycles (especially for the production of secondary metabolites) make the full factorial search impractical for medium optimization when several variables are examined. However, the full factorial search is effective if only a few variables (2–4) are evaluated (32). Rincón *et al.* (33) successfully used full factorial designs (2^4 and 3^2) to optimize the production of L-lactic acid in the fermentation of whey. A total of 29 experimental trials were performed in groups of 16, 4, and 9 to achieve an enhanced lactic acid production rate.

7.2 Statistical search

7.2.1 Screening effects

A search procedure widely used to identify those variables which have a significant effect on the desired response from a larger number of potential variables (> 5) with a minimum of testing was introduced by Plackett and Burman (34). They developed a number of designs for almost every multiple of four experimental trials from 4 to 100. Each design is a fraction of the two-level factorial design. Three of the Plackett and Burman designs frequently used consist of 12, 20, and 28 experimental trials. The maximum number of variables that can be evaluated in one design is equal to one less than the number of individual experiments. An example of a Plackett and Burman design for 12 separate trials is presented in *Table 5*, consisting of seven

Table 5. Plackett–Burman design for 12 trials

Trial	Random order[a]	x_1	x_2	x_3	x_4	x_5	x_6	x_7	'Dummy' variables 1	2	3	4
1		+	+	−	+	+	+	−	−	−	+	−
2		−	+	+	−	+	+	+	−	−	−	+
3		+	−	+	+	−	+	+	+	−	−	−
4		−	+	−	+	+	−	+	+	+	−	−
5		−	−	+	−	+	+	−	+	+	+	−
6		−	−	−	+	−	+	+	−	+	+	+
7		+	−	−	−	+	−	+	+	−	+	+
8		+	+	−	−	−	+	−	+	+	−	+
9		+	+	+	−	−	−	+	−	+	+	−
10		−	+	+	+	−	−	−	+	−	+	+
11		+	−	+	+	+	−	−	−	+	−	+
12		−	−	−	−	−	−	−	−	−	−	−

[a] Use random number table.

assigned variables (such as different nutrients) and four unassigned variables, commonly referred to as the 'dummy' variables, used to estimate the experimental error during analysis of the data. The matrix is designed so that each independent variable is evaluated six times at its high (+) level and six times at its low (−) level. Also, each time independent variable x_1 is evaluated at its high value, independent variable x_2 is evaluated three times at its high value and three times at its low value. The same holds true when variable x_1 is evaluated at its low value. This matrix design cancels the effect of changing variable x_2 in the presence of variable x_1, allowing variable x_1 to be independently evaluated. This characteristic of the design holds as long as there are no apparent interactions between the variables. Other fractional factorial designs (35) can be used when interactions need to be considered.

The search procedure to identify the variables having a significant effect is given in *Protocol 1*.

Protocol 1. Plackett and Burman procedure to identify the most important of seven variables in a system

Method

1. Identify the variables (medium components).
2. Identify the response to be measured, for example, biomass level, product concentration, enzyme activity.
3. Assign each variable a high (+) and a low (−) value. (A large differential is recommended, but too large a differential can mask the effects of the other variables.)
4. Design a matrix as illustrated in *Table 5*.
5. Run the tests in random order to avoid bias in the experimentation.
6. Read the results (i.e. response to be measured, for example biomass level, product concentration, enzyme activity).
7. Determine the effect (E) of the first independent variable (x_1) on the response:

   Ex_1 = (Total of high responses/6) − (Total of low responses/6).
8. Repeat Step 7 for each of the remaining variables (x_2 to x_7).
9. Determine the effect of (E) of each of the 'dummy' variables (1, 2, 3, and 4).
10. If the effect of any of the 'dummy' variables is not close to zero, suspect an experimental error or interactions.
11. Calculate the variance effect (V_{eff}) by averaging the squares of the 'dummy' variable effects:

$$V_{eff} = (E_1^2 + E_2^2 + E_3^2 + E_4^2)/4.$$

12. Calculate the standard error (SE) which is the square root of the variance:

$$SE = \sqrt{V_{eff}}.$$

13. Apply the Student t test for each variable by dividing its effect by the standard error, for example:

$$tx_1 = Ex_1/SE.$$

14. Consult probability tables to decide whether the effect is significant. Consider the effect 'real' (caused by the nutrient and not by chance) when the tx_1 value is greater than the P value (2.8) of the t-distribution at four degrees of freedom and a significance level of 0.95.

15. Select variables which have significant effects and then embark on further optimization of these variables.

The other frequently used designs (20 and 28 trials) may be constructed by shifting the first row of their matrices (*Table 6*) in a cyclic manner one place, 18 and 26 times, respectively (36). The last row consists of only minus signs. The use of Plackett and Burman designs has been made easier by their inclusion in recently developed statistical software, such as JMP® (SAS Institute Inc.).

7.2.2 Exploring the response surface

Once the number of continuous independent variables which have a significant effect on the response is narrowed to only a few (3–5), a method is required for finding the combination of these variables that supports the best or acceptable response in a timely manner. A response surface type of experimental programme is quite popular and effective for this situation (37, 38, 39). The progression towards the optimum is followed by a series of contour lines constructed from a determination of the linear, interaction, and curvature effects of the independent variables, using the following full quadratic polynomial model for three independent variables:

$$Y = b_0 + b_1(x_1) + b_2(x_2) + b_3(x_3) + b_{12}(x_1x_2) + b_{13}(x_1x_3)$$
$$+ b_{23}(x_2x_3) + b_{11}(x_1)^2 + b_{22}(x_2)^2 + b_{33}(x_3)^2;$$

where:

Y = desired response
b_0 = regression coefficient at centre point
b_1, b_2, b_3 = linear coefficients
x_1, x_2, x_3 = independent variables
b_{12}, b_{13}, b_{23} = second-order interaction coefficients
b_{11}, b_{22}, b_{33} = quadratic coefficients.

Since curvature effects are estimated, the experimental design is required to have a minimum of three levels for each independent variable. Although this requirement is achieved with a full three-level factorial design, frequently

Table 6. First row of two Plackett–Burman designs

Number of trials	Elements
20	+ + − − + + + + − + − + − − − − + + −
28	+ − + + + + − − − − − + − − − + − − + + + − + − + + − +

they prove to be impractical. Here again, the use of partial factorial designs are attractive, especially those of Box and Behnken (40). Each of their designs is a fraction of a full three-level factorial. The Box–Behnken design for the three independent variables and 13 experimental trials is presented in *Table 7*. Each column represents an independent variable and each row an experimental trial. The elements, +, 0, and − represent the high, medium, and low levels, respectively, of each independent variable. The geometric character of this three-variable design is a cube (*Figure 1*) with all experimental points at the mid-points of its edges except the centre point (0 0 0). Thus, all experimental points (except the centre one) lie on a single sphere or equal distance from the centre. The values assigned to the levels of independent variable should be equally spaced. Since the centre point is replicated twice (used to provide a measure of the inherent experimental error), a total of 15 experimental trials are performed, again in random order to avoid bias in experimentation. After the trials are completed and the responses determined, the coefficients of the quadratic polynomial model are calculated using regression analysis. These calculations may be made by several computer programs,

Table 7. Box–Behnken design for three independent variables

Trial	Random Order[a]	Independent variables		
		x_1	x_2	x_3
1		+	+	0
2		+	−	0
3		−	+	0
4		−	−	0
5		+	0	−
6		+	0	−
7		−	0	+
8		−	0	−
9		0	+	+
10		0	+	−
11		0	−	+
12		0	−	−
13		0	0	0

[a] Use random number table.

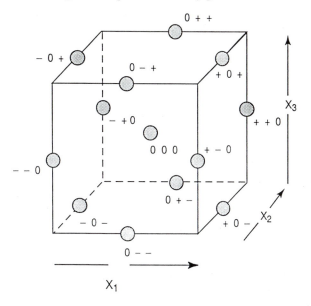

Figure 1. Box–Behnken design.

including the JMP® software which also generates contours of the responses against two independent variables.

An example of a contour plot generated during medium development of one of our product candidates is presented in *Figure 2*. A suggested area of optimal productivity is encircled by the 750 units/L contour. By performing a 'confirmation' fermentation at the suggested optimum conditions (68 g/L glucose and 18 g/L peptonized milk), a high titre of 770 units/L was achieved. A more precise optimum may have been identified by running a second set of similar trials or a pattern search (discussed below) in the optimum region. The use of a screening method that considers first-order effects (such as the Plackett and Burman designs) followed by the response surface type of programme that considers interactions, has proven to be a very efficient medium optimization strategy (41, 42).

7.3 Pattern search

Another popular and easy-to-use optimization strategy is the sequential simplex method (43) in which the optimum area is located through a series of sequential moves towards the better responses. The key component of this method is the simplex, a geometric figure having a number of vertices (experimental points) equal to one more than the number of independent variables (n) to be investigated. For example, the simplex for a two-variable experiment is a triangle, for a three-variable experiment it is a tetrahedron, etc. This search is initiated with only $n + 1$ experimental trials and followed by

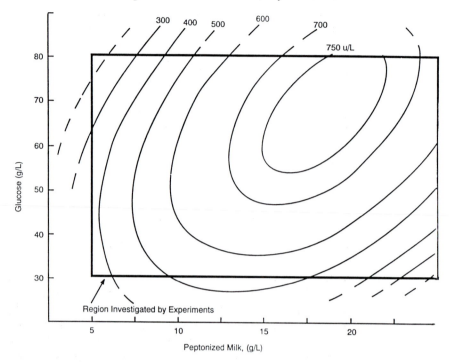

Figure 2. Contour plot for two independent variables.

one additional trial each time the simplex is moved, in accordance with the 'rules' of this procedure (44). Only the medium components that had a significant effect on the desired response in an initial screening/optimization study are examined further. For simplicity, a two-variable example is presented in *Figure 3*. The first vertex (A), is usually equal to the level of variables x_1 and x_2 that gave the best response in an initial screening/optimization study. The location of the next two vertices (B and C) is dependent on the step size (length) selected for each edge of the triangle adjacent to vertex A. Although the step size is arbitrary, it should be large enough to cause a change in the response. Also, initially selecting a large step size usually results in reaching the optimum area more quickly. Long (45) suggested that one side of the first triangle should be parallel to one of the independent variable axes. After vertices B and C are defined, the response at each of the experimental points is determined and ranked. The vertex that produces the least desirable response is discarded and replaced by vertex D, the mirror image of vertex A across face BC. Thus a new simplex, BCD, is formed. The response at the new experimental point is determined and ranked with those previously determined for vertices B and C. Here again the vertex with the least desirable response is discarded, provided it is not the reflected vertex. Discarding this vertex would cause the simplex to reflect back to its original position,

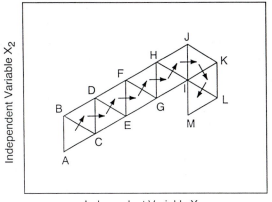

Independent Variable X₁

Figure 3. Simplex optimization for two independent variables.

preventing the simplex from reaching the optimum. Thus, the vertex with the second worst response in the new simplex is discarded, allowing the simplex to continue to seek the optimal response. As the simplex moves, occasionally the reflected vertex may exceed the boundaries of one or more of the variables (such as the solubility of a medium component). The simplex is brought back into the boundaries by assigning a very undesirable response to this experimental point. Once the 'optimum' is located, the simplex circles. A more precise optimum may be located by conducting a second simplex search with smaller step sizes in the region of the previously identified optimum. This procedure is summarized in *Protocol 2*.

Protocol 2. Simplex optimization of a pair of nutrient ingredients

Method

1. Decide upon the two nutrient ingredients to be optimized.
2. Draw two axes (as in *Figure 3*) representing the concentrations of the two ingredients.
3. Choose an initial combination of ingredient concentrations, normally the optimum combination so far demonstrated. Decide on another two combinations such that, when the points are inserted on your figure, an equilateral triangle is constructed (ABC in *Figure 3*).
4. Carry out the growth experiments and read the results (i.e. response to be measured, for example biomass level, product concentration, enzyme activity).
5. Construct a line on your figure from the worst result experiment (A in *Figure 3*) through the mid-point of the line joining the other two

---

Protocol 2. *Continued*

experiments (BC in *Figure 3*). The nutrient combination to be used in the next experiment will be on this line.

6. Determine the precise position of the next combination of concentrations (i.e. the next experiment) along the constructed line as that point (D in *Figure 3*) which allows the construction of an equilateral triangle with the two best previous results (BCD in *Figure 3*).

7. Carry out the growth experiments and read the results.

8. Repeat the procedures described in Steps 5 and 6.

9. Continue the process until the series of triangles 'circle' as in *Figure 3*.

In the previous example of a two-dimensional simplex, the coordinates of the reflected vertex is easily determined graphically. However, with a three-dimensional simplex or higher, the following equation may be used to establish the coordinates of the reflected vertex, R:

$$R = P + (P - W);$$

where W is the coordinates of the discarded vertex, and P is the average coordinates of the retained vertices.

This calculation is simplified by using a worksheet similar to that used by Long (45). As described, reflection is the key operation of the simplex method; however, by modifying this method, Neadler and Mead (46) were able to include two additional operations, expansion and contraction.

This sequential search method is quite attractive for medium optimization when the fermentation cycle is relatively short, as is the case with many recombinant *E. coli* fermentations. This method is also attractive when further medium optimization is required during process scale-up when the number of available fermenters is limited.

Once the medium is optimized for the targeted response(s) employing one or more of the search methods just described, re-optimization may be considered, especially if the optimal response level is below expectation. Re-optimization could include additional independent variables (such as carbon and nitrogen sources) and larger ranges of the previously examined independent variables. Medium re-optimization is usually required when one or more of its constituents is no longer available or becomes too expensive (i.e. economically unattractive). And last, this technique continues to be a critical component of mutation/selection programmes, running parallel to the selection of improved mutants.

Acknowledgement

We thank F. Shen for his critical review of the statistical part of this chapter.

References

1. Atlas, R. M. and Parks, L. C. (1993). *Handbook of microbiological media*. CRC Press, Boca Raton.
2. Demain, A. L. and Solomon, N. A. (1986). *Manual of industrial microbiology and biotechnology*. American Society for Microbiology, Washington, DC.
3. Monaghan, R. L., Alberts, A. W., Hoffman, C. H., and Albers-Schonberg, B. (1980). US Patent 4,231,938.
4. Burg, R. W., Miller, B. M., Baker, E. E., Birnbaum, J., Currie, S. A., Hartman, R., *et al.* (1979). *Antimicrob. Agents Chemother.*, **15**, 361.
5. Maiese, W. M. and Wax, R. G. (1977). US Patent 4,024,251.
6. Kojima, I., Cheng, Y. R., Mohan, V., and Demain, A. L. (1995). *J. Indust. Microbiol.*, **14**, 436.
7. Stephenne, J. (1990). *Vaccine*, **8**, S69.
8. Zhang, J., Marcin, C., Shifflet, M. A., Salmon, P., Brix, T., Greasham, R., *et al.* (1996) *Appl. Microbiol. Biotechnol.*, **44**, 568.
9. Zabriskie, D. W., Armiger, W. B., Phillips, K. H. and Albano, P. A. (1988). In *Trader's guide to fermentation media formulation*. Trader's Protein, Memphis.
10. Verduyn, C. (1991). *Antonie van Leeuwenhock*, **60**, 325.
11. Demain, A. L. (1989). In *Regulation of secondary metabolism in Actinomycetes* (ed. S. Shapiro), p. 127. CRC Press, Boca Raton.
12. Cortés, J., Liras, P., Castro, J. M., and Martín, J. F. (1986). *J. Gen. Microbiol.*, **132**, 1805.
13. Masuma, R., Tanaka, Y., and Ómura, S. (1982). *J. Antibiotics*, **35**, 1184.
14. Young, M. D., Kempe, L. L., and Bader, F. G. (1985). *Biotechnol. Bioeng.*, **27**, 327.
15. Queener, S. and Swartz, R. W. (1979). *Econ. Microbiol.*, **3**, 35.
16. Atkinson, B. and Mavituna, F. (1991). *Biochemical engineering and biotechnology handbook*, p. 703. Stockton Press, NY.
17. Martin, J. F. (1989). In *Regulation of secondary metabolism in Actinomycetes* (ed. S. Shapiro), p. 213. CRC Press, Boca Raton.
18. Inamine, E. and Birnbaum, J. (1973). US Patent 3,770,590.
19. Weinberg, E. D. (1989). In *Regulation of secondary metabolism in Actinomycetes* (ed. S. Shapiro), p. 239. CRC Press, Boca Raton.
20. Scott, R. E., Jones, A., Lam, K. S., and Gaucher, G. M. (1986). *Can. J. Microbiol.*, **32**, 259.
21. Alberts, A. W., Chen, J., Kuron, G., Hunt, V., Huff, J., Hoffman, C., *et al.* (1980). *Proc. Natl Acad. Sci. USA*, **77**, 3957.
22. Jones, R. P. and Greenfield, P. F. (1984). *Process Biochem.*, **April**, 48.
23. Guirard, B. M. and Snell, E. E. (1981). In *Manual of methods for general bacteriology* (eds. P. Gerhardt, R. G. E. Murray, R. N. Costilow, E. W. Nester, W. A. Wood, N. R. Krieg, *et al.*), p. 79. American Society for Microbiology, Washington, DC.
24. Garvie, E. I. (1967). *J. Gen. Microbiol.*, **48**, 429.
25. Sambrook, J., Fritsch, E. F., and Maniatis, T. (1989). In *Molecular cloning: a laboratory manual* (ed. C. Nolan), p. 17.13. Cold Spring Harbor Laboratory Press, NY.
26. Kniskern, P. J., Hagopian, A., Montgomery, D. L., Carty, C. E., Burke, P., *et al.* (1991). In *Expression systems and processes for rDNA products* (ed. R. T. Hatch,

C. Goochee, A. Moreira, and Y. Alroy), p. 65. ACS Symposium Series No. 477. American Chemical Society, Washington DC, USA.

27. Sanchez, S. and Quinto, C. M. (1975). *Appl. Microbiol.*, **30**, 750.
28. Sambrook, J., Fritsch, E. F., and Maniatis, T. (1989). In *Molecular cloning: a laboratory manual* (ed. C. Nolan), p. 1.5. Cold Spring Harbor Laboratory Press, NY.
29. Moat, A. G. and Foster, J. W. (1988). *Microbial physiology*, p. 21. John Wiley & Sons, NY.
30. Silveira, R. G., Kakizo-mo, T., Takemoto, S., Nishio, N., and Nagai, S. (1991). *J. Ferment. Bioeng.*, **72**, 20.
31. Kennedy, M. J., Sarah, L., Reader, R., Davies, J., Rhoades, D. A., and Silby, H. W. (1994). *J. Ind. Microbiol.*, **13**, 212.
32. Haltrich, D., Preiss, M., and Steiner, W. (1993). *Enzyme Microb. Tech.*, **15**, 854.
33. Rincón, J., Fuertes, J., Moya, A., Monteagudo, J. M., and Rodríguez, L. (1993). *Acta Biotechnol.*, **13**, 323.
34. Plackett, R. L. and Burman, J. P. (1946). *Biometrika*, **33**, 305.
35. Box, G. E. P., Hunter, W. G., and Hunter, J. S. (1978). *Statistics for experiments*, p. 373. John Wiley & Sons, NY.
36. Stowe, R. A. and Mayer, R. P. (1966). *Ind. Eng. Chem.*, **58**, 36.
37. Prapulla, S. G., Jacob, Z., Chand, N., Rajalakshmi, D., and Karanth, N. G. (1992). *Biotech. Bioeng.*, **40**, 965.
38. Rao, P. V., Jayaraman, K., and Lakshmanan, C. M. (1993). *Proc. Biochem.*, **28**, 391.
39. Lekha, P. K., Chand, N., and Lonsane, B. K. (1994). *Bioproc. Eng.*, **11**, 7.
40. Box, G. E. P. and Behnken, D. W. (1960). *Technometrics*, **2**, 455.
41. Roseiro, J. C., Esgalhado, M. E., Amaral Collaço, M. T., and Emery, A. N. (1992). *Proc. Biochem.*, **27**, 167.
42. Haltrich, D., Laussamayer, B., and Steiner, W. (1994). *Appl. Microbiol. Biotechnol.*, **42**, 522.
43. Spendley, W., Hext, G. R., and Himsworth, F. R. (1962). *Technometrics*, **4**, 441.
44. Deming, S. N. and Morgan, S. L. (1973). *Anal. Chem.*, **45**, 278.
45. Long, D. E. (1969). *Anal. Chim. Acta*, **46**, 193.
46. Neadler. J. A., and Mead, R. A. (1965). *Comput. J.*, **7**, 308.
47. Bergey's Manual of Determinative Bacteriology, Eighth Edition, (1975) (ed. R. E. Buchanan, N. E. Gibbons). The Williams & Wilkins Co., Baltimore, MD, USA.

4

Working with laboratory fermenters

STEPHEN COLLINS

1. Introduction

Shake flasks are commonly used to grow microbial cells in small quantities at relatively low cell densities (up to 5–10 g/litre). However, the experimenter has little control over the environment experienced by the microorganisms. Process variables such as pH or oxygen concentration are likely to change during the course of the experiment. Terms such as 'late log phase' are commonly used to describe such cultures when there is, in fact, no data to support the assumption of constant growth rate implied in the term. Indeed, it is likely that changes in the environment will affect the physiology of the cells.

The first requirement of a laboratory fermenter is to provide a device in which the environmental variables which are likely to affect culture physiology can be monitored and controlled. It consists essentially of a sterilizable vessel fitted with an agitator and aeration system, into which various measuring probes can be fitted. The vessel and fittings must be designed to maintain aseptic conditions and to permit inoculation, sampling, and other necessary operations with minimal risk of contamination to the culture. In addition to data from the probes further information is obtainable by analysis of the air stream leaving the fermenter ('vent gas') and culture supernatant (see Chapters 6 and 7, respectively).

The range of physiological conditions which can be defined reproducibly is greatly extended by continuous culture methods. In chemostat culture, the limiting nutrient can be defined, and growth rate becomes a parameter under the control of the experimenter when steady state is achieved. This opens the possibility for many types of study not amenable to simple batch techniques. Fed-batch culture is another technique which may be used to control growth rate and define nutrient limitation, although a true steady state is not obtained in this technique. It can be used to achieve very high cell densities, as in the bakers' yeast fermentation, where cell concentration may exceed 100 g/litre. It is also of great value in a number of industrial processes where the product of interest is made after cell proliferation has ceased—examples include the manufacture of several antibiotics, citric acid, and biological polymers.

The intention of this chapter is to provide practical guidance to individuals who have experience of microbiology and aseptic techniques who are starting work with laboratory fermenters. Readers requiring additional detail on the topics dealt with here are referred to the previously published volume in this series (1). It is also assumed that the beginner will not be handling pathogens requiring special containment.

2. Laboratory requirements

If the normal facilities of a microbiology laboratory are available then no additional facilities are necessary for setting up one or two small bench-top fermenters, although the demands placed upon the media make-up facilities (autoclaves and incubators used for inoculum production) will necessarily increase. However, additional services will be required for a specialized fermentation facility. Consider the following points if setting up such a facility:

(a) Cooling water: oxidative fermentations produce heat, approx. 450 J per mmole O_2 consumed. Cooling is therefore essential for intensive aerobic fermentations. Cooling water is also needed for the exit gas condenser.

(b) Compressed air: except for small laboratory fermenters with their own air pump, compressed air is essential. The pressure must be compatible with equipment. Filtration is required to remove particles and oil, minimizing the duty of the sterilizing filter. Compressors are noisy and better housed outside the main laboratory.

(c) Steam: most *in situ* sterilizable fermenters require a steam supply. Steam is also needed for sample valves and may be required for sterilizing connections to ancillary equipment.

(d) Electricity supply: a 3-phase (450 V) supply is required for some types of equipment. A large number of standard electricity sockets will also be needed.

(e) Flooring and drainage: the need for a constant supply of cooling water poses a potential flooding risk, but the use of pressure hosing with 'Swagelock' or similar fittings minimizes it—avoid silicone rubber tubing and 'Jubilee clips'. A waterproof, self-draining floor minimizes the risk of flood damage.

(f) Furniture: adequate provision of normal laboratory fittings for equipment cleaning, preparation, and maintenance is essential. Ensure adequate provision for storage including tools and spares.

3. Choice of vessel

When choosing a fermenter consider the following points:

(a) Size: Small fermenters cost less, require less medium and space, and (if only one or two are required) do not need a special laboratory. However, the miniaturization of components makes them less reliable and more difficult to work with, increasing the risk of breakdown, accidental damage, or contamination. The scale of operation needs to be compatible with sampling requirements to avoid undue perturbation of the process from volume changes. Fermenters of 1–2 litres may be satisfactory for simple batch operation if large or numerous samples are not required. For continuous culture work small fermenters have the considerable advantage of minimizing the medium consumption. However, accurate quantitative work is more difficult at this scale because errors in liquid and gas flow measurements increase. It is much more difficult to obtain precise control over flow rate if the desired value is low, so a working volume of 5–10 litres is usually preferable for fed-batch work. If the fermenter is being used to make product or experimental materials, the scale will, of course, be determined by those requirements.

(b) Top or bottom drive: small bench fermenters are usually top driven. For *in situ* sterilizable equipment most manufacturers offer bottom drive as standard because the free access to the top plate gives greater convenience in use and more scope for the introduction of ports, probes, or other equipment. The risk of sudden total seal failure has been almost eliminated with modern equipment so this arrangement is really only likely to be a disadvantage if the medium contains insoluble and abrasive materials which could damage the seal.

(c) Autoclavable or *in-situ* sterilizable: *in-situ* sterilization is much quicker and more convenient. The main advantage of autoclavable equipment is its lower cost. However, sterilization *in situ* does require attention to safety because of the high temperature and pressure used. A pressure gauge and safety valve are essential. If a probe is insecure then it will fly out causing the vessel's boiling contents to be sprayed all over the laboratory. Use a check-list to ensure that all proper steps are taken to make the vessel secure. If glass vessels are to be used they must be designed to cope with the pressure and protected by a metal shield during sterilization. When purchasing an autoclavable fermenter, check that the assembled vessel, with probes, etc. will fit your autoclave.

(d) Glass or stainless steel: steel in contact with process fluids should be 316L (USA standard) stainless, but it is unlikely that a competent manufacturer will offer anything else. The safety advantage of all steel fermenters is obvious from the above discussion. Other benefits are better simulation of large-scale equipment, and temperature control can be provided by a jacket thus avoiding the need for internal coils. Most manufacturers do not supply steel vessels of less than 5 litres working volume and glass is usually the cheaper alternative. *In-situ* sterilizable glass vessels have steel top and bottom plates, usually held together with tie rods, with the joints sealed with rubber gaskets. The base may be dished or have a short cylindrical section enabling probes and sample ports to be fitted to it. Ensure that the fermenter has sufficient and appropriately sized ports for all probes, gas and liquid inputs and outputs, sampling, and inoculation. Examples of glass and stainless steel vessels are shown in *Figure 1*. A sectional diagram of a fermenter vessel is given in *Figure 2*.

4. Sterilization

Use a check-list to ensure that the necessary pre-sterilization preparation has been carried out. An example is given below, but specific details will depend upon the type of the fermenter being used. The head space and connecting air lines must be sterilized by steam which may either be generated from medium in the vessel or by injection from an external steam line. The temperature of the vessel or the media in it should be monitored, but sterilization times need to allow for all equipment to come up to temperature. Ensure that steam penetrates to all parts to be sterilized, e.g. by venting safety valves. If the vessel contains medium, run the agitator at low speed to ensure even temperature distribution. Sterilize sample valves, etc. at the same time as the main vessel.

Autoclavable vessels must be fully assembled, with all probes calibrated and additive bottles fitted before sterilization. Flexible lines must be clamped to prevent liquids siphoning (or sterilized with all vessels empty and filled

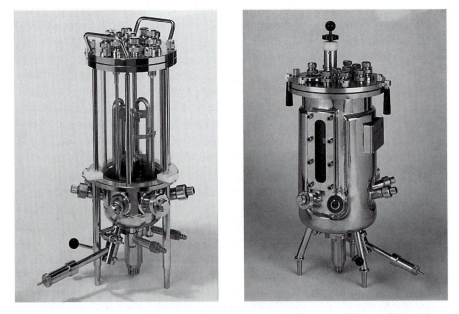

Figure 1. Glass and stainless steel fermenter vessels (Courtesy B. Braun Biotech.).

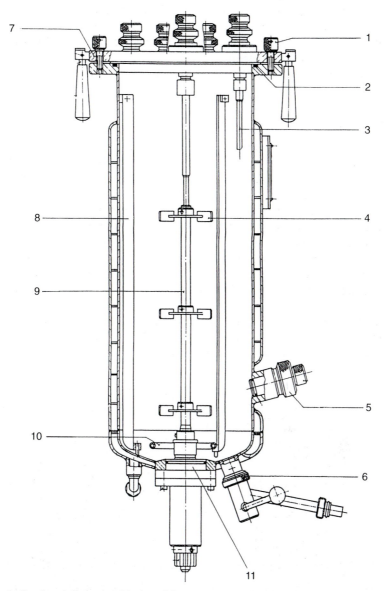

Figure 2. Sectional diagram of jacketed fermenter vessel. 1, Head plate securing bolt; 2, 'O'-ring; 3, air inlet; 4, impeller; 5, probe port; 6, sample valve; 5, head plate; 8, baffle; 9, drive shaft; 10, sparger; 11, seal assembly (Courtesy B. Braun Biotech.).

aseptically afterwards) and each vessel must be vented through a sterilizing filter. A basket or cradle to enable the assembled fermenter to be carried easily to and from the autoclave, minimizing the risk of accidentally breaking a connection, is recommended.

Example check-list for fermenter turn-round

1. **End previous run**
   - stop data logging to computer
   - stop gas analysis
   - clamp all flexible lines
   - kill vessel contents (e.g. 80 °C 30 min)
   - cool vessel
   - disconnect cooling water to condenser

2. **Cleaning**
   - 0.1 M NaOH at 80 °C for 30 min
   - 0.1 M citric acid 80 °C for 30 min
   - clean or replace exit and inlet filters
   - remove and clean probes
   - seal all outlets

3. **Preparation of ancillary equipment**
   - clean and check condition of flexible tubing on: acid, alkali, and antifoam bottles, feed bottle
   - check and clean pump

4. **Prepare and sterilize fermenter**
   - replace probes
   - check sufficient ports for experimental plan
   - check and calibrate electrode
   - renew septa
   - seal all outlets, ensure all ports are secure
   - fit shield to glass vessels
   - electrodes pressurized for sterilization
   - set recorder to monitor sterilization
   - fill thermostat reservoir
   - begin sterilization
   - steam the sample port
   - check DOT probe zero
   - when sterilization is complete set to running temperature
   - refill thermostat reservoir
   - set electrode pressure for fermentation
   - connect air inlet filter
   - check DOT '100%' value
   - zero the mass flow meter
   - complete other probe calibrations
   - fill bottles, prime lines, adjust pH to running value
   - add filter-sterilized ingredients
   - add antifoam
   - add carbon source or other nutrients if sterilized separately
   - set up data logging computer
   - inoculate fermenter
   - set up DOT control system

5. Aeration and agitation

Aeration rates of 0.5–1 volume of gas per volume of liquid per minute (vvm) are commonly used. Inlet air is sterilized by filtration (membrane or depth filters can be used) and enters the broth from a sparger near the bottom of the fermenter. The exit air is usually filtered both to protect the fermenter sterility and to avoid generating microbial aerosols. A condenser is usually fitted to keep the exit filter dry and to reduce evaporative loss. Air flow can be measured with a rotameter, but readings must be corrected for the air pressure at the measuring point. Thermal mass flow meters are preferable and give an electronic readout which can be recorded. Measurement of fermenter air pressure, although not absolutely necessary, is required if the performance of the aeration system is to be understood. Abnormal high pressure, usually the result of an exit filter blockage, may cause problems with titrant, antifoam, or media supply lines.

The major duty of the agitation system is to break up the gas bubbles, which generate a large surface area, to raise the rate of oxygen dissolution. This is essential for aerobic processes since the concentration of oxygen in air-saturated water at 30 °C at atmospheric pressure is only about 200 μM (6.4 mg/litre); at commonly achievable fermentation rates this would be consumed in a few seconds. The maximum achievable oxygen transfer rate determines the upper limit of productivity for many aerobic fermentations.

The major components of the aeration/agitation system are:

(a) **Impellers**: six-blade Rushton turbines are usually supplied for microbial work. They generate high sheer and good bubble break-up. They are most suitable for low viscosity fluids (e.g. yeast or unicellular bacteria), but are less satisfactory with viscous broths produced by filamentous or gum-producing microorganisms. Larger diameter impellers designed to achieve axially directed flow, possibly in combination with a draught tube to improve circulation, provide better mixing and aeration of such cultures.

(b) **Baffles**: are required to prevent rotation of liquid and the formation of a vortex which makes mixing and aeration much less effective. Internal coils and vertically fitted probes may provide sufficient baffling in small vessels.

(c) **Sparger**: this is usually circular and fitted closely below the bottom impeller.

6. Aseptic connections

It is usually necessary to make connections to the fermenter after sterilization, e.g. for antifoam, pH corrective fluids, medium, medium supplements, etc. Various systems can be used. A portable blow torch is better than a Bunsen burner for 'flaming'.

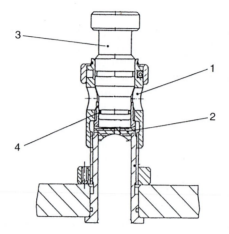

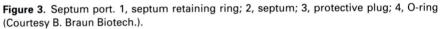

Figure 3. Septum port. 1, septum retaining ring; 2, septum; 3, protective plug; 4, O-ring (Courtesy B. Braun Biotech.).

6.1 Septum ports

A rubber septum is held in place by a ring. When being sterilized or when it is not in use the septum is protected by a plug screwed into the ring (*Figure 3*). The liquid line to be connected terminates in a wide hollow needle (typically 3–10 mm in diameter) which is protected by a cover during sterilization.

Protocol 1. Making a septum port connection

Method

1. Remove the protective plug.
2. Wet the septum surface with about 1–2 ml alcohol or industrial methylated spirits (IMS).
3. Ignite the alcohol and allow to burn out (**NB**: be sure it really is out before proceeding to avoid the risk of burning your hands).
4. Uncover the needle, flame it briefly, insert through the septum and secure.

This makes a permanent connection. Removal and replacement of a needle connection results in a high risk of contamination and is not recommended.

6.2 Line connections

Bayonet- or screw-fitting line connectors are available (*Figure 4*). They are commonly used in continuous culture work for replacing medium and culture receptor bottles. They are simple to use, but there is a slight risk of contamination.

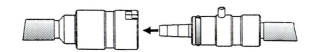

Figure 4. Bayonet fitting line connector (Courtesy B. Braun Biotech.).

Protocol 2. Use of a line connector

Method

1. Drain the line and clamp off the fermenter side.
2. Uncover a new sterile connector piece and flame.
3. Break the connection and flame fermenter side-connection piece.
4. Make the connection and remove the clamp.

Note: It is essential to minimize the time of exposure of the open connector pieces. It is usually easier and quicker with two people—one holding the connecting pieces and the other the blow torch.

6.3 Steam sterilizable connectors

Lines to the fermenter and vessel are closed by valves either side of the connector which may be opened, a new connection made, and re-sterilized. This appears to eliminate the contamination risk associated with making and breaking a line, but it is not foolproof. It is essential to ensure that steam fills all parts of the connector between the isolating valves displacing all air and condensate, and that sufficient time is allowed for the equipment to reach the sterilizing temperature and for sterilization to occur. Typically, this means that the line cannot be used for at least 30 minutes.

7. Inoculation

The simplest system is to inoculate using a hypodermic syringe via a septum port.

Protocol 3. Inoculation using a syringe

Method

1. Take up an inoculum from the shake flask (or other vessel in which it has been grown) into a sterile hypodermic syringe.
2. Replace the protective covers on the needle and carry the syringe to the fermenter.

Protocol 3. *Continued*

3. Sterilize the septum surface as described in *Protocol 1*.

4. Inject the inoculum.

5. Flame the septum and protective plug again and replace the plug.

The procedure carries a significant risk of contamination. This can be reduced by using a laminar-flow cabinet while taking the inoculum from the flask, but much depends upon the skill of the operator. There is also a potential safety hazard in using hypodermic needles and syringes with live organisms so the procedure is unacceptable for use with potential pathogens.

These problems can largely be overcome by growing the inoculum in a flask fitted with a side arm near the bottom. A flexible tube connects the flask to a septum-port connecting needle (or other appropriate connection system) and is closed by a clip. The use of a steam-sterilizable connector or special inoculation port (provided by some manufacturers) permits the inoculation system to be removed—otherwise the flask must be connected to the fermenter following *Protocol 1* and left in place after transfer of the contents.

8. Sampling

8.1 Syringe

The simplest method is to use a hypodermic syringe and a septum port. There is an obvious contamination hazard in repeatedly puncturing a septum. Flaming the surface after use and replacing the covering plug reduces the risk, but it is impossible to eliminate it. It is the most rapid technique and can be used with a stopping solution in the syringe (e.g. perchloric acid) to permit the measurement of concentrations of intermediates or substrates which would otherwise change in the few seconds required for other techniques. If this speed of sampling is not required use a hood or sampling valve to avoid the contamination risk.

8.2 Hoods

Autoclavable fermenters are commonly supplied with a sample hood designed to take a screw-fitting glass bottle. The hood is connected to the fermenter through a flexible tube ending in a dip pipe immersed in the culture. The flexible tube is normally closed with a clip—taking a sample normally only requires the clip to be opened when the positive pressure of the aeration system will be sufficient to cause the culture to flow into the sample bottle. Note that the tube will contain some culture which may not be typical of what is in the fermenter. It may be necessary to remove this, e.g. by taking two samples and discarding the first. When sufficient culture has been collected the tube is clamped, the sample bottle removed and replaced with a clean sterile bottle (remembering to flame the bottle neck and hood).

8.3 Sample valves

Stainless steel fermenters are normally fitted with a re-sterilizable sample valve (*Figure 5*). These are of various designs, but the usual arrangement is that they fit into the vessel so that the inner surface of the valve fits flush with the vessel wall and is sealed by an 'O' ring. The valve is designed so that

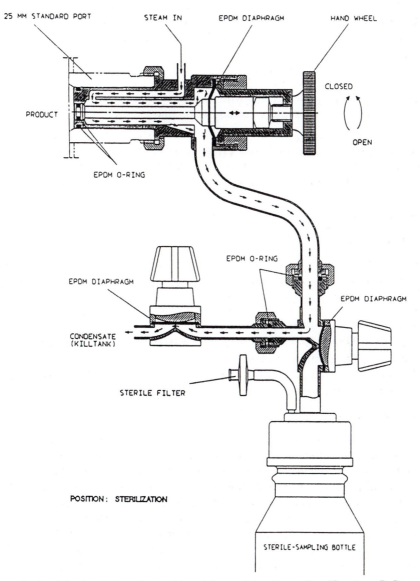

25 MM STANDARD PORT   STEAM IN   EPDM DIAPHRAGM   HAND WHEEL

CLOSED

PRODUCT

OPEN

EPDM O-RING

EPDM DIAPHRAGM

EPDM O-RING

EPDM DIAPHRAGM

CONDENSATE (KILLTANK)

STERILE FILTER

POSITION: STERILIZATION

STERILE-SAMPLING BOTTLE

Figure 5. Combined sample valve and hood for contained sampling (Courtesy B. Braun Biotech.).

steam can circulate everywhere beyond this seal. The valve is opened by moving it into the fermenter broth allowing the culture to flow out. The valve should be re-sterilized immediately after use. A slow stream of steam can be allowed to pass through the valve continuously to ensure maintenance of sterility, but this is inconvenient because the valve is always hot and will need to be cooled before a live sample can be taken. It is normally preferable to allow the valve to cool and to protect it with a removable cover or a length of tubing.

9. Media

The design of media is dealt with in Chapter 3. However, there are some specific points which require consideration here.

9.1 Sterilization of large volumes

There is no problem if the media can be sterilized in the fermenter, but if it is necessary to heat-sterilize volumes of 5 litres or more in an autoclave it can take a very long time for the unmixed contents to reach 120°C. Long autoclave cycles are likely to result in caramelization of a carbohydrate substrate and damage to vitamins and other delicate components. It may be necessary to compromise on less rigorous heat sterilization protocols or to use filtration to avoid medium damage. In continuous culture work filtration also has the advantage that filter-sterilizing into a sterile reservoir reduces the need to make and break medium lines.

9.2 Microbial growth in media supply lines

If the medium being pumped into a fermenter can support growth then the organism will eventually grow back up the supply line and contaminate the reservoir. A system to heat the inflowing stream can be effective in preventing grow-back of mesophilic organisms. (A simple device consists of a hot-water jacket surrounding a central tube, rather like a small Liebeg condenser with an abnormally narrow centre. Medium break systems (see Chapter 5 in ref. 1) can also be used, but the requirement to divert some of the incoming air through the device complicates interpretation of the gas analysis.) However, it is usually better to avoid the problem by careful consideration of the media design. For example, if the main source of nitrogen in the fermentation is supplied as ammonium ions, this can conveniently be achieved by using an ammonia solution to control the pH and providing some of the phosphate and sulfate as the respective acids. This will result in a medium of low pH which will not support growth. Another possibility is to provide a separate supply of the carbon source so that the fermenter is supplied with two streams, neither of which will support growth.

9.3 Salt balance

Common practice in continuous culture work is to design media so that one nutrient is limiting and all others are present in excess. This approach is unlikely to cause problems if biomass concentrations of up to 10 g/litre are required. However, if a higher biomass is needed (and densities up to 100 g/ litre are readily achievable with many organisms in fed-batch or continuous culture) excess salt may result in growth inhibition by high ionic strength. For example, if ammonium sulfate is used as the nitrogen source and sodium hydroxide for pH control, consumption of the ammonia would result in the accumulation of sodium sulfate which, in fed-batch culture, would eventually inhibit growth.

If it is unacceptable to use ammonia for pH control (e.g. because a nitrogen-limited culture is required) urea may provide the nitrogen source which would avoid these problems (but note that most microbial ureases require nickel and this element is not commonly included in trace element recipes). Knowledge of the composition of the microbial biomass in terms of the major elements (C, N, P, K, Mg, and S) enables media compositions to be calculated to avoid the accumulation of gross excesses (see Chapter 3).

10. Process measurement and control

As was stated in the introduction a major reason for using laboratory fermenters is to be able to monitor and control process variables. Only a brief survey can be provided here—readers are referred to Chapters 1 and 7 in ref. 1 for further information. The simplest form of control is on–off control as used in a simple thermostat. This may be acceptable for the control of temperature or pH if the variable tends to move in one direction only and the rate does not vary too greatly. However, if the response time of the measurement or the effect of corrective action is slow it is liable to result in overshoot or 'hunting'. It is totally unsatisfactory for dissolved oxygen control. Most fermenter manufacturers now supply equipment with proportional integral differential (PID) controllers where the degree of corrective action is a function of three values: the proportional error (i.e. the size of the error as a fraction of the proportional band—decreasing the proportional band increases the system sensitivity); the integral of the error as a function of time (i.e. the larger the duration of the error, the greater the corrective action taken); and the rate of change in the error (i.e. the corrective action increases the more rapidly the value is moving away from the set point and decreases if it is moving towards it).

10.1 pH

10.1.1 Measurement

pH Sensors measure the potential developed across a glass membrane as a result of the difference in concentration of hydrogen ions, to which the

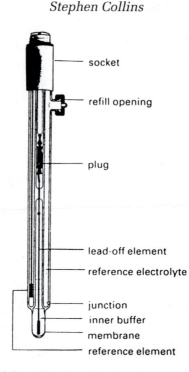

socket

refill opening

plug

lead-off element

reference electrolyte

junction
inner buffer
membrane
reference element

Figure 6. 'Ingold' combination pH probe (Courtesy Mettler Toledo).

membrane is selectively permeable. This is compared with a reference electrode contained in a separate compartment making electrical contact with the culture via a porous plug (*Figure 6*). The probe must be calibrated prior to each sterilization and the electrolyte topped up at the same time if necessary. Two buffer solutions should be used for calibration to ensure that the slope is correct (theoretically 59 mV per pH unit at 25 °C). It is usual to use a buffer near pH 7 to calibrate and one near pH 4 for the slope check—the use of a lower pH buffer is normally preferred since high pH buffers may be subject to change due to CO_2 absorption.

Since both the pH of the buffer and the response of the probe are temperature dependent but the meter's temperature compensator only allows for the latter effect, attention to this detail is needed when calibrating. Unless a special retractable housing is used, it is impossible to remove the pH probe during a run to check the calibration. Some indication of instrument drift can be obtained by checking the pH of samples, but the pH is prone to change during sampling as a result of CO_2 desorption. The effect may be quite large if the fermenter is pressurized.

Conventional electrolyte-filled probes on larger fermenters are fitted inside pressurized housings (*Figure 7*) to keep a positive pressure over the fermenter (this prevents chemical contamination of the electrolyte and reduces

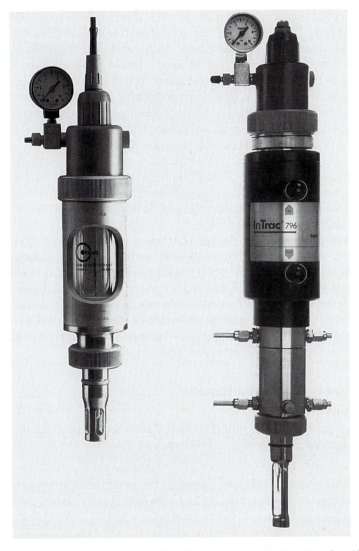

Figure 7. Conventional (left) and retractable (right) pressurizable housings for pH probes (Courtesy Mettler Toledo).

the risk of plug blockage). Sealed gel-filled probes provide a convenient alternative.

10.1.2 Control agents

The direction of pH movement is determined by the overall stoichiometry of the growth reaction. For an organism growing on a neutral substrate (e.g. carbohydrate) in a medium containing ammonium salts, the uptake of ammonia will cause a reduction in pH even if no acidic fermentation products accumulate. Therefore if nitrogen limitation is not required it is best to control the downward pH movement with ammonia. Conversely, use of nitrate as the nitrogen source results in an upward pH movement and here nitric acid is the appropriate control agent. If the carbon is supplied as the salt of an organic acid (e.g. acetate or succinate) the pH movement will be upward as the acidic substrate is oxidized leaving the alkaline counter ion in solution. Similarly, oxidation of an amino acid also causes an upward pH movement because this leaves ammonia in solution. Sulfuric acid is usually preferred to control upward pH movements because hydrochloric acid is highly corrosive to stainless steel. Phosphoric acid is usually best if sulfuric acid must be avoided since many organisms reduce nitrate; this may complicate the microbial physiology, therefore nitric acid should only be used when nitrate metabolism is intended.

It is usual practice to set the pH controllers with a dead band (i.e. separated upper and lower pH limits) to avoid setting up a salt making device! Acids and alkalis at the strengths normally used (typically 2–6 M) are often regarded as self-sterilizing. Ammonia solutions cannot be autoclaved, thus filtration is the only option if a sterilization process is considered necessary.

Monitoring the quantity and rate of usage of the titrant provides valuable information both in constructing a mass balance and in detecting changes in the rate of production or consumption of acidic metabolites.

10.2 Dissolved oxygen tension

10.2.1 Measurement

All oxygen probes consist of a detection system separated from the culture by a gas-permeable membrane. Two types of detection system are in common use:

(a) Galvanic probes where one measures the potential developed by a cell. These consist of a lead cathode and a silver (oxygen reducing) anode.

(b) Polarographic probes where a constant potential is applied and the current (determined by the oxygen reduction rate) is measured.

Halling's recommendation of the Ingold polarographic type (1) because of its superior stability, reliability, and response time is still good (*Figure 8*). DOT is normally expressed as a percentage of air saturation. The concentration represented as '100%' is dependent upon temperature and pressure, so precise interpretation of DOT data requires that the temperature should be held at the normal fermentation value and the pressure recorded at calibration. The 100% value should be checked after sterilization prior to inoculation. The zero point can be determined by sparging with nitrogen. It is also possible to 'zero' the meter during *in-situ* sterilization (a small correction to the zero value is necessary in this case). The zero point can be checked during (or

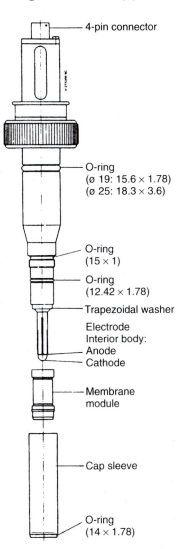

4-pin connector

O-ring
(ø 19: 15.6 × 1.78)
(ø 25: 18.3 × 3.6)

O-ring
(15 × 1)

O-ring
(12.42 × 1.78)

Trapezoidal washer

Electrode
Interior body:
Anode
Cathode

Membrane
module

Cap sleeve

O-ring
(14 × 1.78)

Figure 8. 'Ingold' dissolved oxygen probe (Courtesy Mettler Toledo).

at the end of) a fermentation, provided that the perturbation of the system can be tolerated; if there is a substantial respiring biomass present, the aeration is cut off and the agitation rate reduced, then the DOT will fall rapidly to zero.

Since DOT probes consume oxygen the value is only meaningful if the culture is agitated, otherwise the liquid layer adjacent to the probe becomes depleted. Furthermore, probe outputs are highly temperature sensitive—if the temperature oscillates, a similar oscillation may be observed on the DOT measurement.

10.2.2 Control

The DOT value can be controlled to a desired value provided there is a sufficient biomass present so that a balance can be achieved between supply and consumption of oxygen. Control by the adjustment of agitation is much more flexible than by aeration rate and is usually preferred. There are a number of possible problems in achieving control of DOT:

(a) Probe response times are at best around 5–10 sec. If the controller is set to respond too rapidly 'hunting' will result.

(b) If the oxygen uptake rate is low (e.g. when there is little biomass) small changes in a relatively low agitation speed cause great variation in the oxygen transfer rate making stable control difficult to achieve.

(c) When the biomass is high the DOT will change very rapidly if the system is perturbed.

Therefore if it is necessary to tune the controller, it should be set up to make gradual changes. The control is then achieved largely through finding appropriate values for the proportional and differential terms of the DOT controller—the rapid potential response of the system means that a large integral action term is undesirable.

Since the K_m of microbial cytochrome oxidase is normally around 10 μM, choice of any set-point in the normal measuring range will mean that the oxygen supply is unlikely to be limiting provided that the culture is homogeneous and well mixed. However, these conditions may not be true if the broth is viscous or contains organisms growing in pellets.

10.3 Temperature

10.3.1 Measurement

Temperature is normally measured and recorded using a platinum resistance thermometer. These are usually reliable, although many workers like to use a mercury thermometer as well. This can provide a useful check against instrument failure. Thermometers can be contained in housings allowing them to be replaced during a run.

10.3.2 Control

Heating is normally needed during the early stages of growth when the biomass is low. As the oxygen-uptake rate increases metabolic heating becomes significant and cooling is then required to maintain the correct temperature. Temperature control is most conveniently achieved with a jacket (or internal coils) through which water is circulated from a reservoir fitted with both a heater and a cooling coil. The jacket also serves to circulate steam or superheated water during *in-situ* sterilization. Other heating systems can be used on small autoclavable fermenters, e.g. band heaters or infra-red lamps, but this only makes sense if it is intended to operate under conditions of relatively low oxygen uptake when cooling is not required.

10.4 Foam

10.4.1 Detection

A foam probe usually consists of a metal rod surrounded by insulating material connected via the foam detection instrument to the body of the fermenter. A low voltage electrical potential is applied. If foam in the fermenter reaches the probe the electrical circuit is completed. This is a very simple device—the only problems are damage to the insulating material (which is fragile in some instances) and ensuring the probe is properly secured so that the pressure of *in-situ* sterilization does not cause it to fly out.

10.4.2 Control

Foam is usually controlled by the addition of an antifoaming agent. Silicone emulsions and polypropylene glycol (PPG) are commonly used. PPG is often preferred because its solubility in water at low temperature makes it more compatible with membranes and chromatographic processes used in downstream processing. Special proprietary antifoam agents are available having better temperature/solubility characteristics than PPG and, in some cases, achieving foam control with much smaller amounts of additive. Timed or metered additions of antifoam are preferable to addition in response to a probe for fed-batch work if the volume change is large, or for continuous culture work if a weir is used as the constant volume device. Agitation of the culture contributes to foam breakdown so, paradoxically, foam may sometimes be reduced by *increasing* agitation speed.

10.5 Dissolved CO_2

Probes are available for measuring dissolved CO_2 concentrations. They consist of a pH electrode surrounded by a bicarbonate buffer which is contained within a CO_2 permeable membrane. If the physiological effects of CO_2 are the objects of study this device is obviously useful. Control of dissolved CO_2 can be achieved by blending CO_2 with the inlet air to achieve a desired value.

10.6 Redox

A redox probe consists of a platinum electrode (at which redox reactions occur) and a reference electrode housed in a separate compartment making contact via a porous plug (just as for a pH electrode). The problem is to know what the signal means, since the electrode can respond to any oxidation/reduction system present and it cannot be assumed that they are at equilibrium in a fermenter broth. Since the reduction of oxygen is likely to be the dominant reaction if traces of the gas are present, it can be useful for monitoring oxygen concentrations at values below the useful range of DOT probes. However, interference from other species may be a confounding factor.

10.7 Vent-gas analysis

Knowledge of oxygen uptake and CO_2 evolution can be of great value in monitoring and controlling fermentations. This topic is dealt with in depth in Chapter 6. An important practical point is to ensure that the gas analyser cannot be damaged by a foam-out. A combination of a foam trap followed by a hydrophobic filter is recommended.

10.8 Biomass

The main difficulty with on-line biomass measurement is that many devices proposed for this purpose have been subject to interference by gas bubbles. However, the light-scattering system of Wedgwood and the latest version of the 'Bugmeter' (Aber Instruments) appear to have overcome this problem. The topic of biomass measurement is also dealt with in Chapter 5 of this volume.

11. Continuous culture

It is commonly said that continuous culture is a means of keeping a cell in exponential growth phase indefinitely. This statement is misleading since the physiological state of an exponentially growing batch culture is only achievable continuously in a turbidostat. Most continuous culture work is done with chemostats where the dilution rate is set at a value below the maximum growth rate and the medium is usually designed so that a particular nutrient is limiting. This defines steady-state conditions which can be maintained indefinitely (but the experimenter must beware of the possibility of genetic change). This ability to choose and define physiological conditions makes the technique much more powerful than simply maintaining 'exponential phase'. Continuous culture work commonly involves examining the effect of the range of different nutrient limitations and dilution rates on a process or product of interest. Consider the following points in setting up a continuous culture:

- sterilization and storage of medium;
- prevention of line growth;
- control and measurement of flow;
- maintenance of constant volume.

11.1 Sterilization and the storage of media

Reservoir bottles are required for the storage of media and reception of culture. They need to be large to minimize the frequency of bottle changing, with the associated risk of making and breaking a wet line, but the weight of a full bottle means that vessels much over 20 litres are not commonly used. Handling is safer and easier if bottles are contained in carriers with handles.

11.2 Control and measurement of flow

Peristaltic pumps are commonly used. Flow rate is determined by the rotational speed and the diameter of the tubing. Tubing is the only component in contact with the medium, thus sterilization is simple and the pump can be changed easily if necessary. Use only the tubing recommended by the manufacturers. The main disadvantage of the peristaltic pump is that tube distortion can cause the flow-rate to change. Diaphragm pumps (such as the Braun FE211 described in ref. 1) are preferred by some workers. The volume delivered per stroke is determined by the displacement of the pump head, making it a more reproducible device. Even so, flow-rate variation can occur. The main disadvantage is that there is a major risk of contamination if the pump diaphragm or tubing fails (the latter is a common problem with the FE211 if the valves are set incorrectly). Nevertheless, it is possible to run continuous culture experiments for periods of several months using either type of pump. Note also that pumps may not produce the perfect smooth flow postulated in the simple theory of the chemostat. If the flow is discontinuous, if only because it falls dropwise from an input needle, the concentration of limiting nutrient will oscillate. There may be little effect if the pulse period is comparable to the fermenter circulation time (1–2 sec) but longer pulses may result in the loss of biomass yield.

Flow measurement is essential. A simple and commonly used device consists of a 'T'-piece in the tubing upstream of the pump with a sterile burette attached to the side arm which is clamped off when not in use. To measure flow rate, remove the clamp, draw liquid into the burette, clamp the reservoir supply line, and determine the rate of liquid flow from the burette. Check the flow rate at least once every 24 hours. An alternative is to place the reservoir on a balance and measure the rate of weight loss. This avoids the complication of a junction in a sterile line; the use of an electronic balance linked to a supervisory computer can provide continuous monitoring of flow.

11.3 Measurement and control of volume

The simplest constant volume device is a weir consisting of a tube rising from the bottom of the fermenter to the desired liquid height. Alternatively, the tube may descend from a fitting in the top plate. Weirs are commonly used, but there are two problems associated with them:

(a) Variation in gas hold-up or agitation speed may mean that a constant level device does not give a constant volume. It is essential to check the volume at least daily. Common practice is to turn off the agitator, air flow, and pump briefly and to compare the volume against graduations on the outside of the vessel (or sight-glass).

(b) The liquid being drawn off may not be representative of the culture. This is especially a problem with filamentous fungi growing in pellets, therefore weir systems are not recommended for this application. If the weir consists of a tube dipping down into the liquid with the culture being pumped upwards, gravitational separation can occur (especially if the organisms tend to flocculate)—a 'J'-tube is preferable. If there is foam the weir will take liquid from the foam, not the main bulk of the liquid. It is therefore better, even with downwardly directed weirs, to pump the culture away; if the exit pump is set at about 2–3 times the rate of the feed pump then if there is a foam head it will rise well above the weir lip. The use of a pump to control the weir exit also ensures that the vent gas leaves the fermenter by the proper route (essential for the proper operation of the condenser and gas analyser).

The alternative to a weir is an exit line in the main liquid bulk connected to a pump which is activated by some other device sensing the culture volume. The use of conductivity or capacitance level probes overcomes the problem of organism separation, but variations in volume due to change in agitation speed, gas hold-up, or foam can still occur. Technically, the best solution (although alas by far the most expensive) is to control to constant fermenter weight, monitored using load cells, although in this case care is required to ensure that movement of the flexible tubing cannot cause an apparent change.

11.4 Interruption of steady state

Many organisms will remain viable for periods of a week or more if the medium supply is interrupted, provided that the aeration is turned off, agitation set to a low value, and the culture is cooled as far as possible. 'Boxing-up' in this way is a useful procedure enabling mechanical breakdowns to be corrected without losing valuable experiments.

12. Computer data logging and control

Historically, the outputs of the various instruments used to monitor a fermentation were recorded on paper using chart recorders. However, with the growth in the capability of computers (especially PCs) over recent years, a computer system for data logging would now be considered as a normal part of any well-equipped fermentation laboratory.

Conventional recorders are still useful as a back-up and can help validate the computer record, but the PC provides a much more convenient means of data storage, access, and display. The effective display of information and ease of comparison with other fermentation profiles provide a major benefit to the operator in diagnosing process problems and determining appropriate action.

12.1 Typical facilities of fermentation software

Different software packages specifically written for fermentation applications are available from many fermenter suppliers. One should expect to see the following features:

(a) ability to control instruments, switching on or off as required or changing control set points;

(b) convenient alphanumeric listing of measured values;

(c) configurable graphical display of historical data;

(d) system for off-line data recording (e.g. spreadsheet);

(e) word processing package for recording operator comments;

(f) calculation package enabling the user to write algorithms for derived process variables and control functions;

(g) configurable alarm system highlighting variables outside 'normal' range;

(h) secure system for data back-up and retrieval.

12.2 Remote access

Using a modem and telephone link, it is possible to set up a computer so that an operator at a distant site can view or control the process. Its main use is to enable the process to be monitored and controlled remotely (e.g. start of a new phase of fermentation or shut-down on process completion) outside normal working hours. Password protection to prevent unauthorized access is essential. An improved level of security can be provided by 'dial-back', whereby once an incoming caller has been identified the line is disconnected and communication re-established by the laboratory computer dialling a pre-configured number.

12.3 Alarms

Most systems written for fermentation processes include provision to flag values outside the normal range. In addition, it may be desirable to set up a system to activate an external alarm. It is possible to configure an output to activate an alarm device in the event of a process variable going outside its normal range. This could be used to call a site security number or to operate a telephone pager requesting the remote operator to call in. A simple algorithm to operate an external alarm could have this form:

> Represent any variable in the normal range to the value 1.
> Represent any variable in the alarm range to the value 0.
> Multiply all values together.
> If result is zero, switch alarm on.

Choose variables for inclusion and alarm values carefully—alarm systems generating unnecessary or false alarms are worse than useless.

12.4 What to monitor

The simple answer is to record everything you can—pH, DOT, temperature, stirrer speed, titrant and antifoam usage, gas analysis data, air flow rate, nutrient feed rate, and the results of any other on-line equipment, e.g. balances, biomass measuring device, HPLC, redox, and dissolved CO_2. Analysis of trends in different variables and comparisons between gas exchange rates, alkali usage rates, and substrate feed rates can be very important in process diagnosis. Apparent inconsistencies from a 'normal' pattern may well be the consequence of an equipment malfunction rather than a biological change.

12.5 What to control

Where the fermenter is equipped with its own local controllers it is usually better to use them as the primary control system. The computer is then used as a supervisory system which will permit changes in set points (for example) in pH or temperature. If values too far from the set points occur, the computer may be configured to shut down the process automatically as well as sending an alarm. This can be of great value in saving what would otherwise be a lost fermentation. For example, if a pH controller fails then setting the computer to stop a chemostat's feed and air supply whilst sending an alarm may give the operator time to correct the fault with only minor disturbance when otherwise the continuing pH movement would have killed the culture. Apparatus for which no local controller is provided can be controlled by the computer, provided that there is a measuring device sending an electronic system and the controller is also activated electronically. An example might be an air flow system with separate mass flow meter and electronically controlled needle valve. This will give much more constant control of the air flow than can be achieved by periodic checking and manual adjustment. Similarly, the rate of change of mass in a media supply bottle can be used to calculate the feed rate and make corrections to a pump, compensating for calibration drift.

12.6 Example: control of a fed-batch process

It is likely that the experimenter will also wish to use the computer to control the fermentation process. A good example is fed-batch work where control of the feed profile is likely to be critical. The objective might be to define particular feed profiles and to study the effect on formation of a product. Consistent achievement of a desired profile is much more likely if the process is automated (and of course it avoids the need for operator attendance out of normal working hours).

Fed-batch culture is also used when the objective is to maximize biomass production. A well-known example is baker's yeast fermentation for which a number of control systems have been described. The objective in this case is to minimize or avoid the formation of ethanol which occurs if carbohydrate is supplied too fast (the so-called 'Crabtree effect') by maintaining a carbon-limited feed.

Feedback control can be achieved either by measuring the ethanol concentration directly and attempting to control it to a particular (low) concentration or indirectly by analysing the vent gas and controlling the feed from the respiratory quotient (RQ) = ratio of CO_2 evolution rate to oxygen uptake rate. Ethanolic fermentation generates CO_2 but uses no oxygen, whereas the oxidation of carbohydrate consumes one mole of oxygen per mole CO_2 consumed. The following is a fed-batch control protocol adapted from Wang *et al.* (2) which has been found to be effective in controlling yeast fermentations. It is given here in descriptive form and would need to be converted into a set of algorithms appropriate to the particular software package used.

Protocol 4.   Computer control of fed-batch *Saccharomyces cerevisiae* fermentation

Method

Let feed rate (*FR*) be given by:
$$FR = FR_0.e^{\mu t};$$
when t is a variable having the units of time, FR_0 is the value when $t = 0$, and μ is the nominal growth rate—FR_0 and μ are parameters chosen by the experimenter. Control of the process is achieved by manipulation of t. If the computer calculates output values at a time interval of δt a number of conditions can be combined together thus:

1. Add δt to the previous value t.

2. If RQ exceeds the set point and if 10 minutes have elapsed since the last reading of RQ subtract 20 min (0.333 h).

3. If DOT is below the minimum value subtract $2 \times \delta t$.

4. If DOT has risen by 15% in the previous 30 min and the pump is not already started, start the pump and set $t = 0$.

5. If the pH or temperature enters the alarm range set $FR = 0$.

12.6.1 Explanation of *Protocol 4*

(a) Condition 1: gives the normal increment required for an exponential feed.

(b) Condition 2: there is a time lag between any changes in the feed rate and its detection by the gas analyser. This is a function of the time required to equilibrate the gas and liquid phases and to reach a new steady state in the gas phase. Time must also be allowed for the gas to travel to the analyser and (if it is measuring streams from more than one fermenter) for the value for the particular fermenter to be updated. The choice of 10 minutes is somewhat arbitrary. The effect is that if the RQ remains high the combined effect of conditions (1) and (2) is to give a stepwise decline in t with the average rate of decline being equal to the normal rate of increase. In carbon-limited growth without ethanol formation the RQ is slightly higher than 1.0 (usually about 1.07) so the RQ limit must be above this; a value of 1.2 works well.

(c) Condition 3: this is included to prevent the culture becoming oxygen limited. If the DOT controller works by increasing the stirrer speed to maintain a particular value, then as the feed rate increases the stirrer speed will also increase. Eventually maximum speed is reached and the DOT must begin to fall. If some minimum value is set below the normal control point then the combined effect of conditions (1) and (3) is to cause t to decline at the same rate as it would normally increase when the DOT is below the minimum. In practice, this results in the feed rate being controlled to achieve the minimum DOT.

(d) Condition 4: in carbon-limited fed-batch fermentation it is normally desirable to start the pump at the point where the originally supplied carbon source is exhausted. The rise in DOT is characteristic of a batch culture which has run out of oxidizable substrate. One way of achieving the desired effect is to give an initial large negative value to t (so that the resulting feed rate is well below the stalling speed of the pump) and multiplying the previous value of t by zero when the condition is met.

(e) Condition 5: this is the emergency shut-down condition.

This set of simple conditions can be adapted in various ways, for example: the parameter μ is the maximum growth rate—if it is set at a value above μ_{crit} (above which the Crabtree effect occurs) then the RQ control function will result in a culture growing at μ_{crit}.

RQ may be used to control other fermentations where an undesired product accumulates, but this requires that the substrate and product are significantly different in oxidation state. If the conversion is from carbohydrate to (say) acetic acid, both of which have the empirical formula CH_2O, the RQ for this conversion is 1 so it cannot be detected by this system. Other approaches to detecting acetic acid formation could be to look for a higher ratio of alkali consumption to the feed addition and/or a low ratio of CO_2 evolution to the feed rate, but neither would be as sensitive as the detection of ethanolic fermentation by RQ.

If the maximum transfer of heat, rather than oxygen, is limiting in a particular system the process could be set to run at a maximum temperature slightly above the local controller set point using another condition similar to (3).

Note also that if the original nutrient contained more than one substrate and diauxic growth occurs, condition (4) may cause the feed to be started prematurely. It should be possible to identify appropriate conditions by running a few pilot experiments and determining characteristics which enable the differentiation of diauxic transition from substrate exhaustion. Thus, although this protocol was originally written for *S. cerevisae* fermentations it can be adapted for a number of other uses.

References

1. McNeil, B. and Harvey, L. M. (ed.) (1990). *Fermentation: a practical approach.* Oxford University Press, Oxford.
2. Wang, H. Y., Cooney, C. L., and Wang, D. I. C. (1979). *Biotechnol. Bioeng.*, **21**, 975.

Further reading

Pirt, S. J. (1975). *Principles of microbe and cell cultivation* Blackwell Scientific, Oxford.
Norris, J. R. and Ribbons, D. W. (ed.) (1970). *Methods in microbiology*, Vol. 2. Academic Press, London.

5

Measurement of biomass

ANDREW P. ISON and GAVIN B. MATTHEW

1. Introduction

1.1 General remarks

The on-line measurement of some physical parameters in fermentation broths, such as pH and temperature, is relatively easy and commonplace (see Chapter 4). This has been made possible by the advanced technology that has now become standard.

As yet, on-line monitoring of biomass in the fermenter has not become routine. However, there are many techniques available for biomass determination. This chapter gives detailed protocols for those techniques likely to be used by microbiologists, biochemists, microbial physiologists, and biochemical engineers. For those requiring substantial investment and specialist equipment, a strategy for the application of the technique is given. In these cases it is necessary to assume that the operator has gained some experience with the equipment and is familiar with the operating manuals of commercially available equipment. Most techniques will require some investment of time, dependent on the experience of the researcher, to personalize the technique for the specific application and to ensure its reproducibility.

1.2 What is biomass?

In a recent article, Fiechter and Seghezzi (1) indicated that many of the terms used in the description of processes based on the utilization of organisms are still misused, with no consistency of definition. They stated that 'fermentation' is just such an example, indicating that a taxonomist would use the term to describe the production of ethanol by microorganisms, whereas the microbiologist would use the term to refer to the phenomena of repression, and the process engineer would refer to the process itself as a 'fermentation'. It is this latter definition that will predominate throughout this chapter.

A similar problem arises with the term 'biomass' which would initially appear to be a simple issue, but what is actually meant by this term is subject to conjecture and the answer to the question 'what is biomass'? will be dependent on the objectives of the researcher involved. Biomass, for example, could be the number of cells visible under a microscope. However, this, too, is difficult to determine if filamentous cells were to be considered. It could also mean the number of cells possessing an intact membrane, but then again other issues are raised such as viability. Does a cell with an intact membrane have the necessary cellular machinery for carrying out the desired task? Or it could very simply mean the mass of cells present. The arguments are endless, but it is clear that, before establishing which method to utilize, the criteria necessary for any particular application should be assessed.

1.3 Specific and volumetric rates

If there is so much confusion about what exactly biomass is, then why is the measurement of such a variable so important and why is it beneficial to achieve this measurement rapidly? The key to this is how a researcher would utilize knowledge of the biomass concentration, however defined, when this is available. Fermentation technologists frequently discuss performance in terms of volumetric rates (units/ml/h) and specific rates (units/g biomass/h). Volumetric rates are used in design studies and calculations. Specific rates, on the other hand, are indicative of fermentation performance and, as such, are important parameters for monitoring fermentations and, in combination with other parameters, will improve decision making. This, in turn, can lead to improved monitoring and control which will lead to the ability of a researcher to gain more information more rapidly and, in the case of industrial fermentations, reduce costs and speed new processes into production.

1.4 Off-line and on-line measurement

The majority of techniques for determining biomass are off-line systems, that is to say, they require a sample to be taken and processed away from the fermentation. This generally involves some time delay before the result is available, by which time the fermentation has progressed and is out of step with the newly acquired information. A number of systems have employed predictive tools to establish some sort of control mechanism, but in many cases the information only provides assurance that the fermentation is not deviating from a desired profile. The ability to measure biomass, however it is described, on-line, would be an extremely valuable asset to a fermentation technologist because it would remove the necessity for predictive controls by providing instantaneous values.

2. Chemical methods

2.1 Bioluminescence and chemiluminescence

These methods are all indirect and work by relating the amount of growth to ATP. Bioluminescence uses the firefly catalase-catalysed reaction of ATP and luciferin which, in the presence of oxygen, produces light that can be monitored, i.e.:

$$ATP + luciferin + O_2 = oxyluciferin + AMP + PP_i + CO_2 + light. \quad [1]$$

Biomass is expressed in terms of the ATP concentration, and the assumption is that living cells contain a reasonably constant amount of ATP which is lost when the cell dies. As a consequence, it should also be a good measure of viability. Bioluminescence is reasonably sensitive, with values as low as 10^5 cells/ml detectable, and is also suitable for immobilized systems (2). However, the assumption that biomass contains a constant amount of ATP is perhaps one of the biggest sources of error when estimating biomass. This anomaly has resulted in the development of an alternative technique which measures the total ATP, ADP, and AMP present (3). This is believed to be consistent from cell to cell irrespective of the physiological state of the cell. ATP is measured by the firefly luciferase reaction and ADP and AMP by independent enzyme reactions, therefore, it is more time consuming. Other errors in both techniques are a result of selectivity and degradation in the analytical procedures which have been reported by Harris and Kell (4). *Protocol 1* gives the method employed for intracellular ATP analysis. The resultant ATP concentration should then be correlated with the dry weight of the cells grown in a chemically defined medium.

Protocol 1. Determination of intracellular ATP analysis as a basis for biomass concentration

Equipment and reagents

- Bio-Orbit ATP monitoring kit (Labsystems). Follow all instructions given in the kit manual to obtain the correct concentrations. The kit comprises the following four components:
  (i) *monitoring reagent*, a lyophilized mixture of: firefly luciferase; D-Luciferin, 50 mg bovine serum albumin, 0.5 mmol magnesium acetate, 0.1 μmol inorganic pyrophosphate. Store at $-18°C$ and reconstitute by adding 10 ml of the Tris buffer
  (ii) *releasing reagent*: undisclosed ionic surfactant for permeabilizing microbial membranes for the release of ATP, mixed with ATPase inhibitors. Store at 4°C

(iii) *ATP standard*: 0.1 μmol ATP, 2 μmol magnesium sulfate. Store at $-18°C$. Reconstitute by adding 1 ml of the Tris buffer to give a 10^{-5} M ATP solution.
(iv) *Tris buffer*: 100 mM Tris–acetate buffer, 2 mM EDTA pH 7.75 at 25°C
- BioOrbit 1253 luminometer
- 100 and 500 μl pipettes, sterile pipette tips
- 50 mM phosphate buffer pH 7
- Ice and ice bucket

Method

1. Since ATP is heat stable avoid contamination of equipment. Wear examination gloves to insert disposable pipette tips into racks before sterilizing them by autoclaving at 121°C and 1 bar for 20 min.

2. Switch on the luminometer 15 min before use.

Protocol 1. *Continued*

3. Dilute the cell samples with 50 mM phosphate buffer to a cell concentration of 0–1 g/litre dry weight.

4. Pipette 500 μl of the monitoring reagent into a cuvette. Insert into the measuring chamber, close the cover, press the 'Background' button to zero the instrument.

5. Determine extracellular ATP as follows:
   (a) Pipette 100 μl of tris buffer into a cuvette.
   (b) Pipette 100 μl of the sample into the cuvette.
   (c) Add 500 μl of the monitoring reagent, agitate manually.
   (d) Place the cuvette into the measuring chamber of luminometer. Press the 'Start' button. Read and note the measurement.
   (e) Repeat steps (a) to (d) three times for accuracy,

6. Determine total ATP as follows:
   (a) Pipette 100 μl of sample into a cuvette.
   (b) Add 100 μl of the releasing agent, agitate for 30 sec.
   (c) Add 500 μl of the monitoring reagent, agitate manually.
   (d) Place the cuvette into the measuring chamber of luminometer. Press the 'Start' button. Read and note the measurement.
   (e) Repeat steps (a) to (d) three times for accuracy.

7. Prepare an ATP standard curve as follows:
   (a) Make an appropriate range of standards by diluting the stock ATP solution with the Tris buffer.
   (b) Pipette 100 μl of buffer into a cuvette.
   (c) Add 100 μl of the ATP standard into the cuvette.
   (d) Add 500 μl of the monitoring reagent, agitate manually.
   (e) Place the cuvette into the measuring chamber of the luminometer. Press the 'Start' button. Read and note measurement.
   (f) Repeat steps (a) to (e) three times for accuracy.

8. Calculate the intracellular levels of ATP as follows:
   (a) Subtract the extracellular reading from the total to give the intracellular ATP.
   (b) Read from a standard curve to convert 0 M ATP.

In the case of chemiluminescence the heme protein-catalysed reaction between ATP and luminol in the presence of hydrogen peroxide again produces light which can be monitored.

2.2 DNA analysis

The use of DNA analysis as a measurement of microbial biomass is not recommended as a primary method for determining the number of cells present.
While DNA isolation is common in the biochemistry laboratory, the analysis
requires the presence of perchloric acid and its highly oxidative nature means
it falls outside the established safety standard for most laboratories. It should
only be used as a last resort, with considerable care and attention, and with
the approval of the laboratory safety officer. The method, however, has been
used to provide a correlation with another microbial biomass measurement
such as dry weight analysis (5) where the complex medium contains undissolved solids. The method known as the diphenylamine method was pioneered by Burton (6) and developed for DNA by Gurtler and Schulein (7).
The assay is colorimetric, depending on the reaction between deoxyribose
and the diphenylamine reagent and is summarized in *Protocol 2*. Further
details of biomass fractionation, DNA and RNA analysis are given in Chapter 7 (Section 4).

Protocol 2. Determination of DNA for biomass measurement

Equipment and reagents

- Stock DNA solution (1 g DNA sodium salt dissolved in reverse osmosis water)
- 0.4 M and 0.2 M perchloric acid[a]
- Ice
- 10 ml centrifuge tubes
- Centrifuge

- Glass test tubes and marbles to rest on top of the tubes
- Spectrophotometer with deuterium lamp
- Eppendorf tubes
- Microcentrifuge
- Quartz cuvettes

Method

1. Create a range of standards by diluting the stock DNA solution with reverse osmosis water to obtain a range from 0.01 mg/ml to 1 mg/ml.

2. Take 2 ml of cold 0.4 M perchloric acid and add to 2 ml of the standard in a 10 ml centrifuge tube. Mix the mixture gently.

3. Centrifuge at 6–8000 *g* for 10 min at 4°C. Discard the supernatant and resuspend the pellet in 2 ml of 0.2 M perchloric acid in glass test tubes.

4. Place the test tubes containing the resuspended pellet in a water-bath set at 100°C for 20 min, cover the tops of the tubes with the marbles to prevent evaporation.

5. Decant the sample into Eppendorf tubes and centrifuge at 8–10000 *g* for 10 min.

6. Decant the supernatant into a 1 ml quartz cuvette and read the absorbance at 280 nm (deuterium lamp on) against reverse osmosis water as a blank.

Protocol 2. *Continued*

7. Repeat for each of the standard dilutions to create the standard curve.

8. Repeat Steps 1–6 for broth samples, and determine the DNA content by checking the absorbance against the standard curve. If it is impossible to assay the broth samples immediately, mix these samples with an equal volume of 0.4 M perchloric acid and store at $-4°C$ until required. When processing stored samples, omit Step 2 and follow the other steps as normal.

[a] **NB**: Perchloric acid is an extremely hazardous chemical. This is chiefly due to its powerful oxidative nature and as such it will react violently with a large number of carbonaceous materials. In general, it is not covered under standard laboratory safety and the Safety Officer should be informed if this method is to be used.

2.3 Fluorescence

Fluorescence utilizes the ability of some chemical compounds to be excited by light waves with the subsequent emission at different frequencies. The ability to produce a spectral shift, known as Stokes' shift, can therefore be exploited in the measurement of biomass. It is necessary to establish the correct wavelength which corresponds to the maximal absorbance of the sample. The light is passed through the sample and the re-emitted light is filtered to minimize the influence of scattered light.

There are many examples of this technique and methods based on enzymes, other proteins, pigments, and metabolites have been presented. The most advanced technique is perhaps monitoring the fluorescence of NADH and NADPH in the hope that this can be related to biomass concentration. NADH is present in every cell and, thus, this measurement is applicable to every kind of cell. In contrast, the amount of NADPH per cell is very variable and therefore difficulties can be observed at low cell concentrations. The results obtained using NADH as a measure of biomass will depend on the activity of the redox reactions in the cell, most notably those in the cytosol and mitochondria.

The technique stems from work published in the late 1970s and early 1980s based on the key research performed by Harrison and Chance (8) and Zabriskie and Humphrey (9). *Table 1* shows some of the organisms where fluorescence has been utilized for biomass determination.

As with a number of spectrophotometric techniques described here the measurement is relatively easy but it is the interpretation of the data that is difficult, necessitating some investment of time. The data are influenced by a number of parameters such as the metabolic state of the cell, its viability, and the extracellular and intracellular environments of the cell. An examination of the data can be simplified since changes in cellular metabolism are relatively rapid when compared with the accretion rate of biomass. However,

Table 1. Biomass measurement using fluorescence

Organism	Reference
Yeasts	
Saccharomyces cerevisiae	Zabriske (10) (11)
	Zabriskie and Humphrey (9)
	Beyeler *et al.* (12)
	Beyeler and Meyer (13)
	Scheper and Schugerl (14)
	Arminger *et al.* (15)
Candida sp.	Einsele *et al.* (16)
Zymononas mobilis	Scheper and Schugerl (14)
Bacteria	
Escherichia coli	Scheper (17)
	Walker and Dhurjati (18)
	Brandis *et al.* (19)
Bacillus subtilis	Meyer *et al.* (20)
Pseudomonas putida	Boyer and Humphrey (21)
	Li and Humphrey (22)
Corynebacterium glutamicum	Winter *et al.* (23)
Filamentous organisms	
Penicillium chrysogenum	Scheper and Schugerl (14)
Streptomyces sp.	Zabriskie and Humphrey (9)

there may also be some contribution to the fluorescence signal by other background components and it is necessary to subtract this from the original measurement. Zabriskie (11) was able to correlate baker's yeast biomass using this technique, but found that it was necessary to control the pH and temperature carefully and to ensure that all nutrients were in excess. Zabriskie (11) obtained a linear relationship between the fluorescence (measured in net mV from the probe) and the biomass concentration on a log–log plot under these conditions. In examining the effectiveness of fluorescence to monitor *Bacillus subtilis* cell density, Meyer *et al.* (20) found that an optical density (see Section 4.3) of 2.0 was the detection limit of the system employed, but they concluded that fluorescence was a suitable measuring device for this organism. In monitoring a recombinant *E. coli* strain, however, they found that the results were at the detection limit of the system, and for *E. coli* K12 they found no correlation with biomass concentration.

2.4 Near infrared spectroscopy

Near infrared (NIR) spectroscopy was originally pioneered for use in the food industry because of its ability to carry out non-invasive multi-component analysis. Its application in fermentation processes is a relatively recent development pioneered by a research group at Pfizer in the United Kingdom.

Publications on this method are still scarce, but they have reported on its use for biomass determination (24, 25), metabolite concentration determination (24, 25), and antibiotic concentration (26).

The major drawbacks with this technique are the expense of the equipment and the data analysis. However, as more research is carried out and the technique becomes more established equipment prices are likely to fall and data interpretation is likely to get easier. At this stage, though, additional equipment such as HPLC is necessary for calibration and validation of the system. As a consequence, this necessitates the measurements of large numbers of samples in order to statistically substantiate the results. Currently, analysis can be performed off-line or on-line with *in-situ* probes. Spectra are available in published tables (27).

The technique is based on the absorption of energy in the range 700 nm to 2500 nm being related to the chemical or physical characteristics of the sample examined. Certain chemical groups absorb at given wavelengths, and it is the deconvolution of these patterns that is the key to relating them to components, for example biomass. The main bands studied relate to —OH, —NH, and —CH groups. Clearly the deconvolution process is complicated and requires the application of regression analysis to achieve quantitative results. The general approach to data acquisition, calibration, and analysis using NIR spectroscopy has been described by Hall and Pollard (28) who, in using the technique in clinical applications, required both accuracy and reliability. This publication has examined serum proteins, trigylcerides, and glucose and gives an extensive review of the theory, variate analysis, and validation. It is recommended as a starting point for further studies in the use of NIR technology.

3. Microscopic methods

These methods require a sample of the fermentation broth to be removed from the system before analysis can take place. Such methods include direct count microscopy, viable cell counts, epifluorescence, and image analysis.

3.1 Direct count microscopy

The manual measurement of cells after staining is an established, if somewhat laborious technique. Perhaps one of the greatest advantages of such methods is the ability of the staining to differentiate between living and dead cells. It is also the technique that requires the least hardware, with the microscope the most expensive piece of equipment needed. The choice of stain is perhaps the most difficult part of the procedure. The common stains are methylene blue, phenolphthalein, and neutral red which are pH indicators and show the difference between intracellular and extracellular pH in living cells. There are other stains which are specific to certain cell components but their use is less common. *Protocol 3* shows the method used for methylene blue staining. If an alternative stain is required then the further reading section indicates good sources for various methods.

3.2 Viable cell counts

The method of viable cell counts can be a slow method since it relies on measuring growth of microorganisms by counting colony formation. The delay in obtaining the results from this method means that it is ineffective in providing data for process control and evaluation. However, it is commonly used as 'back-up' information, validating results obtained more rapidly by an alternative technique. The technique requires good microbiological skills in order to avoid contamination during the dilution and plating out steps. *Protocol 4* details the serial dilution method for the determination of colony formation. However, the technique is suitable for unicellular microorganisms and spore suspensions only.

Protocol 3. Direct microscopy counts for biomass concentration determination

Equipment and reagents

- Universal bottles
- Vortex mixer
- Bijou bottles
- Methylene blue or other suitable stain
- Light microscope set for bright field illumination, 40 × and 100 × lenses
- Pasteur pipettes
- Haemocytometer and coverslips. For bacterial cultures a chamber of 0.02 mm depth is used and for yeasts and fungal spores, a depth of 0.1 mm is used

Method

1. Pipette 1 ml of the well-mixed fermentation broth sample into 9 ml sterile water aseptically into a Universal bottle. Repeat to reach the required dilution. (The precise dilution will have to be determined prior to actual measurement, but there should be between 5 and 200 cells per square in the haemocytometer, see below.)

2. Agitate the Universal bottle on the vortex mixer.

3. Pipette 2 ml of the contents of the Universal bottle into a Bijou bottle and add a drop of the appropriate stain. Mix the suspension using the vortex mixer.

4. Press the coverslip on to the surface of the haemocytometer over the graduated area. Use a Pasteur pipette to introduce the stained cells' solution to the edge of the coverslip. The counting chamber should fill by capillary action. Take care not to under- or overfill the chamber as this invalidates the results (culture fluid should not enter the channels surrounding the graduated zone).

111

Protocol 3. *Continued*

5. Place the haemocytometer on the microscope stage and treat as a normal slide. Select the appropriate objective lens for the cells to be counted and focus the microscope.

6. For speed of measurement count the number of stained and unstained cells in five squares, i.e. each of the four corners of the measuring area and a central square.

7. If accuracy is more important than speed, count the number of stained and unstained cells in every square. The number of squares counted will affect the statistical accuracy of the measurement, the more squares counted the more accurate the count. In either case, the total number of cells counted should be over 100 to obtain an accurate cell count.

8. Remove the coverslip and wash the slide and coverslip with ethanol. Dry and repeat the procedure from Step 1.

9. Calculate the number of stained and unstained cells per mm^3 based on the number of squares counted, the volume of each square counted, and the dilution used, i.e. (number of cells counted/number of squares) $\times$ dilution $\times$ volume of 1 square.

10. Convert to cells/ml by multiplying by 1000.

Protocol 4. **Serial dilution counts for biomass concentration determination**[a]

Equipment and reagents

- Universal bottles
- 50 mM phosphate buffer pH 7
- Sterile pipette tips
- Vortex mixer
- Bunsen burner

- Suitable agar plates (media used will depend on the microorganism), dried at 40°C for at least 30 min prior to use
- Incubator

Method

1. Fill 11 Universal bottles with 9 ml of 50 mM phosphate buffer per sample. Seal the lids and sterilize in an autoclave.

2. Take one cooled Universal bottle and loosen the cap. Remove the cap and pass the neck of the bottle through a flame. Vortex mix the fermentation broth sample and, using a pipette with a sterile tip, remove 1 ml and add to the Universal bottle. Flame the neck again and replace the cap.

3. Take another Universal bottle and loosen the cap. Remove the cap and pass the neck through the flame. Keep the neck near the flame.

Vortex mix the previous Universal and loosen the cap. Remove the cap and pass the neck through the flame. Using a pipette with a new sterile tip remove 1 ml of the initial dilution and add to the second Universal bottle.

4. Repeat the above steps until all the Universals have been used. A dilution series of 10^{-1} to 10^{-11} has now been created.

5. Prepare three suitable agar plates per dilution.

6. Take the first required dilution Universal bottle and mix on the vortex mixer. Remove the cap and pass the neck through the flame. Using a pipette with a fresh sterile tip remove 0.1 ml and pipette on to the surface of the agar. Keep the agar plate and lid close to the flame. Remove the lid and spread the 0.1 ml aliquot across the surface of the agar plate using a glass spreader (sterilized by dipping in ethanol, burning the remaining ethanol off in the Bunsen flame, and then allowing to cool).

7. Repeat the above procedure twice more for the dilution.

8. Repeat Steps 1–7 for each required dilution.

9. Mark the plates with the relevant details and incubate at the appropriate temperature for 24 h.

10. Following incubation remove the plates and count the number of colonies per plate. Plates with more than 250 or less than 30 colonies should be discarded.

11. The average cell count per dilution should be calculated from the three plates.

12. Calculate the original number of viable cells per ml dependent on the dilution used.

[a] This method is suitable for most unicellular organisms.

3.3 Epifluorescence

Epifluorescence technology examines cells after staining with a range of fluorochromes such as acridine orange, this reacts with intact RNA and DNA leading to a fluorescence. The samples must be observed under ultraviolet light such that single-stranded DNA or RNA fluoresces orange/red and double-stranded DNA fluoresces green. The technique, however, is really only suitable for unicellular organisms.

3.4 Image analysis

Image analysis is a useful tool for biomass determination but is really dependent on the ability of the user to automate it for a specific application. The use of image analysis to count cells is feasible, but the necessity to prepare the

Table 2. The use of image analysis for biomass characterization

Microorganism	Reference
Penicillium chrysogenum	Adams and Thomas (29)
	Packer and Thomas (30)
	van Suijdam and Metz (31)
Streptomyces clavuligerus	Packer *et al.* (32)
Streptomyces tendae	Reichl and Gilles (33)
Saccharomyces cerevisiae	Costello and Monk (34)
Escherichia coli	Singh *et al.* (35)
Pseudomonas aeruginosa	Singh *et al.* (35)
Pseudomonas fluorescens	Lawrence *et al.* (36)
	Metz *et al.* (37)

sample and the cost of the hardware prevents it from becoming an established technique. The technique uses grey levels and computer automation to determine cell mass. The main advantages are in the ability to adapt the software element of the computer programs to extract information on the morphology of filamentous organisms. It can also distinguish between undissolved solids, cells with an intact cytoplasm, and degenerated cells which does yield significantly more data than just a quantity of biomass. Such systems have been employed for a number of organisms and these are given in *Table 2*. The reader is referred to the original article for further reading on a specific application.

4. Physical methods

4.1 Dry weight methods

The determination of microbial cell mass by removing the liquid component from a sample and back-calculating the cellular concentration is perhaps one of the most common methods for biomass determination, although it is a very slow procedure requiring up to 24 hours for an accurate measurement. However, recent instrument developments called moisture balances have allowed procedures to be adapted to provide dry weight values in approximately 30 min. The general technique is, however, inaccurate when the fermentation medium contains undissolved solids. In addition, the method measures dead cellular material, which will again render the result inaccurate (38). There are a number of ways of achieving a dry weight measurement. *Protocols 5* and *6* give methods based on centrifugation followed by drying. *Protocol 7* gives a method based on the filtration of a sample. When using the filtration technique the washing step can be very important and some of the undissolved solids can be removed by selection of the wash solvent, e.g. calcium carbonate can be removed using mineral acids. However, the choice of solvent should not allow leaching or the lysis of the biomass. Stone *et al.* (39) have reported methods for the dry weight analysis of a *Penicillium chrysogenum* culture; they also reported on the variability of those measurements by analysing multiple samples and the reader is referred to this paper for the rigorous statistical analysis.

Protocol 5. Eppendorf method for dry weight analysis

Equipment and reagents
- Three Eppendorf tubes per sample
- 90°C oven
- Microcentrifuge
- Five-decimal place balance
- Reverse osmosis water

Method

1. Dry the Eppendorf tubes at 90°C for 1 h.
2. Label the tubes appropriately. Weigh the tubes on a five-decimal place balance and note the weight of each tube.
3. Pipette 1 ml of a well-mixed sample of the broth into each of the tubes.
4. Seal the tube lids and place into a balanced microcentrifuge rotor.
5. Spin the samples down for 10 min at 8–10 000 *g* in the microcentrifuge.
6. Once the microcentrifuge has stopped rotating, remove the tubes and pour off the supernatant (this may be kept for other analyses).
7. Resuspend the pellet in 1 ml reverse osmosis water and repeat the centrifugation procedure.
8. Place the labelled tubes in a rack and dry in an oven at 90°C for 25 h.[a]
9. Remove the rack from the oven (wear heat-resistant gloves), place in a desiccator, and allow to cool.
10. Weigh the tubes to five-decimal places. Replace the labelled tubes in a rack and dry in an oven at 90°C, reweigh the tubes until the mass is constant.
11. Subtract the initial mass of the Eppendorf tube from the final weight and calculate the dry weight for each tube. The differences in recorded weight will determine the accuracy of the measurements.

[a] A microwave oven (650 watt) may be used as an alternative, set at 'defrost' for 20 minutes.

Protocol 6. Glass tube method for dry weight analysis[a]

Equipment and reagents
- Three Pyrex tubes per sample
- 90°C oven
- Bench-top centrifuge
- Five-decimal place balance
- Reverse osmosis water

Protocol 6. *Continued*

Method

1. Dry the glass tubes at 90°C for 1 hour.

2. Label the tubes appropriately. Weigh the tubes on a five-decimal place balance and note the weight of each tube.

3. Pipette 10 ml of a well-mixed sample of the broth into each of the tubes.

4. Seal the tube lids and place into a balanced centrifuge rotor.

5. Spin the samples down for 10 min at 3–4000 *g* in the bench-top centrifuge.

6. Once the centrifuge has stopped rotating, remove the tubes and pour off the supernatant (this may be kept for other analyses).

7. Resuspend the pellet in 10 ml reverse osmosis water and repeat the centrifugation procedure.

8. Place the labelled tubes in a rack and dry in an oven at 90°C for 24 h.[b]

9. Remove the rack from the oven (wear heat-resistant gloves), place in a desiccator, and allow to cool.

10. Weigh the tubes to five-decimal places. Replace the labelled tubes in a rack and dry in an oven at 90°C, reweigh the tubes until the mass is constant.

11. Subtract the initial mass of the glass tube from the final weight and calculate the dry weight for each tube. The differences in recorded weight will determine the accuracy of the measurements.

[a] This method is suitable when larger sample volumes are available and the cell concentration is low.
[b] A microwave oven may also be used (see *Protocol 5*).

Protocol 7. Filtration method for dry weight determination of biomass concentration[a]

Equipment and reagents

- Whatman glass microfibre filters (three per sample)
- Five-decimal place balance
- 90°C oven
- Vacuum supply
- Sartorious SM vacuum filter holder or similar, e.g. Buchner flask and filter funnel
- Reverse osmosis water

Method

1. Pre-dry the filters in an oven at 90°C overnight, label and then weigh on the five-decimal place balance.

2. Place one filter in a Sartorious SM vacuum filter holder connected to a vacuum supply.

3. Pipette 10 ml of well-mixed fermentation broth on to the surface of the filter and apply the vacuum to pull the liquid through the filter. Ensure that the sample is evenly distributed over the filter and avoid the edges.

4. While still applying a vacuum, wash the sample with reverse osmosis water and allow to dry for 2 min. Repeat this operation.

5. Carefully remove the filter from the housing and dry for 24 hours in the 90°C oven.

6. Remove the filters from the oven (wear heat-resistant gloves). It may be better to use forceps to transfer them to a suitable container. Place the container in a desiccator and allow to cool.

7. Weigh the filter on the five-decimal place balance. Note the weight. Replace the filter in the oven and dry. Reweigh until a constant weight is attained.

8. Subtract the initial mass of the clean filter from the final weight and calculate the dry weight for each filter. The differences in recorded weight will determine the accuracy of the measurements. Calculate cell dry weight per unit volume based on the original sample volume.

[a] This method is suitable for mycelial organisms grown in defined media. It can also be used for media containing undissolved samples but will be subject to error. This error can be reduced by calculating the dry weight prior to inoculation, although it should be borne in mind that this pre-inoculation dry weight will change as the organisms grow and break down the media components.
[b] A microwave oven may also be used, see *Protocol 5*.

4.2 Packed cell volume

As the name implies this is a rapid measurement by centrifugation, but the accuracy is poor, particularly at low cell concentrations. It is also known as the wet weight method. It is useful when the volumes available are large. The method is best employed when a rapid measurement is required and accuracy is not the major issue. It measures cell volume rather than cell mass and the centrifugation conditions must be standardized. The major drawback to this method is the manner in which the cells pack down. This is particularly noticeable with filamentous organisms where the packing can be influenced by the cell morphology.

Protocol 8. Packed cell volume method for biomass determination[a]

Equipment
- Graduated glass centrifuge tubes
- Bench-top centrifuge with swing-out rotor

Protocol 8. *Continued*

Method

1. Decant a suitable amount of the well-mixed sample into the centrifuge tubes. Use three tubes per sample to give good statistical repro-ducibility. Maximize the volume of the glass tubes as the amount of packed cell material must be clearly discernible. Note the volume.

2. Spin down the samples in the bench-top centrifuge at 4–6000 g for 10 min.[b]

3. Using the graduations on the centrifuge tube, calculate the volume of the supernatant. Subtract this from the volume noted in Step 1 to give the packed cell volume.

[a] This method is only suitable for relatively high biomass concentrations.
[b] Check that 10 min is sufficient time for there to be no change in the packed cell volume.

4.3 Turbidimetry

Turbidimetry is one of two light-based techniques for measuring biomass, but is only applicable for unicellular organisms. It is based on the transmission of light through a known path of a cell suspension, but it has a narrow range where sensible results can be obtained. The technique is restrictive, being affected by gas bubbles and undissolved solids, although robust *in-situ* probes have been developed.

The theory is based on the Beer–Lambert law for light absorption:

$$I = I_0\, e(-c\tau l); \qquad [2]$$

where I is the intensity of the beam after attenuation by scattering, I_0 is the intensity of the incident light, c is the concentration of suspended particles (biomass), τ is the 'turbidity coefficient', and l is the light path length of the sample. However, this is usually expressed in terms of the measured parameter known as the turbidity or optical density:

$$\text{Turbidity} = \log_{10}[I_0/I] = (\tau c l)/2.303 = \text{apparent absorbance.} \qquad [3]$$

In most cases, the path length and the 'turbidity coefficient' are constant such that there is a constant relationship with particle (biomass) concentration.

The amount and angular distribution of the scattered light can frequently be described by precise or approximate solutions. The most simple cases are with bacteria whose dimensions are similar to the wavelength used and whose refractive index is less than 5% greater than that of the suspending solution. In these cases, the degree of scattering can be described by either the Rayleigh–Gens or Jobst approximations. The main elements of these approximations are that: (i) the amount of scattering is inversely proportional to λ^n where λ is the wavelength and n varies in the range 2 to 4 and is dependent on the shape and orientation of the bacterial cells, and (ii) that measured turbidity is usually less than the true turbidity due to forward scattering as a result of the type of device used.

As the cell concentration increases, and, thus, the apparent absorbance, the Beer–Lambert law deviates from its linear dependence on concentration as a result of the destructive interference between suspended particles (bacterial cells) and the increased complexity of the scattered light. The relationship described in the equations should therefore only be used for samples where the absorbance is below 0.5. Samples may, of course, be diluted to bring them into this range. *Protocol 9* details the procedure necessary for the turbidimetric determination of biomass concentration.

Protocol 9. Turbidimetric determination of biomass concentration

Equipment and reagents
- Single or dual beam laboratory light spectrophotometer
- Plastic disposable cuvettes
- Vortex mixer
- Reverse osmosis water

Method

1. Pipette 1 ml of a well-mixed sample into 9 ml reverse osmosis water and mix using the vortex mixer.

2. Pipette 3 ml reverse osmosis water[a] into a disposable cuvette and place in the spectrophotometer at the established wavelength[b]. Use this to set the zero for instrument.

3. Pipette 3 ml of the mixed sample into a 3 ml plastic disposable cuvette.

4. Place the sample cuvette in the spectrophotometer and read absorbance set against the blank. If absorbance is outside the range 0.3–0.5 absorbance units, then the sample requires further dilution.

5. If the sample is outside the range, dilute 1:10 with reverse osmosis water and read absorbance again. Repeat again if necessary.

6. Calculate the actual absorbance as a result of the dilution. For light in the 600 nm to 700 nm range one absorbance unit approximately corresponds to 1.5 g dry cell weight per litre.

---

[a] If the medium is turbid this should be used as a blank in place of reverse osmosis water.
[b] It may be necessary to scan through a range of wavelengths, 400 nm to 700 nm, to establish the optimal wavelength for absorbance measurement. Established wavelengths are between 600 nm and 700 nm for yeast and bacterial cultures. This method is suitable for most unicellular organisms.

The use of the spectrophotometric method for high biomass concentrations has also been investigated as process intensification increases the demand for reliable monitoring methods. Thatipamala *et al.* (40) have reported an adaptation of the technique suitable for concentrations of baker's yeast up to 100 g/l dry cell weight. The method utilizes a cell mixture of a known concentration as a reference rather than the customary analyte blank.

A number of commercial probes are available on the market, at a price, but all require some study and assessment before their use can become routine. The usual problems are: (i) an inability to dilute the sample or account for this at the higher biomass concentrations achieved in fermenters; (ii) growth on the surface of the probe, (iii) the problems associated with gas bubbles, and (iv) the problems associated with other suspended particles in the fermenter broth, i.e. solid medium components.

4.4 Nephelometry

This is the second technique employing light as the means of measurement. This method uses a measure of the scattered light rather than the transmission of light seen in turbidimetry. The light is scattered in a direction perpendicular to the incident beam of light. This scattered component is directly proportional to the cell concentration and is given by the following equation:

$$I_s/I_0 = Kc; \tag{4}$$

where I_s is the intensity of light scattered within a given solid angle, I_0 is the incident light intensity, K is the proportionality constant dependent of the geometry of the system employed, and c is the concentration of suspended particles (cells). The technique is more suitable for low cell concentrations than turbidimetry, with detection limits as low as 10^4 cells per ml with best results obtained in the range 10^6 to 10^9 cells per ml. However, the technique is susceptible from interference from small particles and is generally more expensive, in terms of equipment, than turbidimetry.

4.5 Electrical counting and sizing

Although this chapter is concerned with measurements of biomass one of the advantages of this technique is that the equipment utilized also allows cells to be sized. The equipment required is quite expensive to purchase but it will have a number of other uses in the laboratory; the most well-established machine for this is the Coulter Counter. The technique is based on measuring the effect of an electric field on microorganisms. It is dependent on the cells being suspended in a conducting medium but, since growth media generally fulfil this requirement, this is not a restriction. However, it does limit measurement to cells growing in defined media.

In the instrument the cells are forced to flow through a small aperture across which a constant current electrical field is applied. As cells are generally non-conducting they cause the voltage to increase as they pass through the aperture since they increase the electrical resistance across the aperture. The cells have to be at such a concentration that two cells cannot pass through the aperture at the same time; this naturally eliminates the use of this technique for filamentous organisms or any other cell not present as a single cell.

Earlier, it was indicated that cell size, in addition to cell number, can be obtained from this instrument since the change in resistance is a function of cell size. This is useful when the cell size and shape change during a culture.

4.6 Flow cytometry

The principle of flow cytometry is similar to that of electrical counting, but utilizes light rather than electrical resistance. The technique can be used in a number of ways, but the normal method is to direct a laser source on one side of a tube through which the cells pass singly and monitor the interruption of the signal by some detection equipment. This signal is then computed to an absorbance which is calibrated against cell number. The basic technique can be adapted for other cell components and the use of fluorescence emission. Scheper *et al.* (41, 42) have reported the use of flow cytometry for both *Saccharomyces cerevisiae* and *Escherichia coli* combined with fluorescence to yield data on cell size, protein concentration, RNA and DNA content. Kaprelyants and Kell (43) have also demonstrated the use of this technique combined with dye staining to quantitatively determine viable and non-viable bacteria, including an adaptation to allow its use for Gram-negative bacteria.

4.7 Dielectric permittivity

In Section 1.2, it was indicated that a clear and unambiguous definition of biomass is difficult, but that the most generally useful biomass measurement is the number of viable cells. Measuring the dielectric properties (the electrical capacitance and conductance) of a cell suspension to indicate the amount of microbial cells present would appear to offer an excellent measurement of the number of viable cells.

Upon the application of an electrical field of radio frequencies, the induced-charge polarization (measured as capacitance) in a cell suspension differs from that of the suspending medium alone by an amount which is directly proportional to the volume fraction of the solution enclosed within the selectively permeable cell membranes. This is because the charge separation induced in the solution also occurs in the cytoplasm of the cells. The ions in the cytoplasm are prevented from fully migrating to their respective poles by the selectively permeable cell membrane and thus cause a polarization across the cell, measured as capacitance.

The dielectric properties of cell suspensions are strongly dependent on the frequency (44). At low frequencies (about 0.5 MHz), the capacitance measured is that of the cells and the suspending solution. At higher frequencies (about

10 MHz), the direction of the electrical field switches too rapidly for the cytoplasmic ions to polarize across the cell, thus the capacitance measured is solely that of the suspending solution. As these dielectric properties are dependent on the possession of an intact cell membrane, this technique can be said to measure viable cells only, the possession of an intact cell membrane being a reasonable definition of viability. Unfortunately, this technique requires some sophisticated and expensive equipment. However, if it is available then much information can be gained about the cells for a small investment in time. A strategy for the rapid assessment of the suitability of the equipment offered by Aber Instruments is given as *Protocol 10*. This method is relatively new and significant improvements have occurred over the last few years in removing some of the problems initially associated with this measurement. Other equipment is becoming available and Hewlett-Packard offer an alternative, although less sophisticated system. Such a system has been employed by Mishima *et al.* (45, 46) for application on a variety of cell systems including human leukaemia cells and plant cells.

Protocol 10. Strategy for the evaluation of capacitance measurement for biomass determination

Equipment and reagents

- Biomass monitor (or similar capacitance measuring system)
- Magnetic stirrer and stirrer bar
- 100 ml Duran bottle and cap
- Retort stand and clamps
- Plastic water-bath and thermometer

- 0.1 M KCl solution
- Sterile (uninoculated) medium of interest
- A concentrated suspension of cells of interest (of known dry weight and/or viable cell concentration), suspended in the above medium

Method

1. Drill out the Duran bottle cap to allow a snug fit for the Biomass monitor probe. This ensures the reproducibility of the relative positioning of the probe in the bottle.

2. Set the water-bath to 26°C.

3. Add 100 ml of 0.1 M KCl and the stirrer bar to the Duran bottle, insert and secure the probe,

4. Clamp the Duran/probe assembly in position in the water-bath. Place the water-bath itself on a magnetic stirrer such that the stirrer bar is centralized. Apply one clean pulse and allow to equilibrate.

5. Set the frequency of Biomass monitor to 0.2 MHz, note the capacitance and conductance.

6. Repeat Step 6 for 0.3, 0.4, 0.5, 0.6, 0.7, 0.8, 0.9, 1, 2, 4, 6, 8, and 9,5 MHz.

7. Remove and drain the Duran bottle and wipe the probe clean.

8. Set the water-bath to the growth temperature of the organism used.

9. Repeat Steps 4–8 with 0.1 M KCl, with the uninoculated medium, and with the concentrated cell suspension.

10. Plot the frequency scans for the solutions as capacitance against log frequency.

11. Calculate the capacitance due to the cells (ΔC) at low frequencies by subtracting the capacitance of the medium from that of the medium plus cells. From the dry weight or viable cell concentration, calculate the capacitance per gram dry weight or per cell number. If the ΔC of the normal maximum biomass concentration relates to less than 5 pF then this may make the use of the Biomass monitor troublesome.

12. Compare the capacitance of the medium to that of the KCl at the growth temperature of the microorganism. Note any ΔC at low frequencies as these may effect the biomass measurement.

13. From the above plots, select an appropriate low frequency at which to measure biomass. This should be above 0.3 MHz to avoid the probe-related problems at very low frequencies.

14. To characterize the Biomass monitor set-up, calculate the cell constant at the measuring frequency selected from the tables in the manual using the data from the 26°C, 0.1 M KCl frequency scan.

The objective of the biomass probe is its ability to be used on-line; Harris and Kell (4) have listed those characteristics that would be desirable for the on-line measurement of biomass and these are given in *Table 3*. Clearly, in comparison with the other techniques described here, the use of the dielectric properties matches most of the requirements. The technique also has many off-line applications, such as measuring the solvent tolerance of cells (47) and

---

Table 3. Characteristics of an on-line biomass probe (adapted from ref. 4)

1. Continuous, real-time measurement
2. Sensitive to significant changes
3. Biologically inert
4. Non-destructive assay with no added reagent
5. Compatibility (i.e. many probes using the same equipment)
6. Long lifetime
7. Low cost
8. Use in opaque and turbid solutions
9. Cleanable *in situ*
10. Sterilizable *in situ*
11. Ability to distinguish between biomass and dead cells
12. Ability to operate in media containing undissolved solids
13. Able to measure filamentous and unicellular organisms

Table 4. Culture conditions used for biomass probe evaluation (adapted from ref. 48)

Organism	Biomass concentration (g DCW/L)[a]	Scale operation (litres)
S. virginae	30	2000
S. cerevisiae	106	20/1500
P. pastoris	89	20

[a] DCW = Dry cell weight.

cell disruption, but in terms of biomass monitoring it is probably limited by the absence of a databank of information which would allow rapid data interpretation. However, Fehrenbach *et al.* (48) reported results for a variety of culture conditions and organisms. A summary of the results obtained are shown in *Table 4*. Although the system works best with large organisms at high concentrations, such as *Saccharomyces cerevisiae*, and its initial success has been in the brewing industry (49), research at University College London has extended this work and its applicability with a range of organisms and fermentation conditions has been established. These are reported in *Table 5*. The studies show that for very small microorganisms such as *Pseudomonas putida* the signal obtained from a relatively large cell concentration (> 10 g/L dry cell weight) gave a capacitance signal below the manufacturer's recommended level. Reasonable results were obtained, but in a defined medium an optical method would be more appropriate. Use of the technique has most benefit in systems where the medium contains undissolved solids, which would be assumed to be biomass in some of the other techniques described, and where filamentous organisms are present. The technique was found to be more reliable in larger scale reactors due to the greater cell concentration and reduced changes that occurred in agitation and aeration. It has also been shown to be effective in fed-batch cultures. One important result has shown that a residual capacitance of approximately 5% is observed with totally disrupted cells indicating that cell debris also contributes to the signal.

Table 5. Effective biomass measurement by capacitance

Organism	Medium Defined	Operating mode Complex	Batch	Fed-batch
Saccharomyces cerevisiae	Yes	Yes	Yes	Yes
Pseudomonas putida	Yes[a]	Yes	Yes	Yes
Penicillium chrysogenum	Yes	Yes	Yes	Yes
Streptomycetes	Yes	Yes	Yes	Yes

[a] Optical density measurement preferable.

For on-line use the recent introduction of a multiplexer for this system will help reduce costs substantially since it will now only be necessary to purchase a probe and head amplifier for each vessel. However, the necessity for some preliminary experiments should be remembered and it would probably take at least one full week of effort before some results could be obtained.

4.8 Other techniques

4.8.1 Filtration probe

This is a method that has received little attention since the appearance of articles introducing it during the early 1980s (50–52). This is a simple device that samples the fermentation broth and filters it. The filter-cake depth is then determined by an optical sensor and the filtrate is measured by a load cell. Clearly, with a knowledge of the original sample and using suitable calibration the cell mass can be determined.

This method has been improved by other researchers (53) for mycelial *Penicillium chrysogenum* to give an on-line computer interfaced method. Little has been reported since the publication of this paper and this technique would only be recommended for those who wish to develop it and for a culture system where little change is expected in the coming future.

5. Mathematical modelling methods

5.1 Mass balance analysis

This method can be tedious and is based on a complete knowledge of the system under study. It is, therefore, only applicable in systems employing defined medium and it requires the measurement of as many parameters as possible, including an elemental composition of the biomass. It is based on being able to measure all the inputs and outputs of a fermentation (or process) to evaluate the biomass concentration based on the measurements. It is not on-line and requires a good computational model of the system but it does yield a comprehensive picture of the fermentation. Further details can be obtained by reading Chapter 9 in this book, and for a comprehensive study of mass balancing the reader is referred to the book by Roels (54).

5.2 Mass spectrometry

The measurement of fermenter vent-gas analysis is covered in Chapter 6 of this book; a method for the estimation of biomass by derivation from the carbon dioxide evolution rate (*CER*) and oxygen uptake rate (*OUR*) has been developed. Using *OUR* as an example, the general approach is to assume that oxygen utilization can be described as a simple linear sum of growth-related and maintenance terms:

$$OUR = \mu \, X \, / \, Y_{x/o}^{\,max} + m \, X; \qquad [5]$$

where OUR is the oxygen uptake rate (mmol/L/h); X is the biomass concentration (g/L); μ is the specific growth rate (1/h); $Y_{x/o}^{max}$ is the maximum yield of biomass on oxygen (g cells/mmol O_2 consumed), i.e. when $m = 0$ and m is the maintenance coefficient (mmol O_2/g cell h).

Then, using the midpoint rule for numerical quadrature, the biomass concentration can be progressively evaluated as the fermentation proceeds using the following expression.

$$X = X_{n-1} + \frac{(1/2)\, \Delta t_n \{X_{n-1} \cdot \mu_{n-1} + Y_{x/o}^{max} \cdot OUR_n\}}{1 + (1/2)\, \Delta t_n m\, Y_{x/o}^{max}} \qquad [6]$$

$$\mu_n = Y_{x/o}^{max}\, [(OUR_n/X_n) - m]; \qquad [7]$$

where X_n is the biomass concentration (g/L) value at the nth vent-gas sample; OUR_n is the oxygen uptake rate (mmol/L/h) at the nth vent-gas sample; μ_n is the specific growth rate at the nth vent-gas sample (L/h) and Δt_n is the time interval between $(n-1)$th vent-gas sample and the nth sample (h). The constants $Y_{x/o}^{max}$ and m need to be estimated from experiments using an alternative method for biomass determination. It is also adequate to assume that m is approximately zero for the initial growth phase of many fermentations and as a result only one parameter, $Y_{x/o}^{max}$ is required.

This method does require the on-line use of a mass spectrometer for the rapid calculation of the CER and OUR. Most mass spectrometers have a valve system that allows the sampling of the vent-gas from many fermenters and although each sample can be analysed rapidly the number of fermenters will determine the frequency of sampling from a given fermenter, i.e. the Δt_n in Equation 6. A good computer is then necessary to carry out the required computations. Once initialized, the system works well. However, the use of this method for the estimation of biomass is only as good as the model used. The initial article on the subject details all the necessary calculations (55) and a further publication has demonstrated its use at the pilot scale (56).

6. Conclusions

In an article published some years ago Carleysmith and Fox (57) stated 'the single most vital yet most problematical value sought during fermentation is the biomass concentration'. In this chapter a number of techniques that were in existence prior to that statement have been described. Those that have been developed since then have, for the most part, reflected the advancements in microelectronics with the expected costs associated with improved instrumentation. The measurement of biomass is still, however, dependent on three main questions: what is your definition of biomass?; how much time are you prepared to spend obtaining the data?, and, finally, how much money are you prepared to spend?

References

1. Fiechter, A. and Seghezzi, W. (1992). *J. Biotechnol.*, **27**, 27.
2. Gikas, P. and Livingston, A. G. (1993). *Biotechnol. Bioeng.*, **42**, 1337.
3. Karl, D. M. and Holm-Hansen, O. (1978). *Marine Biol.*, **48**, 185.
4. Harris, C. M. and Kell, D. B. (1985). *Biosensors*, **1**, 17.
5. Suphantharika, M., Ison, A. P., Lilly, M. D., and Buckland, B. C. (1994). *Biotechnol. Bioeng.*, **44** (8), 1007.
6. Burton, R. (1956). *Biochem J.*, **62**, 315.
7. Gurtler, H. and Schulein, C. (1980). Paper F63.7 presented at IFS conference, London, Canada. August 1980.
8. Harrison, D. E. F. and Chance, B. (1970). *Appl. Microbiol.*, **19**, 446.
9. Zabriskie, D. W. and Humphrey, A. E. (1978). *Appl. Environ. Microbiol.*, **35** (2), 337.
10. Zabriskie, D. W. (1976). PhD dissertation, University of Pennsylvania, USA.
11. Zabriskie, D. W. (1979). *Biotechnol. Bioeng. Symp.*, No. 9, 117.
12. Beyeler, W., Einsele, A., and Fiechter, A. (1981). *Eur. J. Appl. Microbiol. Biotechnol.*, **13**, 10.
13. Beyeler, W. and Meyer, C. (1984). *Biotechnol. Bioeng.*, **26**, 916.
14. Scheper, T. H. and Schugerl, K. (1986). *Appl. Microbiol. Biotechnol.*, **23**, 440.
15. Armiger, W. B., Forro, J. F., Montalvo, L. M., Lee, J. F., and Zabriskie, D. W. (1986). *Chem. Eng. Commun.*, **45**, 197.
16. Einsele, A., Ristroph, D. L., and Humphrey, A. E. (1979). *Eur. J. Appl. Microbiol. Biotechnol.*, **6**, 335.
17. Scheper, T. H., Gebauer, A., and Schugerl, K. (1987). *Chem. Eng. J.*, **34**, B7.
18. Walker, C. C. and Dhurjati, P. (1989). *Biotechnol. Bioeng.*, **33**, 500.
19. Brandis, J. W., Ditullio, D. F., Lee, J. F., and Armiger, W. B. (1989). In *Computer applications in fermentation technology* (ed N. M. Fish, R. I. Fox, and N. F. Thornhill), p. 235. Elsevier Applied Science, London.
20. Meyer, H-P., Beyeler, W., and Fiechter, A. (1984). *J. Biotechnol.*, **1**, 341.
21. Boyer, P. M. and Humphrey, A. E. (1988). *Biotechnol. Techniques*, **2** (3), 193.
22. Li, J. and Humphrey, A. E. (1989). *Biotechnol. Lett.*, **11** (3), 177.
23. Winter, E. L., Rao, G., and Cadman, T. W. (1988). *Biotechnol. Tech.*, **2** (4), 233.
24. Macaloney, G., Hall, J. W., Rollins, M. J., Draper, I., Thompson, B. G., and McNeil, B. (1994). *Biotechnol. Tech.*, **8** (4), 281.
25. Vaccari, G., Dosi, E., Campi, A. L., Gonzalez-Vara y R., A., Matteuzzi, D., and Mantovani, G. (1994). *Biotechnol. Bioeng.*, **43**, 913.
26. Hammond, S. V. and Brookes, I. K. (1992). *9th International Biotechnology Symposium*, p. 325. August 1992, ACS, Washington.
27. Burns, D. A. and Ciurczak, E. W. (ed.) (1992). *Handbook of near-infrared analysis*. Practical Spectroscopy Series, Volume 13. Marcel Dekker, NY.
28. Hall, J. W. and Pollard, A. (1992). *Clin. Chem.*, **38** (9), 1623.
29. Adams, H. L. and Thomas, C. R. (1988). *Biotechnol. Bioeng.*, **32**, 707.
30. Packer, H. L. and Thomas, C. R. (1990). *Biotechnol. Bioeng.*, **35**, 870.
31. van Suijdam, J. C. and Metz, B. (1981). *Bioprocess Eng.*, **23**, 111.
32. Packer, H. L., Belmar Campero, M. T., and Thomas, C. R. (1989). *Computer applications in fermentation technology* (ed. N. M. Fish, R. I. Fox, and N. F. Thornhill), p. 23. Elsevier Applied Science, London.

33. Reichl, U. and Gilles, E. D. (1991). In *Biochemical Engineering—Stuttgart* (ed. M. Reuss, H. Chmiel, E. D. Gilles, and H. J. Knackmuss), p. 340. Carl Fischer, Stuttgart.
34. Costello, P. J. and Monk, P. R. (1985). *Appl. Environ. Microbiol.*, **49**, 836.
35. Singh, A., Pyle, B. H., and McFeters, G. A. (1989). *J. Microbiol. Meth.*, **9**, 73.
36. Lawrence, J. R., Korber, D. R., and Caldwell, D. E. (1989). *J. Microbiol. Meth.*, **10**, 123.
37. Metz, B., de Bruijn, E. W., and van Suijdam, J. C. (1981). *Biotechnol. Bioeng.*, **23**, 149.
38. Mallette, M. F. (1969). In *Methods in Microbiology* (ed. J. R. Norris, and D. W. Robbins), vol. 1, p. 521. Academic Press, London.
39. Stone, K. M., Roche, F. W., and Thornhill, N. F. (1992). *Biotechnol. Tech.*, **6** (3), 207.
40. Thatipamala, R., Rohani, S., and Hill, G. A. (1991). *Biotechnol. Bioeng.*, **38**, 1007.
41. Scheper, T., Hitzmann, B., Rinas, U., and Schugerl, K. (1987). *J. Biotechnol.*, **5**, 139.
42. Scheper, T., Hoffmann, H., and Schugerl, K. (1987). *Enzyme Microbiol. Technol.*, **9**, 399.
43. Kaprelyants, A. S. and Kell, D. B. (1992). *J. Appl. Bacteriol.*, **72**, 410.
44. Harris, C. M., Todd, R. W., Bungard, S. J., Lovitt, R. B., Morris, G., and Kell, D. B. (1987). *Enzyme Microbiol. Technol.*, **9**, 181.
45. Mishima, K., Mimura, A., Tokahara, Y., Asami, K., and Hanai, T. (1991). *J. Ferment. Technol.*, **72**, 291.
46. Mishima, K., Mimura, A., and Tokahara, Y. (1991). *J. Ferment. Technol.*, **72**, 296.
47. Kell, D. B., Markx, G. H., Davey, C. L., and Todd, R. W. (1990). *Trends Anal. Chem.*, **9** (6), 190.
48. Fehrenbach, R., Comberbach, M., and Petre, J. O. (1992). *J. Biotechnol.*, **23**, 303.
49. Austin, G. D., Watson, R. W. J., and D'Amore, T. (1994). *Biotechnol. Bioeng.*, **43**, 337.
50. Nestaas, E. and Wang, D. I. C. (1981). *Biotechnol. Bioeng.*, **23**, 2803.
51. Nestaas, E. and Wang, D. I. C. (1981). *Biotechnol. Bioeng.*, **23**, 2815.
52. Nestaas, E. and Wang, D. I. C. (1983). *Biotechnol. Bioeng.*, **25**, 781.
53. Thomas, D. C., Chitter, V. K., Cagney, J. W., and Lim, H. C. (1985). *Biotechnol. Bioeng.*, **27**, 729.
54. Roels, J. A. (1983). *Energetics and kinetics in biotechnology.* Elsevier, Amsterdam.
55. Buckland, B. C., Brix, T., Fastert, H., Gbewonyo, K., Hunt, G., and Jain, D. (1985). *Bio/Technology*, **3**, 982.
56. Gbewonyo, K., Jain, D., Hunt, G., Drew, S. W., and Buckland, B. C. (1989). *Biotechnol. Bioeng.*, **34**, 234.
57. Carleysmith, S. W. and Fox, R. I. (1984). *Adv. Biotechnol. Process*, **4**, 1.

Further reading

General biomass measurement

Clarke, D. J., Blake-Coleman, B. C., Carr, R. J. G., Calder, M. R., and Atkinson, T. (1986). *Tibtech.*, **July**, 173. (Monitoring reactor biomass)
Fry, J. C. (1988). Determination of biomass. In *Methods in aquatic bacteriology* (ed. B. Austin), p. 27. John Wiley & Sons, Chichester.

Sonnleitner, B., Locher, G., and Fiechter, A. (1992). *J. Biotechnol.*, **25**, 5. (Biomass determination)

Pons, M.-N. (ed) (1992). *Bioprocess monitoring and control.* Hanser Press, Munich.

Chemical methods

Gerhardt, P., Murray, R. G. E., Costilow, R. N., Nester, E. W., Wood, W. A., Krieg, N. R., *et al.* (1981). *Manual of methods for general bacteriology.* American Society of Microbiology, Washington.

Microscopical methods

Postgate, J. R. (1969). *Methods Microbiol.*, **1**, 611. (Viable counts and viability)

Physical methods

Agar, D. W. (1985). Microbial growth rate measurement techniques. In *Comprehensive biotechnology* (ed. C. W. Robinson and J. Howell), p. 305. Pergamon Press, Oxford.

Cox, R. P., Miller, M., Nielsen, J. B., Nielsen, M., and Thomsen, J. K. (1989). *J. Microbiol. Meth.*, **10**, 25. (Continuous turbidometric measurements of microbial cell density in bioreactors using a light emitting diode and a photodiode)

Ebina, Y., Ekida, M., and Hashimoto, H. (1989). *Biotechnol. Bioeng.*, **33**, 1290. (Origin of changes in electrical impedance during the growth and fermentation process of yeast in batch culture)

Endo, H., Sode, K., Ogura, K., Ohya, K., and Karube, I. (1989). *J. Biotechnol.*, **12**, 307. (Determination of microbial concentration with a piezoelectric gum sensor)

Gordon, S. H., Greene, R. V., Freer, S. N., and James, C. (1990). *Biotechnol. Appl. Biochem.*, **12**, 1. (Measurement of protein biomass by Fourier Transform Infrared–Photoacoustic spectroscopy)

Groot, W. J., Mijnhart, R. A., van der Lans, R. G. J. M., and Luyben, K. Ch. A. M. (1991). *Biotechnol. Tech.*, **5** (5), 371. (A simple capillary viscosity meter for the on-line measurement and control of the biomass concentration in high density cultures)

Kilburn, D. G., Fitzpatrick, P., Blake-Coleman, B. C., Clarke, D. J., and Griffiths, J. B. (1989). *Biotechnol. Bioeng.*, **33**, 1379. (On-line monitoring of cell mass in mammalian cell cultures by acoustic densitometry)

Seydel, J. K. and Wempe, E. (1980). *Drug Res.*, **30** (1), 298. (A simple, fast and inexpensive kinetic method to differentiate between total and viable bacteria using Coulter counter technique)

Yasouri, F. N. and Foster, H. A. (1991). *Biotechnol. Tech.*, **5** (4), 237. (Measurement of myxobacterial growth using conductivity)

Zips, A. and Faust, U. (1989). *Appl. Environ. Microbiol.*, **55** (7), 1801. (Determination of biomass by ultrasonic measurements)

Mathematical methods

Rodin, J. B., Lyberatos, G. K., and Svoronos, S. A. (1991). *Biotechnol. Bioeng.*, **37**, 127. (A simple model to describe transient differences between cell number and biomass growth rates of *Escherichia coli*)

Fermenter vent-gas analysis

PETER M. SALMON and BARRY C. BUCKLAND

1. Introduction

Almost any microbial process involves the consumption or evolution of gases, and vent-gas analysis therefore provides a convenient means to monitor microbial activity. In contrast to other monitoring techniques for which the culture medium must be placed in direct contact with a sampling device or probe, vent-gas analysis poses no risk to sterile operation and has consequently become indispensable in both research and manufacturing (1).

Vent-gas analysis provides information on the rates of utilization or production of gases such as oxygen, carbon dioxide, hydrogen, and methane. Using suitable models, the concentration of these species in aqueous solution can also be estimated. The concentration of dissolved CO_2 is of particular importance in microbial physiology (2, 3). In addition to the permanent gases, the aqueous concentrations of many organic species can be determined by analysis of the vent gas (4). Volatile organic species are important as products (e.g. ethanol, butanol, fragrances, and flavours), as substrates (e.g. ethanol and methanol), and as indicators of the physiological state of a biological culture (1, 5). Vent-gas analysis using a mass spectrometer is also sufficiently sensitive for tracer studies to be performed using isotopes such as oxygen-18 and carbon-13 (6).

2. Methods for vent-gas analysis

The variety of potential techniques for the chemical analysis of gas streams is enormous. Only a few have been used to any extent for fermentation monitoring, however, and these techniques are described here.

2.1 Thermal conductivity

Thermal conductivity has been used for many decades as a method for gas analysis. In the simplest approach, the gas is passed over a heated filament (usually platinum) and the extent of heat removal is determined by measuring the electrical resistance of the filament using a Wheatstone bridge circuit

(7). Simple flow-through cells are very sensitive to variations in sample flow rate. Instruments in which the bulk of the flow bypasses the measurement cell are less sensitive to flow variations but have a much longer response time (typically 20 sec rather than 1 sec). There are several novel commercial designs that are intended to reduce response time while maintaining low sensitivity to changes in the sample flow rate.

The major drawback of thermal conductivity instruments is that they are non-specific. Water, ethanol, and other volatiles in fermentation vent gas affect the measurements. This necessitates extensive sample treatment to remove interfering compounds by condensation or drying. Carbon dioxide has a thermal conductivity that is about two-thirds that for both oxygen and nitrogen, and can consequently be quantified in fermenter vent gas by this technique. Additional selectivity can be imposed by measuring thermal conductivity before and after CO_2 removal by absorption in sodium hydroxide. Contamination of the sample cell does, however, lead to drift and frequent calibration is necessary. Thermal conductivity instruments are inexpensive, but are not recommended for applications where accuracy or long-term reproducibility are important.

2.2 Flame ionization

In a flame-ionization detector, the gas sample is mixed with a hydrogen stream that is burnt in air or oxygen. Ionization of organic compounds in the sample causes a current to flow between two electrodes across which a voltage is applied. Inorganic species such as O_2, N_2, CO_2, Ar, H_2O, and NH_3 elicit no response, and consequently the detector can be used to detect ethanol or other organic compounds in fermenter vent gas (1). Flame-ionization detectors are very sensitive, produce a linear response over a wide range of concentrations, and have a short response time (9). They are, however, rather non-specific and inappropriate for the analysis of complex gas streams unless the various components are first separated by a technique such as gas chromatography.

2.3 Gas chromatography

In gas chromatography (GC), components are separated by distributing them differently between two phases, one stationary and the other mobile. The extent of separation is determined by chemical and physical interactions between the sample components and the stationary phase, which selectively retards different species and thus separates them into narrow bands (8). The stationary phase is contained as a wall coating or a packing within a column (typically several metres in length and up to few millimetres in diameter) and commonly comprises a non-volatile liquid coated on an inert support material (9). For permanent gases, a solid absorbent comprising silica gel, polystyrene, or molecular-sieve materials is generally employed rather than a liquid (10).

A complete GC system comprises a carrier gas supply, sample injector, chromatography column, temperature-controlled oven, gas-component detector, and electronics for signal acquisition and peak integration (8). The detectors most commonly employed are the thermal conductivity and flame-ionization sensors described in Sections 2.1 and 2.2. With a suitable choice of materials and operating conditions, the components of interest can be monitored as separate peaks in the effluent, and accurately quantified despite the non-specific nature of the detector.

Gas chromatography requires precision valves and moving parts, and consequently requires careful operation and maintenance. Moreover, the time required for the analysis of each sample is generally between 1 and 30 minutes, much longer than that required for any other instrument in common use for monitoring fermenter vent gas. There is, however, a commercial instrument fabricated using silicon micromachining technology that allows analysis within 30 sec (1). The device incorporates a miniaturized fused silica column and thermal conductivity detector, and is appropriate for components with concentrations as low as 1–10 p.p.m. (Microsensor Technology, Inc.).

Despite its complexity, GC is used extensively for monitoring fermentation vent gas. The technique has been employed to determine O_2, CO_2, H_2, CH_4, N_2O, and many of the volatile organic compounds of interest. Unless the selectivity and flexibility that GC affords is essential, however, other methods are simpler, less expensive, more rapid and more reliable.

2.4 Electrochemical sensors

The oxygen concentration in gas streams can be measured using electrochemical sensors similar to the probes commonly employed to monitor dissolved oxygen tension. Oxygen diffuses across a permselective membrane (usually of poly(tetrafluoroethylene) (PTFE), silicone rubber, or both) and is reduced electrochemically at the surface of a noble metal cathode. Selectivity is provided by the properties of the membrane (which excludes other reducible species) and by the choice of polarizing voltage. The current is proportional to the oxygen concentration if diffusion across the membrane is rate-limiting. Similar probes can be used for gases such as N_2O (11, 12). The probes have a slow response time because of the membrane, are sensitive to temperature ($\sim$ 4% change in signal per °C), and prone to drift ($\sim$ 0.2% of range per hour) as the result of electrolyte depletion and water loss into the gas stream (13). In consequence, the probes are rarely used for vent-gas monitoring, except as an inexpensive back-up to more accurate instruments.

Yttria-stabilized zirconia ceramic elements are routinely used as specific sensors for oxygen. The ceramic electrolyte is generally formed into a closed-end tube and coated on both sides with thin porous layers of platinum that act as electrodes (8). At temperatures in the 600–800 °C range, vacancies in the crystal lattice permit the passage of oxygen ions. When the two electrodes are in contact with gases of different oxygen content (e.g. reference and sample gases), a voltage is produced that is proportional to the logarithm of the concentration ratio. The response is temperature dependent, and good temperature control of the instrument is essential. The zirconia sensor is simple, inexpensive, and robust, with an accuracy of $\sim 1\%$ of the scale in the range of interest for fermentation monitoring. In consequence, it may be a good choice for applications in which cost rather than versatility or accuracy is paramount (14).

Solid-state sensors are available for a variety of volatile organic species, and their design is often proprietary (e.g. International Sensor Technology). The gas to be analysed is passed over a ceramic or semiconductor material that is, to some extent, specific to the component of interest. Gaseous species diffuse into the material and alter its impedance by modifying the carrier charge density through interactions that include adsorption and in some cases reaction (10). Tin (IV) oxide (SnO_2) sensors are common, and are used to monitor ethanol in fermentation vent gas (13, 15). The rate of response and selectivity of the sensors is generally poor, but they are inexpensive and have good sensitivity in the p.p.m. range.

2.5 Infrared (IR) absorption

When infrared radiation strikes non-symmetrical molecules it causes the bonds to vibrate and rotate, resulting in absorption of energy. The vibrational and rotational frequencies depend on the molecular structure of the compound. Gases such as N_2 and O_2 that contain only one element do not absorb infrared radiation, and consequently IR analysers are widely used to monitor CO_2 and, in some cases, additional components such as water and ethanol in fermenter vent gas (16).

Dispersive photometers that split the electromagnetic spectrum are rarely used in process applications. More common are non-dispersive infrared (NDIR) analysers that are less selective but more sensitive, simple, and reliable (9). Quartz iodide lamps, tungsten filaments, and nichrome wires are used as infrared sources (10), and filters are used to select the desired bands of radiation (e.g. 4200–4400 nm for CO_2). The filters may be fabricated by vapour deposition of multiple coatings on a suitable substrate to obtain the desired transmission characteristics, or more commonly comprise cells containing the gas of interest to selectively isolate the wavelengths needed (8). In some cases, cells containing interfering gases may also be employed to eliminate unwanted wavelengths.

Two basic optical arrangements are commonly employed. In the first, the transmission of radiation in two different wavelength bands is compared, with only one band in the absorbing region of the component of interest. This approach is of somewhat limited utility because it is necessary to identify a

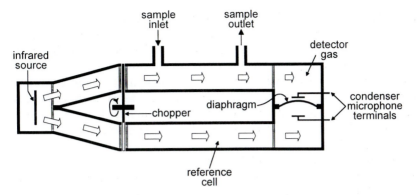

Figure 1. Luft-type non-dispersive infrared analyser with capacitance sensor.

spectral window wherein there is no interference. Moreover, the performance of the source and detector must be similar in the sample and reference
spectral regions. In the second arrangement, a single wavelength band is
used, and infrared transmission through the sample gas is compared with that
through a reference gas (often nitrogen). An instrument based on this
approach is somewhat prone to drift due to contamination or corrosion of the
sample cell, but may be more stable in the event of variations in the performance of the source or detector.

A typical instrument of the so-called Luft type is shown schematically in
Figure 1. Two beams of infrared radiation are generated from two sources or
from a single source with an optical beam splitter. One beam passes through
the sample cell and the other through a reference cell. The detector comprises two compartments containing a gas that absorbs at the desired wavelength—typically the detector gas is the same as the component to be
measured. The compartments are separated by a diaphragm that is distorted
when a pressure imbalance is caused by different levels of infrared absorption in the two paths. A chopper wheel is used to periodically block the
radiation in each path, and this causes oscillation of the diaphragm. The
diaphragm forms part of a condenser microphone whose capacitance can be
measured to determine the amplitude of the oscillations, which in turn can be
correlated with the concentration of the absorbing gas. Luft detectors are
somewhat prone to vibration interference and are subject to failure of the
thin diaphragm. A similar instrument using a microflow sensor in place of the
capacitance detector is available (Siemens AG). The periodic interruption of
the beams by the chopper wheel creates a fluctuating flow through a channel
connecting the two sides of the instrument. This causes a temperature
difference between two heated elements in the flow path. The temperature
difference is quantified from the corresponding variation in the electrical
resistance of the two heating units using a Wheatstone bridge, and correlated
with the sample gas concentration.

135

Alternative detectors are available, the most common of which is a special type of thermocouple comprising blackened gold foil to which wires of dissimilar metals are attached (10). The blackened foil is heated as it absorbs radiation, and the corresponding electromotive force (e.m.f.) from the thermocouple is measured. The assembly is mounted in an evacuated envelope to minimize heat loss to surroundings. Pyroelectric sensors incorporate a small ferroelectric crystal that absorbs infrared radiation. The lattice spacing changes as the crystal is heated, causing changes in electric polarization. The crystal is mounted between two electrodes (one of which must be transparent to infrared radiation), and the voltage needed to counterbalance the polarization potential is measured and related to the concentration of the compound of interest in the sample gas (10). Other solid-state sensors such as the lead selenide photodetector can also be used.

Infrared process analysers are not very selective and are prone to interference from a variety of components in the sample gas, such as water. Extensive sample treatment is generally necessary. Selectivity can be improved by careful design of the filters and by making measurements before and after the removal of different components by condensation or absorption (16). The instruments have an accuracy after calibration of $\sim 1\%$ of the range, but are prone to drift (up to 1% full-scale per day for both the zero and span). This necessitates frequent calibration, which is complicated because the change in detector signal with concentration is often non-linear (17). The time required for a 0–90% response is typically 0.5–5 sec (13) and the analysers are consequently useful for tracking process dynamics, perhaps with a more sophisticated instrument such as a mass spectrometer used intermittently to check and correct the data.

2.6 Paramagnetism

Paramagnetism arises when a substance has a permanent magnetic moment, which generally arises from unpaired electrons. Oxygen is the only gas of interest that is paramagnetic, and analysers that take advantage of this property are consequently very specific (7). The most widely used type of instrument is the thermomagnetic analyser, which makes use of the fact that the magnetic susceptibility is inversely proportional to $T - \theta$, where T is the sample temperature and θ is the so-called Curie temperature (80°C for oxygen). In a typical instrument, the sample is passed through a cell that contains a heated element in a magnetic field. As oxygen in the sample is heated, its susceptibility decreases (i.e. it becomes less paramagnetic). Consequently, cooler oxygen (which is more strongly attracted into the field) moves in, creating a flow often referred to as a 'magnetic wind'. The magnitude of this flow determines the temperature of the heated element, which can be quantified by measuring the resistance of the heating coil using a Wheatstone bridge circuit. A simplified diagram of an instrument of this type is presented in *Figure 2*.

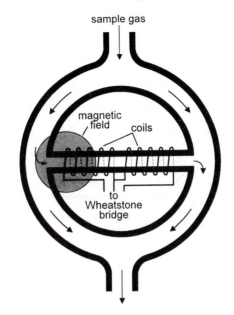

Figure 2. Schematic diagram of a thermomagnetic oxygen analyser.

Thermomagnetic analysers are sensitive to temperature variations and to the thermal properties of the sample gas. Natural convection caused by temperature gradients within the analyser also influences the measurement. Many different designs using the same basic principle have been developed to minimize or compensate for the effects of orientation, sample temperature, and other interferences. Nevertheless, careful instrument installation, sample treatment, and temperature control are essential for acceptable performance from instruments of this type.

A second common type of instrument is the magnetodynamic analyser, which may be preferable when the thermal conductivity of the gas to be analysed varies (perhaps because of changes in the CO_2 content). In the prototypical instrument, two diamagnetic fused-quartz spheres filled with nitrogen are mounted on the ends of a rod to form a dumbbell which is suspended by a stiff fibre (usually of quartz or platinum–iridium) in a cell containing the sample gas (7). The sample cell is mounted in a strong non-uniform magnetic field. The spheres are repelled from the strongest part of the field and rotate until the force produced by twisting the suspending fibre is equal to the magnetic force on the body, which is proportional to the difference in susceptibility between the test body and the surrounding gas. This difference increases as the oxygen concentration increases, causing a change in the deflection which can be measured optically using a mirror mounted on the test body. In other cases, a feedback winding is installed on the dumbbell, and an electromagnet is employed to maintain zero deflection. The electrical current

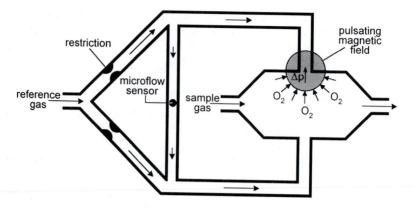

Figure 3. Quincke-type oxygen analyser with microflow sensor (Siemens AG).

required for this purpose is used to calculate the O_2 concentration. This type of unit is not affected by the thermal conductivity of the sample and is not as sensitive to orientation as are instruments that are influenced by natural convection.

A third type of instrument is the so-called Quincke-type analyser, which measures the pressure differential caused by a magnetic field attracting the sample gas (7). In a typical instrument of this type, a rotating magnet is used to generate pressure fluctuations whose amplitude is proportional to the oxygen concentration. Detectors similar to the Luft capacitance sensor or the microflow sensor used in infrared analysers (Section 2.5) can be employed. An instrument using a microflow sensor is depicted in *Figure 3*. A reference gas flows through two channels into the sample cell. One side of the sample cell is subjected to a pulsating magnetic field, which causes a pressure difference between the two reference gas inlets if oxygen is present in the sample gas. This pressure difference causes flow fluctuations through a connecting channel, and these are quantified electronically. The major advantage of these instruments is that the sample gas does not directly contact the detector elements. This reduces the likelihood of drift or failure due to contamination or corrosion by sample components.

Thermomagnetic and magnetodynamic instruments are generally sensitive to vibration, and to the flow rate and moisture content of the sample gas. The Quincke-type analysers are, however, somewhat more robust and have been used successfully in production-scale facilities at Merck & Co. The characteristic response time of paramagnetic analysers ranges from 5 to 100 sec and many of the instruments available are certainly adequate for the tracking of fermentation dynamics. The accuracy of the units is generally ± 1–2% of range (13), and drift is highly dependent on the care taken in analyser installation and maintenance, and on the extent of sample treatment. The cost of the instruments is higher than that of solid-state zirconia sensors, but similar to that for infrared analysers of comparable complexity. Paramagnetic instruments are, to some extent, being displaced in fermentation applications by more robust, more versatile, or less expensive alternatives (see Sections 2.4 and 2.7), but they are still widely used.

2.7 Mass spectrometry

A process mass spectrometer can detect almost any component likely to be encountered in fermenter vent gas, and has a linear response over many orders of magnitude (from sub-p.p.m. levels to 100%). The instrument can simultaneously quantify many different components, including inert compounds used as internal standards. It is insensitive to sample flow rate, and to moisture and other species that interfere with the response of many analysers. The instrument is expensive, but has a rapid response so that large numbers of vessels can be monitored at reasonable sampling intervals. The species commonly measured include O_2, CO_2, N_2, Ar, H_2, CH_4, and volatile organic compounds such as methanol, ethanol, propanol, acetone, and acetaldehyde (4).

The main components of a mass spectrometer are a vacuum system, a sample inlet, an energy source to ionize the various species in the sample, an apparatus for ion separation, and a detector.

2.7.1 Vacuum system

A prerequisite for mass spectrometry is high vacuum (typically between 10^{-8} and 10^{-6} mmHg) to avoid interactions between ions. The mean free path of an ion is a fraction of a centimetre at atmospheric pressure but about 50 m at 10^{-6} mmHg (10). Most mass spectrometers employ two vacuum pumps: a roughing pump to reduce the pressure to less than 1 mmHg, and a high-vacuum pump to further decrease the pressure to the operating level. The roughing pump is typically a reciprocating piston device, and the most common types of high-vacuum pump are the ion pump and the turbomolecular pump (6). The ion pump is quiet, but its pumping action is selective—it may perform poorly with noble gases. The turbomolecular pump is fast and non-selective, but service costs are typically high and it has a high-speed rotor that can cause a high-pitched whine. Some mass spectrometers use oil diffusion pumps but these are less common, perhaps because they are considered more difficult to operate (6).

2.7.2 Sample inlet

Two common types of interface have been used for fermentation monitoring (18). A membrane inlet comprises a permeable membrane, usually of silicone rubber or PTFE, that separates the sample from the vacuum of the mass spectrometer. This type of inlet is desirable when the gas flow rate is limited, or when selective enrichment of particular components is required to increase sensitivity. Moreover, the membrane provides protection against

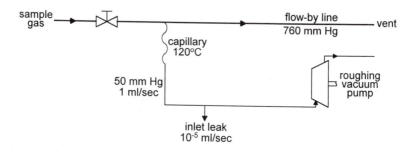

Figure 4. Capillary inlet for a mass spectrometer. Pressure, temperature, and flow rate values are typical for the Perkin-Elmer MGA 1200 (25).

foam and aerosols. In most circumstances, however, the membrane only delays the response of the instrument and complicates calibration (19). The membrane inlet design has been used extensively for direct monitoring of the liquid phase of a fermentation, but is less common for vent-gas monitoring (20, 21). More prevalent is a capillary inlet, such as that depicted in *Figure 4*, which provides a much faster response. The inlet incorporates a flow-by arrangement to ensure that the sampling system is well flushed. The sample is drawn by the roughing pump into the instrument through a capillary, and then enters the high-vacuum chamber of the mass spectrometer through a molecular leak element, which often comprises a glass or metal frit.

The inlet is usually heated to prevent condensation and to reduce adsorption of sample components. The pressure downstream of the capillary is sufficiently low that condensation is no longer an issue, but significant adsorption and even reaction of the sample with surfaces is possible if inappropriate materials are used. To reduce analysis times for polar organic species, adsorption can be minimized by using an inlet probe and capillary constructed of borosilicate glass and fused silica (rather than stainless steel), and by positioning the molecular leak element as close to the ion source as possible (22).

The amount of sample taken into a mass spectrometer is dependent on the pressure at the capillary. All species are, however, equally affected and the concentrations can therefore be corrected using an internal standard or adjusted to mole fractions if all major components are measured. The need for these corrections can be reduced, or even eliminated, if the pressure upstream of the capillary inlet is controlled using a pressure transducer and control valve (1).

2.7.3 Ionization

The standard ionization technique is electron impact (23). In a typical instrument, electrons emitted by a glowing tungsten filament pass through a pair of positively charged slits and are accelerated by an electric field maintained between the slits. Collisions of these electrons with gas molecules produce parent ions (with mass-to-charge ratio equal to the molecular weight) as well as fragments. Positive ions are accelerated by a series of electrostatically charged slits and emerge as a collimated beam of ions (24). Electron impact is stable and reliable but produces extensive fragmentation, which complicates the analysis of complex mixtures. Other so-called soft ionization methods produce only a few ionic species per compound (23). Process instruments using such methods have been developed by several companies, but have not yet seen widespread application for vent-gas analysis (1, 9). An alternative approach for complex sample streams is to use mass spectrometry after an initial separation of components using gas chromatography or even another mass spectrometer.

2.7.4 Ion separation

A number of approaches have been employed for separating ions in mass spectrometers, including time of flight, quadrupoles and hexapoles with voltages comprising DC and radio-frequency (RF) components, electric and magnetic sectors, and the ion cyclotron (23). Of these, the most common are the quadrupole and magnetic sector devices. The quadrupole mass filter is a square array of four electrically conducting rods to which DC and RF potentials are applied. Diagonally opposed rods are connected, and the two pairs are kept $180°$ out of phase, as indicated in *Figure 5*. This arrangement creates crossed, oscillating electric fields perpendicular to the line of travel of the ions between the source and the detector. If the oscillating motion developed by the ions is in resonance with the RF frequency, the ions travel through the quadrupole to the detector. If the oscillating motion is out of resonance, the ions strike the poles and are not detected (10). At a given combination of frequency and potential, ions of only one mass-to-change (m/z) ratio can pass through the rods. To detect different ions, the RF frequency or potential can be scanned. The mass scan can be performed as rapidly as several hundred times a second.

The second common approach for ion separation is the magnetic sector, depicted schematically in *Figure 6*. A uniform magnetic field is used to deflect the ions. The trajectory of a given ion has a radius of curvature that is dependent on the strength of the magnetic field and the m/z ratio of the ion. In some instruments, a permanent magnet is used with four to eight detectors located at appropriate positions to quantify a discrete set of ions (25). An alternative approach is to employ a single detector and to vary the magnetic field through the use of an electromagnet (22, 26). This approach is technically more complicated, but permits the collection of complete spectra and the use of detectors such as secondary electron multiplier devices that are too bulky to be employed in a multicollector instrument. Moreover, compensation for offset or gain drift in the response of a single detector can be provided through the use of internal standards or by the calculation of mole fractions

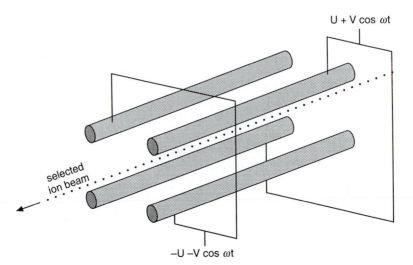

Figure 5. Quadrupole mass filter.

(assuming all components in the sample stream are quantified). Such corrections are less effective when multiple detectors are employed because the calibration drift for various species will differ.

Although quadrupoles are less expensive, smaller, and often faster, magnetic sector instruments are typically more accurate and stable. One reason is that because the separation of ions is dependent on geometry rather than voltage ratios, the magnetic sector instruments produce peak profiles that are much flatter than those obtained with quadrupoles, as indicated in *Figure 7*. In consequence, the magnetic sector analysers are less influenced by temperature or voltage fluctuations, contamination effects, and so on. Quadrupole analysers generally do not have sufficient resolution to discriminate between a peak for a species with a low concentration adjacent to a peak for a species with a high concentration, as might be encountered in monitoring ethanol or methanol at $m/z = 31$ a.m.u. (atomic mass unit) and oxygen at $m/z = 32$ a.m.u. (13). This is the so-called abundance sensitivity problem. VG Gas Analysis Systems Ltd is a leading manufacturer of both quadrupole and magnetic sector mass spectrometers, and has presented data indicating that the accuracy and drift of the magnetic sector instruments is better than that of the quadrupoles by a factor of about two (22, 26). Mass spectrometers have been used for vent-gas analysis at Merck & Co. for two decades, and our experience strongly favours the magnetic sector analysers. Quadrupoles have, however, been successfully used by others in a variety of challenging applications over an equivalent period (1).

2.7.5 Detectors

The ion currents in process mass spectrometers are in the range 10^{-15} to 10^{-9} A, and consequently sensitive ion detectors are required (26). There are two

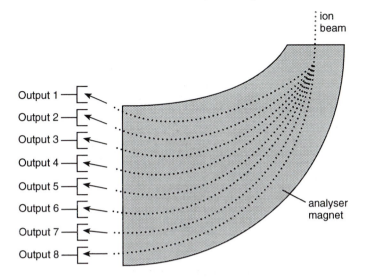

Figure 6. Ion separation in a multicollector magnetic sector mass spectrometer (redrawn from ref. 25, with permission).

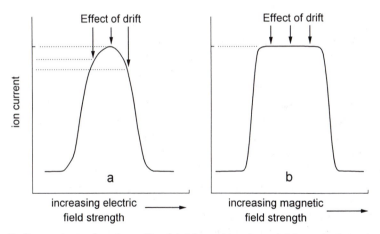

Figure 7. Comparison of peak profiles for (a) quadrupole and (b) magnetic sector mass analysers (redrawn from ref. 22, with permission).

common types of detector: the Faraday cup and the secondary electron multiplier. The Faraday cup comprises a beam-defining slit, a secondary electron suppressor that repels electrons released from the inner surface of the cup by the impinging ions, and the cup itself which collects the ions (10). The current required to neutralize the ions at the surface of the cup is measured using an electrometer, and is directly proportional to the ion concentration. The Faraday cup is rugged and reliable, and is accurate for sample concentrations as low as 1–10 p.p.m. (26).

In a secondary electron multiplier, the ions strike a cathode and cause secondary electrons to be released. The electrons follow a cycloidal path between two glass plates, and additional electrons are released each time an electron strikes one of the plates. In this way, an output about 10^6 times greater than the input ion current is generated. The electrons are collected by an anode, and the current measured to determine the ion concentration. The secondary electron multiplier is less stable than the Faraday cup, but is faster and more sensitive. Most single-collector magnetic sector and quadrupole instruments have both types of detector, and the appropriate assembly can be selected automatically through software (1, 27).

2.7.6 Data analysis

There is generally a small background ion current that must be taken into account during calibration, particularly at low intensities (4). Modern instruments can subtract this background signal automatically. The corrected ion current for each m/z value can then be expressed as the sum of the contributions from the various species in the sample:

$$s_1 = c_1 m_{11} + c_2 m_{12} + \ldots + c_q m_{1q}$$

$$\vdots \qquad \vdots \qquad \vdots \qquad \vdots$$

$$s_p = c_1 m_{p1} + c_2 m_{p2} + \ldots + c_q m_{pq},$$

or

$$s = \mathbf{M}c;$$

where s is the signal vector, $\mathbf{M}$ is the fragmentation pattern or sensitivity factor matrix (determined by calibration), and c is the desired concentration vector (26). Most chemical species produce several peaks due to fragmentation or double ionization (6). Consequently, the linear set of equations is overdetermined, and is generally solved using a least-squares technique. In the case of a multicollector magnetic sector instrument, a limited set of ions with different m/z values is detected and must be carefully selected to allow the desired concentrations to be determined without interference.

2.7.7 Applicability of mass spectrometry

Process mass spectrometers typically can detect ions with m/z values in the range 2 to 200. Magnetic sector instruments have a repeatability of $\pm 0.1\%$ of range at calibration, with zero and gain drift less than 1% of range per month, and a response time of one second or less for permanent gases and for non-absorbing organic species (22, 26, 28). The performance of some quadrupoles may approach these standards. The accuracy achieved in practice is limited largely by imperfect calibration rather than by drift or noise in the measurements. Moreover, the response time is determined by the sampling system and inlet rather than by the mass spectrometer itself.

In consequence of their versatility and performance, mass spectrometers are the most widely applicable instruments available for vent-gas analysis. Their chief drawback is the cost of purchase and maintenance. The primary maintenance issues are related to contamination of the inlet with foreign material (10) and the need for periodic replacement of the filament and ion pump (25).

3. Installation and operation

Vent-gas analysers are typically installed in a central area and shared between many fermenters. The sample system should be designed to remove interfering components and to deliver vent-gas samples to the instruments with minimum delay. The extent of sample treatment necessary is determined by the nature of the components to be monitored and the type of instruments employed. For example, comparatively little sample conditioning is required if the analyser can cope with moisture and variations in pressure and temperature. On the other hand, if moisture or other interfering species must be removed (as is generally the case with thermal conductivity, infrared, and paramagnetic analysers) several sample treatment steps may be needed. To minimize the response time of the sample system, tubing and equipment size should be kept as small as possible, and great care taken to eliminate backmixing and unpurged volumes that will slowly be dispersed into the sample stream.

3.1 Sample probes

The selection of a sampling point for fermenter vent gas requires some care. In many installations, the vent gas passes through a condenser to minimize water loss, through a steam-heated, double-pipe exchanger to prevent growback of contaminating organisms, or through vent filters that are kept dry using steam-heated jackets. Volatile organic compounds are likely to be removed from the vent gas in the condenser, and conversely are likely to be evaporated from any entrained liquids in heated sections of the fermenter vent system. Consequently, the sampling point should be upstream of any such equipment if organic components are to be monitored. The condenser may also be a concern if the concentration of carbon dioxide is to be measured, because the solubility of this species in water is appreciable (and is enhanced by hydration to bicarbonate if residence times are sufficiently long). On the other hand, sampling after the condenser is often advantageous if moisture must subsequently be removed, anyway, for successful operation of the analyser. Moreover, if potentially dangerous organisms are being cultivated it may be desirable to select a sampling point after the vent filters (or to install a separate containment filter for the sample stream). In any case, the sampling point should be located before the fermenter pressure control valve to facilitate transport of the sample stream to the analyser.

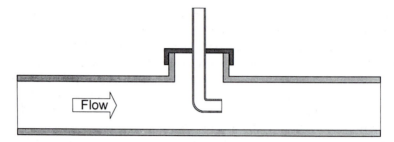

Figure 8. Vent-gas sample probe designed to reduce entrainment of liquids.

In any multipurpose fermentation research or development facility, foaming and entrainment of droplets in the vent gas will be encountered. The sampling system must therefore be designed to cope with this eventuality. Partial elimination of entrained liquid can be effected using a sample probe that faces downstream, as illustrated in *Figure 8*. Probes that force the gas to turn through 180° tend to exclude droplets, which fail to make the turn because of their inertia (24). Such probes may not be practicable for small laboratory fermenters, in which case simple sample taps are employed.

Further protection can be provided using one or more foam sensors, which typically measure the conductivity or capacitance between an insulated element and the tank wall (or between two elements housed in the same probe). Other types of foam detector monitor refractive index, or employ ultrasonic transducers to measure the reflection or transmission of acoustic waves (9). It is desirable in many cases to have two foam sensors: one in the vessel headspace to trigger additions of defoamer or to actuate a mechanical foam-breaker, and another in the vent line to trigger closing of the sample valve if form control is unsuccessful. The sample valve should also be closed if the temperature in the vessel is too high (perhaps > 50°C) to prevent sampling during cleaning and sterilization operations. These interlocks are generally easy to configure in a modern programable controller.

3.2 Sample transport

The fermenter headspace pressure is usually sufficient to deliver the gas to the analyser. A lute (or bubbler) is often used to safely maintain a slight back-pressure in small glass vessels. If the vessel pressure is too low, however, a simple gas membrane or piston pump can be employed. Tubing with a diameter of 2–6 mm is typically used. For the permanent gases, stainless steel or polypropylene tubing is convenient and robust. For volatile organic compounds, poly(tetrafluoroethylene) (PTFE) is preferable to stainless steel, polyvinyl chloride, polyvinylidine fluoride, and polypropylene because the adsorption of sample components (and consequently the lag in response to changes in sample composition) is reduced (4, 29, 30). To further diminish equilibration time and prevent condensation, the tubing should be heated if organic components are to be monitored. Sample decomposition is generally not an issue, and the limits on the temperature of the sample delivery system are set by the physical properties of the tubing, valves, and other equipment. A temperature between 60 °C and 160 °C is typically employed (4, 29), and can be achieved using electric or steam tracing (8, 31), or a jacket of hot water (30). If appropriate materials are used and if the sample conditioning and transfer equipment is adequately heated, the system response time for common volatile organic compounds such as ethanol and acetoin is limited by the residence time of the fermenter headspace and the transfer line, rather than by the kinetics of adsorption and desorption (4).

3.3 Knock-out pots, coolers, filters, dryers, and absorbers

In a heated system used when volatile organic components are to be monitored, obviously moisture and other condensable components are not removed. The sample gas in this case is typically passed through a final 0.2 μm hydrophobic filter (often PTFE) to provide protection for the instrument. In unheated systems, some moisture is generally removed during sample delivery by condensation. Many analysers require further moisture removal, and this can be achieved through the use of small concentric-tube or coil-in-shell heat exchangers with water or a refrigerated coolant (32). Also common are solid-state thermoelectric gas sample coolers that exploit the Peltier effect, which is the cooling that occurs at the contact of two dissimilar conductors when current flows from one conductor to the other. Sample coolers are available that have heat exchangers in the form of impingers, which rapidly separate the condensate from the gas stream thereby avoiding an excessive loss of components, such as carbon dioxide, that are slowly hydrated in solution. For example, the thermoelectric coolers from Universal Analyzers Inc. are rated for less than a 2% loss of CO_2 with an inlet dewpoint of 70 °C and an outlet dewpoint of 5 °C. The bulk of the sample stream is often vented upstream of the chilled surface. This ensures that the lag due to long transfer lines between the fermenters and the analyser area is kept to a minimum, without putting an excessive load on the cooler and subsequent sample conditioning equipment.

Condensate can be removed by a knock-out pot, often in combination with a coalescing filter in which small droplets conglomerate into drops large enough to separate by gravity. Such a filter comprises a graded-porosity hydrophilic matrix through which the fluid takes a tortuous path, with a drain layer to direct coalesced liquids into a sump at the bottom of the housing. The size of a knock-out pot or filter housing should be sufficient to avoid carry-over of liquid, but should not be so large as to significantly add to the response time of the system. An automatic method of draining accumulated liquid is desirable. Float traps generally perform poorly at low pressures, but simple manometer traps which operate without moving parts can be used. Alternatively, a solenoid or air-actuated valve can be installed, and automatically opened periodically or when liquid is detected.

Where required for analysers that are extremely sensitive to moisture, additional drying can be achieved using a desiccant or by diffusion drying. Common desiccants include anhydrous calcium chloride or sulfate, alumina, silica gel, and molecular-sieve materials. The desiccant should be replaced regularly or some mechanism for regeneration should be implemented. Typically, two or more packed beds of desiccant are installed, and each is periodically regenerated by heating and perfusion with dry air or nitrogen. Desiccants are rarely if ever necessary, and should be used with caution because they may absorb desired sample components, such as carbon dioxide, and thus delay the response of the system. Diffusion dryers employ polymeric membranes that are selectively permeable to water (10, 24). The membranes are typically used in a shell-and-tube configuration, with dry air or nitrogen passed through the shell side and the sample gas through the tube side. The apparatus is often operated at high temperature (up to 150°C) to improve the rate of moisture removal.

3.4 Multistream sample manifolds

Each vent-gas analyser is often used to monitor 15 or more fermenters. Under these circumstances, a manifold should be installed with automated switching between the various sample streams and calibration gases. Careful design of the sample manifold is necessary to minimize unpurged volumes and to avoid cross-contamination of the sample streams if a valve should leak. A simple layout is illustrated in *Figure 9*. Three-way valves are employed to eliminate dead-ends, and two valves per stream are used in a configuration which ensures that sample gas is vented to atmosphere rather than contaminating other streams even if both valves leak. Unselected sample streams are continuously vented at the first three-way valve to ensure that the transfer lines are well flushed. The three-way valves for the calibration streams, on the other hand, are configured to conserve the gases when not in use. The pressure of calibration streams should be reduced (using non-bleed regulators) to a value similar to that of the sample streams.

Solenoid valves are most commonly used in sample manifolds because they are compact and inexpensive. They generate heat, but this is not a concern when sampling fermenter vent gas. Direct-operated solenoid valves must necessarily contain magnetic materials that are not as corrosion-resistant as stainless steel, but this is rarely a concern with suitably conditioned sample streams (32). Air-actuated ball valves can be used for greater reliability, but their cost is higher. Multistream rotary valves have been used, but conventional types are prone to leakage and cross-sample contamination. VG Gas Analysis Systems Ltd has designed a multistream rotary valve specifically to avoid these prob-

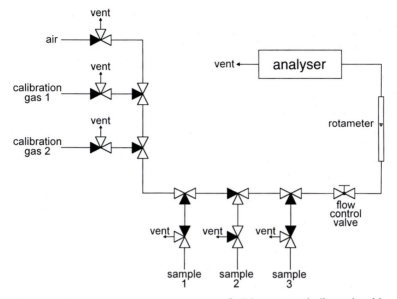

Figure 9. Multistream sample switching system. Solid segments indicate the sides of the valves that are closed.

lems (30). The sample streams discharge into a common vented chamber. A rotary arm with a spring-loaded seal is positioned over the stream to be analysed, and the sample is directed through the arm to the outlet tube. Positive flow through the tube into the common vented chamber provides assurance that no other streams will contaminate the sample of interest (1).

To ensure a rapid response after switching to a new stream, the tubing in the sample manifold should be kept as small as possible. If volatile organic compounds are to be monitored, the system should be heated. Balzers AG provides a special-purpose sample manifold with a low dead-volume, which is heated to 110°C to minimize the equilibration time (4). As a rule of thumb, the time allowed to completely flush the sample lines should be four times the gas residence time (1). This time can be estimated assuming plug flow through the system, but is better determined experimentally because of back-mixing in valves and regulators (32). If a mass spectrometer is employed, the purge time can be reduced by repeatedly evacuating the sample system using the roughing pump (33). This is particularly beneficial if volatile organic compounds are being monitored.

3.5 Pressure, temperature, and flow control

Most vent-gas analysers provide a signal that is proportional to the volumetric concentration of the component of interest. Consequently, variations in sample pressure will directly influence the results. This situation can be addressed by measuring the concentrations of inert species (typically N_2 or Ar) for use as internal standards, by measuring the concentrations of all major components and converting to mole fractions, by measuring the pressure so that the data can be corrected using the ideal gas law, or by controlling the pressure at a fixed value.

The most common method of pressure control is to simply vent the instrument outlet to atmosphere. The discharge tubing should be of large enough diameter to ensure that the instrument is at atmospheric pressure. The pressure is typically reduced across an upstream needle valve that is used to control the sample flow rate through the instrument. Because gas velocities are higher after the pressure is reduced, the response time of the system can be decreased by installing the valve as far upstream as possible. This approach does leave a 2–3% variation due to atmospheric pressure changes (32), and if an error of this magnitude is unacceptable an absolute back-pressure regulator on the instrument outlet can be employed. An alternative is to employ a reducing regulator upstream of the instrument, and to control the flow with a needle valve downstream. A disadvantage of this approach is that the volume of the regulator introduces an additional lag. Another alternative is to use a flow-by line similar to that in *Figure 4*, with a back-pressure regulator downstream of the inlet to the analyser. This approach is useful when the instrument requires a limited flow rate, because the flow-by line allows rapid flushing of most of the sample system.

Variations in temperature can also cause problems. Temperature is often controlled internally or taken into account by the instrument, but it is nevertheless advisable to enclose the entire sample manifold adjacent to the analyser (including pressure and flow control devices and valves) in a temperature-controlled cabinet with an electric heater. Unless moisture has been removed, the temperature should be kept at 60°C or higher to avoid condensation and to minimize adsorption of sample components.

Most analysers require a reasonably constant flow rate for predictable performance. If the pressure is controlled, a simple manual needle valve and rotameter will usually suffice. In other cases, it may be necessary to install a thermal sensor and automatic control valve to ensure that the flow rate is stable. Highly accurate flow and absolute pressure transducers, control valves, and controllers can be purchased commercially in integrated packages (e.g. MKS Instruments).

3.6 Monitoring an analyser system

To ensure that accurate data are collected reliably, simple instrumentation for monitoring the system should be installed. A U-shaped liquid trap with an electric conductivity sensor is often employed to detect water in the sample lines. Pure condensate has a very low electrical conductivity, however, and it is preferable to use a sensor that responds to the dielectric constant or refractive index of the stream or to the extent of thermal dissipation from a self-heated thermistor or electric coil (34). For analysers that cannot tolerate high moisture levels, aluminium oxide hygrometers can be employed to monitor the sample stream. A mechanical gauge can be employed to monitor sample pressure, but its type and location should be selected carefully because the stem and Bourdon tube of a standard gauge can introduce an unpurged volume that will increase the response time of the system (24). Flow rates are typically measured using rotameters, which are available with photoelectric sensors to allow remote monitoring of the float position. Inexpensive thermal or reed-type flow switches are also commonly used to provide an alarm if a sample stream is interrupted.

Leaks in the sample manifold can be diagnosed by monitoring the pressure after admitting instrument air and then closing the valves. Alternatively, the pressure can be monitored while the sample system is evacuated if this step is employed as part of the switching sequence (33).

Many analysers have their own diagnostic capabilities. For example, mass spectrometers typically provide alarms for problems with the capillary, filament, vacuum system, and power supply. Remote monitoring of these alarms can help to minimize instrument downtime.

3.7 Fermenter pressure, volume, air flow, and dissolved oxygen

In addition to the compositional data from the analyser, measurements of pressure, volume, air flow, and dissolved oxygen are required to calculate rates and concentrations in a fermenter. Pressure is usually monitored using strain gauge, piezoresistive, capacitance or resonant-wire transducers. Broth volume can be determined using similar transducers in the form of differential pressure sensors or load cells. The air flow rate should preferably be measured using a mass flow meter. Alternatively, temperature and pressure measurements can be used to convert a volumetric flow rate to standard conditions. The most commonly used flow meters are of the thermal dispersion type, which determine the flow rate by quantifying the rate of heat loss from a heated element (35). The dissolved oxygen concentration can be measured using a polarographic probe, whose response should be checked systematically by varying the headspace pressure (36).

3.8 Data collection

When an analyser is used to monitor many fermenters, it is important to balance the need to rapidly switch between streams with the desire to collect accurate noise-free data. When a new sample stream has been selected, data acquisition should start after an empirically-determined minimum purge time (Section 3.4). Multiple measurements can then be obtained, and filtered or smoothed to reduce noise. Some instruments take hundreds of measurements to provide results with a user-selectable precision (37). To ensure that the sample manifold has been adequately flushed, it is worth tracking the trend in the measurements as data are acquired. A convenient approach is to use a linear exponential filter, in which each successive measured value, c_t, is used to update a smoothed estimate as $\hat{c}_t = \kappa c_t + (1 - \kappa)\hat{c}_{t-1}$ where κ is a filtering parameter. An estimate of the trend in the smoothed data can be obtained as $\hat{S}_t = \lambda(\hat{c}_t - \hat{c}_{t-1}) + (1 - \lambda)\hat{S}_{t-1}$, where λ is another parameter. A typical algorithm is to acquire at least $1/\kappa$ values and then to continue until the absolute value of the trend, $\hat{S}_t$, is less than a target tolerance, δ, indicating that a stable result has been obtained. Appropriate values of κ, λ, and δ depend on the attainable rate of data acquisition and on the performance of the instrument. These values can be selected empirically when the analyser system is commissioned to optimize the rate at which adequately smoothed data can be collected.

The values obtained from any vent-gas analyser are generally expressed on a dry gas basis. Within a fermenter, however, the gas phase can safely be assumed to be saturated with water vapour, and the measurements should therefore be corrected using data available in standard handbooks (e.g. ref. 38). Unless expressed as mole fractions (as is often the case with a mass spectrometer), the results should also be adjusted using the ideal gas law to standard conditions of temperature and pressure to allow mass balances to be performed.

Most of the noise in calculated variables obtained from vent-gas data is a consequence of noise in the measurements of other variables such as the air flow rate and dissolved oxygen concentration. This noise can be reduced by smoothing the data using a low-pass filter. The ability to track process dynamics is not compromised if the filter has a time constant somewhat smaller than the cumulative lag due to gas hold-up in the fermentation broth, the vessel headspace and the sample delivery system, together with the response time of the vent-gas analyser. Many data acquisition systems include a user-configurable analog filter that can be used for this purpose. Alternatively, a simple first-order filter or other smoothing algorithm can be implemented in the software used to collect and manage the data.

4. Calculated variables

Compositional data obtained from vent-gas analysis are generally of limited utility unless interpreted in terms of the rates of consumption and utilization of the relevant species in the fermentation broth. This interpretation of the raw data requires the use of balance equations for both the gas and liquid phases.

4.1 Well-mixed liquid and gas phases

As a first approximation, it is conventional to assume that both gas and liquid phases in a fermenter are well mixed. This assumption implies that concentrations are uniform throughout the liquid phase, and that mole fractions are uniform throughout the gas phase. There will, however, be axial gradients in the volumetric concentrations of species in the gas phase as a direct consequence of the hydrostatic pressure gradient. Experimental and theoretical studies have demonstrated that this assumption is reasonable, at least for small mechanically agitated fermenters. Alternatives that may be more appropriate for large vessels are briefly considered in Section 4.2. For simplicity, we also assume here that the fermenter is isothermal and has a uniform cross-sectional area. The ideal gas law and the simplest form of Henry's law (which relates equilibrium gas- and liquid-phase concentrations through a simple proportionality constant) can be used for the low pressures and dilute concentrations of interest (39). The equations for this case have been given by Heinzle and Dunn (1), and are presented with a few modifications here. The balance equations for species 'i' in the gas and liquid phases can be written as follows:

$$\frac{dV_G C_{Ge,i}}{dt} = G_o C_{Go,i} - G_e C_{Ge,i} - k_{Li}aV_L(C^*_{Le,i} - C_{Le,i}), \qquad [1]$$

$$\frac{dV_L C_{Le,i}}{dt} = L_o C_{Lo,i} - L_e C_{Le,i} + k_{Li}aV_L(C^*_{Le,i} - C_{Le,i}) - V_L\Sigma r_i, \qquad [2]$$

where subscripts 'o' and 'e' refer to the influent and effluent, and subscripts 'G' and 'L' refer to the gas and liquid phases. $C_{Go,i}$, $C_{Ge,i}$, $C_{Lo,i}$, and $C_{Le,i}$ are the gas- and liquid-phase concentrations, V_G and V_L are the gas- and liquid-phase volumes, G_o, G_e, L_o, and L_e are the influent and effluent gas and liquid flow rates, $k_{Li}a$ is a mass transfer coefficient, $C_{Le,i}$ is the liquid-phase concentration that would be in equilibrium with $C_{Ge,i}$, and Σr_i is the total consumption rate of species 'i' in the liquid phase. It is important to note that the gas-phase concentrations, volumes, and flow rates are all considered to have been converted to standard conditions of pressure and temperature (typically $P_{ref} = 1$ atmosphere, $T_{ref} = 25\,°C$).

Using Henry's law and integrating over the fermentation broth volume, one can write:

$$C^*_{Le,i} - (RT_{ref}/H_i\,P_{ref})\,(P_h + V_L\rho_L g/2A)\,C_{Ge,i};$$

where H_i is the Henry coefficient, P_h is the headspace pressure, ρ_L is the liquid phase density, and A is the cross-sectional area of the fermenter.

For gases such as oxygen that have a low aqueous solubility, the liquid-phase supply, removal and accumulation terms in *Equation 2* are negligible. It is also conventional to ignore the gas-phase accumulation term in *Equation 1*, based on the assumption that the gas hold-up is small and that changes in oxygen utilization occur slowly. This simplification may not be valid for rapidly growing cultures (40) or when sudden metabolic changes occur (41), in which case the calculated results will lag actual events in the fermenter.

With these approximations, *Equations 1* and *2* can be added and rearranged to obtain:

$$OUR = G_o(C_{Go,O2} - G_e/G_o\, C_{Ge,O2})/V_L; \qquad [3]$$

where $OUR = r_{O2}$ is the net oxygen utilization rate. *Equation 1* can also be rearranged after simplification to give an expression for the mass transfer coefficient in dimensionless form:

$$\alpha_{O2} = \frac{k_{Lo2}aV_L}{G_o} = \frac{C_{G,O2} - G_e/G_o\, C_{Ge,O2}}{\beta_{O2}(1 + \gamma/2)C_{Ge,O2} - C_{Le,O2}}; \qquad [4]$$

where $\beta_{O2} = RT_{ref}P_h/H_{O2}P_{ref}$, and $\gamma = V_L\rho_Lg/AP_h$. Values of the Henry co-efficient, H_{O2}, can be obtained from the literature (42–44). The aqueous oxygen concentration, $C_{Le,O2}$, employed in *Equation 4* can be measured online using a polarographic probe calibrated to read $\beta_{O2}(1 + \gamma/2)C_{Go,O2}$ before inoculation.

The concentrations of inert species (such as Ar or N_2 in most fermenta-tions) can be used to calculate the ratio G_e/G_o if the simplifications used for oxygen are employed. In this case, the net utilization is zero and conse-quently $G_e/G_o = C_{Go,inert}/C_{Ge,inert}$. If inert species are not monitored, a rough estimate of G_e/G_o can be obtained by considering an overall mass balance using whatever measurements are available.

The solubility of carbon dioxide is sufficiently high that the liquid-phase accu-mulation term cannot generally be neglected. Moreover, in addition to CO_2 pro-duction by the cells, hydration of dissolved CO_2 to bicarbonate must be considered, particularly when the value of the pH is higher than about 6.5 (45):

$$CO_2 \underset{k_b}{\overset{k_f}{\rightleftharpoons}} H_2CO_3 \overset{K_a}{\longleftrightarrow} H^+ + HCO_3^-. \qquad [5]$$

The value of the rate constant k_f at 25 °C is about 1 min^{-1} (46), indicating that hydration of CO_2 to H_2CO_3 is comparatively slow and cannot always be assumed to be at equilibrium. On the other hand, dissociation of H_2CO_3 to HCO_3^- is very rapid. The concentration of H_2CO_3 is always low compared with CO_2 and this (together with the rapid dissociation to HCO_3^-) means that accumulation of H_2CO_3 can be neglected.

Further dissociation to carbonate is negligible in the pH range typically encountered in fermentations (3). Mass balances for CO_2 and HCO_3^- in the liquid phase can therefore be written from *Equation 2* as :

$$\frac{dV_LC_{LeCO2}}{dt} = L_oC_{Lo,CO2} - L_eC_{Le,CO2} + k_{LCO2}aV_L(C^*_{Le,CO2} - C_{Le,CO2})$$
$$+ V_L(CER - r_{HCO_3^-}) \qquad [6]$$

$$\frac{dV_LC_{LeHCO_3^-}}{dt} = L_oC_{Lo,HCO_3^-} - L_eC_{Le,HCO_3^-} + V_Lr_{HCO_3^-}; \qquad [7]$$

where $CER = -r_{CO_2}$ is the net carbon dioxide evolution rate from the biomass, and $r_{HCO_3^-}$ is the net rate of bicarbonate formation given by:

$$r_{HCO_3^-} = k_f C_{Le,CO_2} - k_b/K_a \, C_{Le,H^+} C_{Le,HCO_3^-} \qquad [8]$$

Values for the constants k_f, k_b, and K_a can be obtained from the literature (47).

The gas-phase balance (*Equation 1*) can be rearranged, neglecting accumulation terms as before, to yield:

$$k_{LCO_2} aV_L(C^*_{Le,CO_2} - C_{Le,CO_2}) = G_o C_{Go,CO_2} - G_e C_{Ge,CO_2} \qquad [9]$$

This can be solved for the liquid-phase CO_2 concentration:

$$C_{Le,CO_2} = \left\{ \frac{1}{\alpha_{CO_2}} \frac{G_e}{G_o} + \beta_{CO_2} (1 + \gamma/2) \right\} C_{Ge,CO_2} - \frac{1}{\alpha_{CO_2}} C_{Go,CO_2} \qquad [10]$$

where $\alpha_{CO_2} = k_{LCO_2} aV_L/G_o$, and $\beta_{CO_2} = RT_{ref}P_h/H_{CO_2}P_{ref}$. Estimates of the Henry coefficient H_{CO_2} can be obtained from the literature (42). C_{Le,CO_2} can therefore be evaluated if the value of $k_{LCO_2}a$ is known. Under circumstances where the mechanisms of transport are similar, k_La should vary in a consistent manner with the diffusivity of the solute, D_i. Simple film theory predicts $k_La \propto D_i$, boundary layer theory predicts $k_La \propto D_{i2/3}$, and the surface renewal and penetration theories predict $k_La \propto D_i^{1/2}$ (48). With the exception of one set of results (49), the range of experimental data is consistent with any of these predictions (46). The exponent of 2/3 can therefore be used as a compromise until more results are available, yielding $k_{LCO_2}a/k_{LO_2}a \approx (D_{CO_2}/D_{O_2})^{2/3} \approx 0.88$.

Addition of *Equations 6, 7* and *9* and rearrangement gives:

$$CER = \frac{1}{V_L} \left\{ \frac{\frac{dV_L(C_{Le,CO_2} + C_{Le,HCO_3^-})}{dt} - L_o(C_{Lo,CO_2} + C_{Lo,HCO_3^-})}{+ L_e(C_{Le,CO_2} + C_{Le,HCO_3^-}) - G_o(C_{Go,CO_2} - G_e/G_o C_{Ge,CO_2})} \right\} \qquad [11]$$

Three algorithms of increasing simplicity for the evaluation of C_{Le,HCO_3^-} and CER can be considered. The first is to progressively solve *Equations 7* and *11* numerically as the fermentation proceeds using current and past data. This approach avoids additional assumptions and allows one to track CO_2 evolution under dynamic conditions, assuming that the rate of data collection from the analyser is sufficiently rapid (which is a particular concern when acid is introduced intermittently for pH control because the CO_2 concentration in the vent gas will increase for a short period after each addition). A level of simplification is possible if the time scale for changes in the process is greater than about five minutes. In this case, the hydration reaction can be assumed to be at equilibrium, yielding $C_{Le,HCO_3^-} \approx (k_f/k_b)K_a \, 10^{pH} C_{Le,CO_2}$. Substituting this expression into *Equation 11* allows the value of CER to be calculated directly if the rate of change of the dissolved CO_2 concentration is estimated using current and past data. The final level of approximation is obtained by ignoring the transient terms entirely. This approach is very commonly employed, but is valid only if changes in both the pH and the carbon dioxide evolution rate are slow.

4.2 Alternative mixing models

The assumption that both liquid and gas phases are well mixed is adequate for small agitated vessels (less than about 100 litres), but questionable for large fermenters in which axial concentration gradients may exist. This issue has been examined by residence-time distribution experiments and other studies using variations in temperature, pH, conductivity, or the concentrations of tracers such as helium or acetone to characterize mixing conditions in fermenters (50, 51). The results can generally be described using models in which the extent of axial backmixing is quantified either by the use of dispersion theory or by approximating the fermenter as a set of tanks in series (52). By extending these models to include the lag due to the vessel headspace and sampling system, the relationship between fermentation dynamics and the measured vent-gas concentrations can be described accurately. These models are beyond the scope of this chapter, but a useful simplification for large fermenters is to assume that the liquid phase is well mixed (as in Section 4.1) but that the gas phase moves in plug flow (without backmixing) from inlet to outlet. Variations in the value of $k_L a$ as a result of bubble compression due to hydrostatic pressure, coalescence, and changes in the local shear rate are ignored. The gas-phase concentration of species 'i' is described by:

$$\frac{dC_{Gi}}{dx} - \alpha_i\{\beta_i[1 + \gamma(1 + x)]C_{Gi} - C_{Le,i}\} = 0 \qquad [12]$$

where α_i, β_i, and γ are defined in Section 4.1. A closed-form analytical solution to this equation with inlet condition $C_{Gi}(0) = C_{Go,i}$ can be obtained and used to calculate $C_{Ge,i} = C_{Gi}(1)$. The solutions for the oxygen concentrations are compared in *Figure 10* with those obtained assuming that the gas phase is well mixed. The left panel shows the results for a 0.15 m^3 fermenter and the right panel those for a 60 m^3 fermenter—the difference between the two cases is entirely a consequence of the influence of hydrostatic pressure. For a given value of the dimensionless mass transfer coefficient, α_i, the predicted liquid-phase concentrations are closer to equilibrium with the effluent gas for the plug-flow model, and the difference is accentuated for the large vessel (wherein the hydrostatic pressure gradient is significant). This phenomenon is significant in scale-up because the mass transfer coefficient required to achieve a desired liquid-phase concentration is lower for a large production vessel than for a small laboratory fermenter. Conversely, for a given mass

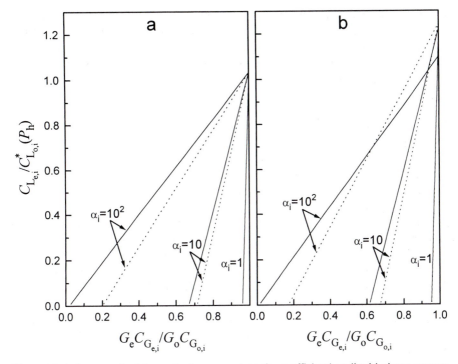

Figure 10. Influence of α_i (dimensionless mass transfer coefficient) on liquid-phase oxygen concentration (normalized to value at equilibrium with influent gas at headspace pressure) for a fermenter sparged with air. H_{O_2} = 857 litre bar mol^{-1}, P_h = 1.5 bar. (a) V_L = 0.15 m^3, A = 0.15 m^2. (b) V_L = 60 m^3, A = 8 m^2. Dotted lines: both gas and liquid phase well mixed. Solid lines: plug flow for gas phase.

transfer coefficient, the gas-phase and liquid-phase concentrations in a large vessel will be closer to equilibrium than those in a small vessel. This is the basis for the common observation that the dissolved carbon dioxide concentration in a large tank can be calculated by presuming equilibrium with the vent gas, whereas this assumption is often not appropriate for small fermenters (3).

4.3 Estimation of aqueous concentrations of volatile organic compounds

Assuming that both gas and liquid phases are well mixed, an expression analogous to *Equation 10* can be written for a volatile organic compound, with the simplification that the inlet gas-phase concentration is zero:

$$C_{Le,i} = \beta_i \left\{ \frac{1}{\alpha_i \beta_i} \frac{G_e}{G_o} + (1 + \gamma/2) \right\} C_{Ge,i}. \qquad [13]$$

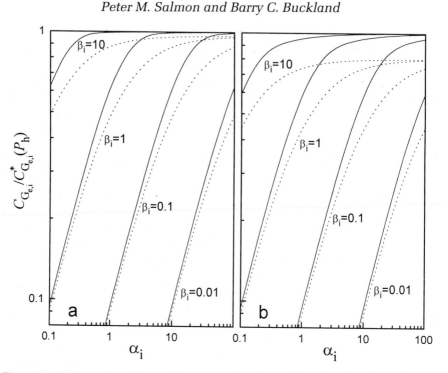

Figure 11. Influence of α_i (dimensionless mass transfer coefficient) and β_i (dimensionless partition coefficient) on gas-phase concentration (normalized to value at equilibrium with effluent gas at headspace pressure). P_h = 1.5 bar. (a) V_L = 0.15 m³, A = 0.15 m². (b) V_L = 60 m³, A = 8 m². Dotted lines: both gas and liquid phase well mixed. Solid lines: plug flow for gas phase.

As $\alpha_i \beta_i \rightarrow \infty$, the liquid-phase concentration approaches $\beta_i(1 + \gamma/2)\, C_{Ge,i}$, which is the concentration in equilibrium with the gas phase at the average fermenter pressure. Oeggerli and Heinzle (4) have shown that the equilibrium limit is attained for any volatile compound of interest under all realistic circumstances. This result is a direct consequence of the high affinity of these compounds for the liquid phase (and hence low Henry coefficient) compared with the permanent gases. For example, the Henry coefficient for ethanol at 30°C is about 10^{-2} bar litre/mol, and for a typical situation where G_e/V_L = 0.5/min, $k_L a$ = 100/h, and P_h = 1.5 bar, the value $\alpha_i \beta_i$ is about 10^4. Camelbeeck *et al.* (53) have experimentally confirmed this conclusion by demonstrating that changes in the rates of agitation and aeration have no influence on the vent-gas measurements.

Figure 11 shows values calculated from *Equation 13* for the 0.15 m³ and 60 m³ fermenters considered in Section 4.2, together with the analogous values from the plug-flow model. The results are presented as the calculated gas-phase concentration normalized against the concentration that would be obtained if equilibrium were attained. For either model, the gas-phase concentration approaches a constant value when $\alpha_i\beta_i \gg 1$. For the plug-flow model, this value corresponds to the equilibrium concentration at the headspace pressure; for the well-mixed model, this value corresponds to the equilibrium concentration at the mean pressure in the fermenter. The difference between these two values for the large fermenter indicates that care must be taken in the selection of a model when the hydrostatic pressure gradient is significant.

Whether a particular volatile compound can be monitored by vent-gas analysis depends on its concentration and volatility, and on the sensitivity of the analyser. Oeggerli and Heinzle (4) have shown that an appropriate criterion is $C_{Le,i}H_i/p_{min} > 1$, where $C_{Le,i}$ is the expected aqueous concentration, H_i is the Henry coefficient, and p_{min} is the minimum partial pressure that can be quantified in fermenter vent gas by the instrument. For example, p_{min} for the Balzers PGM 407 mass spectrometer is estimated to be about 10^{-6} bar, and using $H_{ethanol} = 10^{-2}$ bar litre/mol, $H_{butanediol} = 1.5 \times 10^{-5}$ bar litre/mol, and a typical aqueous concentration of 2 mM, the criterion can be evaluated to give $C_{Le,ethanol}H_{ethanol}/p_{min} = 20$, and $C_{Le,butanediol}H_{butanediol}/p_{min} = 0.03$, indicating that the aqueous concentration of ethanol, but not that of butanediol, can be monitored using vent-gas analysis.

Instrument calibration for volatile organic compounds is best performed empirically, rather than by relying on values of H_i reported in the literature. Calibration factors are typically obtained by adding a known amount of the compound of interest to the fermenter before inoculation and measuring the

---

Table 1. Generalized degree of reduction of various compounds

Compound	Formula	γ'
Formic acid	CH_2O_2	2.0
Citric acid	$C_6H_8O_7$	3.0
Pyruvic acid	$C_3H_4O_3$	3.3
Succinic acid	$C_4H_6O_4$	3.5
Glutamic acid	$C_5H_9NO_4$	3.6
Acetic acid	$C_2H_4O_2$	4.0
Glucose	$C_6H_{12}O_6$	4.0
Lactic acid	$C_3H_6O_3$	4.0
Biomass	$CH_{1.8}O_{0.5}N_{0.2}$	4.2
Mannitol	$C_6H_{14}O_6$	4.3
Glycerol	$C_3H_8O_3$	4.7
Butyric acid	$C_4H_8O_2$	5.0
Toluene	C_7H_8	5.1
Soybean oil	$C_{56}H_{102}O_3$	5.7
Methanol	CH_4O	6.0
Ethanol	C_2H_6O	6.0
Methane	CH_4	8.0

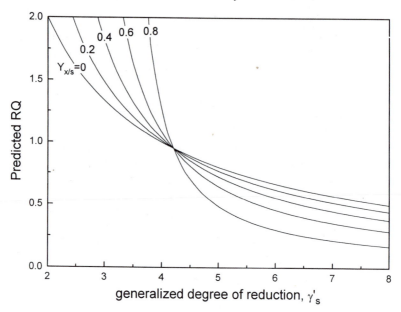

Figure 12. Variation of *RQ* as a function of generalized degree of reduction of substrate, γ'_s, with the yield of biomass on glucose, $Y_{X/S}$ (*C*-mol/*C*-mol), as a parameter.

response, or by withdrawing liquid-phase samples intermittently during a fermentation and analysing them offline by GC or HPLC.

4.4 The respiratory quotient

Perhaps the most frequently used variable calculated from vent-gas data is the respiratory quotient, which is defined as the ratio between the rates of carbon dioxide evolution and oxygen utilization, $RQ = CER/OUR$. The *RQ* value can provide some indication of the nature of substrates being consumed and products being formed in a fermentation. For example, consider the formation of biomass, $CH_{hx}N_{nx}O_{ox}$, and a product, $CH_{hp}N_{np}N_{op}$, from a substrate, $CH_{hs}N_{ns}O_{os}$

$$CH_{hs}N_{ns}O_{os} + aNH_3 + bO_2 \rightarrow Y_{X/S}\,CH_{hx}N_{nx}O_{ox} + Y_{P/S}\,CH_{hp}N_{np}O_{op} + cCO_2 + dH_2O.$$

Elemental balances for carbon, hydrogen, nitrogen, and oxygen can be written and solved in a straightforward fashion for the coefficients *a*, *b*, *c*, and *d*. The coefficients for oxygen and carbon dioxide are $b = (\gamma'_s - Y_{X/S}\,\gamma'_x - Y_{P/S}\,\gamma'_p)/4$ and $c = 1 - Y_{X/S} - Y_{P/S}$, where $\gamma'_i = 4 + h_i - 3n_i - 2o_i$ is the so-called generalized degree of reduction for compound $CH_{h_i}\,N_{n_i}\,O_{o_i}$. The value of γ' for biomass is consistently about 4.2, and the values for some common substrates and products are listed in *Table 1*. The respiratory quotient can then be

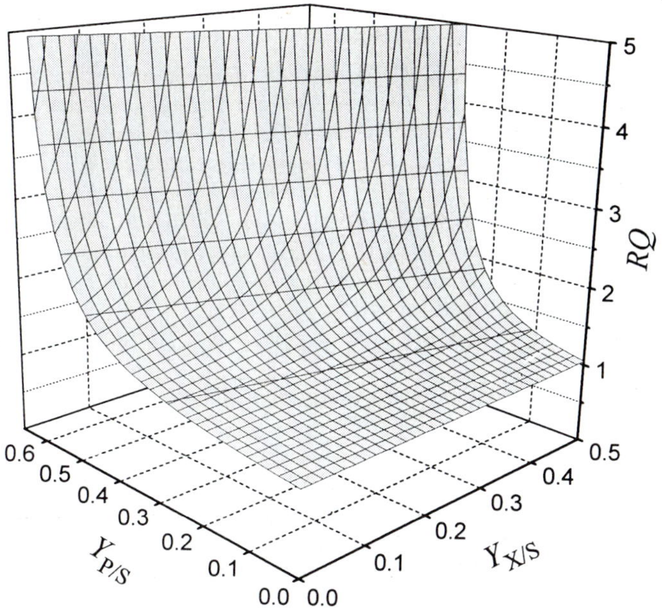

Figure 13. Variation of RQ as a function of $Y_{X/S}$ and $Y_{P/S}$ (C-mol/C-mol) for a fermentation in which glucose is converted to biomass and ethanol.

expressed as $RQ = 4 (1 - Y_{X/S} - Y_{P/S})/(\gamma'_s - Y_{X/S} \gamma'_x - Y_{P/S} \gamma'_p)$. This expression can easily be extended to include other substrates and products, as well as nitrogen sources other than NH_3 (54).

Figure 12 shows the variation of RQ as a function of γ'_s, with $Y_{X/S}$ as a parameter, for a case where no products (other than biomass) are produced. This plot reveals the basis for the observation (28) that the RQ value is about 1.3 for citric acid ($\gamma' = 3.0$), about 1.0 for glucose ($\gamma' = 4$), and about 0.7 for vegetable oil ($\gamma' = 5.7$). In general, the formation of products cannot be neglected and a given RQ value cannot unambiguously reveal the extent to which a particular substrate is being utilized. Consider for example the growth of yeast on glucose with the production of ethanol. For simplicity, the formation of other products such as glycerol is ignored. *Figure 13* shows the RQ for this case as a function of the yield coefficients for biomass and ethanol on glucose, $Y_{X/S}$ and $Y_{P/S}$. It is often useful to consider a given RQ value as defining a contour on such a surface, particularly when the generalized degree of reduction is markedly different for the substrates and products, as in this case. By combining RQ data with other information (including knowledge of the biochemical pathways involved) the progress of a fermentation can be tracked, and appropriate control actions taken to achieve a desired trajectory.

References

1. Heinzle, E. and Dunn, I. J. (1991). In *Biotechnology* (ed. H.-J. Rehm, G. Reed, and K. Schügerl) (2nd edn), Vol. 4, p. 27. VCH Verlagsgesellschaft, Weinheim.
2. Ho, C. S. and Smith, M. D. (1986). *Biotechnol. Bioeng.*, **28**, 668.
3. Royce, P. N. C. and Thornhill, N. F. (1991). *AIChE J.*, **37**, 1680.
4. Oeggerli, A. and Heinzle, E. (1994). *Biotechnol. Progr.*, **10**, 284.
5. Linton, C. J. and Wright, S. J. L. (1993). *J. Appl. Bacteriol.*, **75**, 1.
6. Degn, H., Cox, R. P., and Lloyd, D. (1985). *Meth. Biochem. Anal.*, **31**, 165.
7. Huskins, D. J. (1982). *Quality measuring instruments in on-line process analysis.* Ellis Horwood, Chichester, England.
8. Mix, P. E. (1984). *The design and application of process analyzer systems.* J. Wiley, NY.
9. Pons, M.-N. (1992). *Bioprocess monitoring and control.* Carl Hanser Verlag, Munich.
10. Nichols, G. D. (1988). *On-line process analyzers.* J. Wiley, NY.
11. Bailey, P. L. and Riley, M. (1975). *Analyst*, **100**, 145.
12. Van Niel, E. W. J., Robertson, L. A., Cox, R. P., and Kuenen, J. G. (1992). *J. Gen. Appl. Microbiol.*, **38**, 553.
13. Phillips, J. A. (1990). In *Computer control of fermentation processes* (ed. D. R. Omstead), p. 15. CRC Press, Boca Raton, FL.
14. Anders, K.-D., Müller, W., Kammeyer, R., and Scheper, Th. (1992). *Biotechnol. Tech.*, **6**, 97.
15. Mühlemann, H. M. and Bungay, H. R. (1993). *Biotechnol. Tech.*, **7**, 575.
16. Röttenbacher, L., Behlau, L., and Bauer, W. (1985). *J. Biotechnol.*, **2**, 137.
17. Durham, R. M. (1985). In *Process instruments and controls handbook* (ed. D. M. Considine and G. D. Considine), (3rd edn), p. 6.72. McGraw Hill, NY.
18. Heinzle, E., Furukawa, K., Dunn, I. J., and Bourne, J. R. (1983). *Bio/Technology*, **1**, 181.
19. Cox, R. P. (1987). In *Mass spectrometry in biotechnological process analysis and control* (ed. E. Heinzle and M. Reuss), p. 63. Plenum Press, NY.
20. Pungor, Jr., E., Perley, C. R., Cooney, C. L., and Weaver, J. C. (1980). *Biotechnol. Lett.*, **2**, 409.
21. Bohátka, S., Futó, I., Gál, I., Gál, J., Langer, G., Molnár, J., *et al.* (1993). *Vacuum*, **44**, 669.
22. Dadd, A. T. (1990). *Am. Biotechnol. Lab.*, **8**, 35.
23. Schmid, E. R. (1987). In *Mass spectrometry in biotechnological process analysis and control* (ed. E. Heinzle and M. Reuss), p. 7. Plenum Press, NY.
24. Clevett, K. J. (1986). *Process analyzer technology.* J. Wiley, NY.
25. Schaefer, K. and Schultis, M. (1987). In *Mass spectrometry in biotechnological process analysis and control* (ed. E. Heinzle and M. Reuss), p. 39. Plenum Press, NY.
26. Winter, M. J. (1987). In *Mass spectrometry in biotechnological process analysis and control* (ed. E. Heinzle and M. Reuss), p. 17. Plenum Press, NY.
27. Bartman, C. D. (1987). In *Mass spectrometry in biotechnological process analysis and control* (ed. E. Heinzle and M. Reuss), p. 49. Plenum Press, NY.
28. Buckland, B., Brix, T., Fastert, H., Gbewonyo, K., Hunt, G., and Jain, D. (1985). *Bio/Technology*, **3**, 982.

29. Camelbeeck, J. P., Comberbach, D. M., Orval, M., Pêtre, J. O., and Roelants, P. (1991). *Biotechnol. Tech.*, **5**, 443.
30. Camelbeeck, J. P., Comberbach, D. M., Goossens, J., and Roelants, P. (1988). *Biotechnol. Tech.*, **2**, 183.
31. Coppella, S. J. and Dhurjati, P. (1987). *Biotechnol. Bioeng.*, **29**, 679.
32. Houser, E. A. (1985). In *Process instruments and controls handbook* (ed. D. M. Considine, and G. D. Considine) (3rd edn), p. 6.20. McGraw Hill, NY.
33. Heinzle, E., Oeggerli, A., and Dettwiler, B. (1990). *Anal. Chim. Acta*, **238**, 101.
34. Miller Jr, T. E. (1982). In *Automated stream analysis for process control* (ed. D. P. Manka), p. 1. Academic Press, NY.
35. Ginesi, D. (1991). *Chem. Eng.*, **98**, 146.
36. Kässer, R. (1986). *IFAC Proc. Ser.*, **10**, 127.
37. Todd, D. (1989). *Bio/Technology*, **7**, 1182.
38. Perry, R. H., Green, D. W., and Maloney, J. O. (1984). *Chemical engineers' handbook* (6th edn). McGraw-Hill, NY.
39. Carroll, J. J. (1991). *Chem. Eng. Prog.*, **87**, 48.
40. Aiba, S. and Furuse, H. (1990). *Biotechnol. Bioeng.*, **36**, 534.
41. Dekkers, R. M. (1982). *Proceedings of the 1st IFAC workshop on modelling and control of biotechnical processes* (ed. A. Halme), p. 211. Pergamon Press, Oxford.
42. Schumpe, A. and Quicker, G. (1982). *Adv. Biochem. Eng.*, **24**, 1.
43. Iwai, Y., Eya, H., Itoh, Y., Arai, Y., and Takeuchi, K. (1993). *Fluid Phase Equilib.*, **83**, 271.
44. Eya, H., Mishima, K., Nagatani, M., Iwai, Y., and Arai, Y. (1994). *Fluid Phase Equilib.*, **97**, 201.
45. Yegneswaran, P. K., Gray, M. R., and Thompson, B. G. (1990). *Biotechnol. Bioeng.*, **36**, 92.
46. Smith, J. M., Davison, S. W., and Payne, G. F. (1990). *Biotechnol. Bioeng.*, **35**, 1088.
47. Harned, H. S. and Owen, B. B. (1958). *The physical chemistry of electrolyte solutions*. Reinhold, NY.
48. Cussler, E. L. (1984). *Diffusion: mass transfer in liquid systems*. Cambridge Univ. Press, Cambridge, UK.
49. Dahod, S. K. (1993). *Biotechnol. Prog.*, **9**, 655.
50. Mayr, B., Nagy, E., Horvat, P., and Moser, A. (1994). *Biotechnol. Bioeng.*, **43**, 195.
51. Lübbert, A. (1991). In *Biotechnology* (ed. H.-J. Rehm, G. Reed, and K. Schügerl), (2nd edn), Vol. 4, p. 107. VCH Verlagsgesellschaft, Weinheim.
52. Nocentini, M. (1990). *Chem. Eng. Res. Des.*, **68**, 287.
53. Camelbeeck, J.-P., Comberbach, D. M., Orval, M., Pêtre, J. O., and Roelants, P. (1990). *40th Canadian Chemical Engineering Conference*. Halifax, Canada.
54. Roels, J. A. (1983). *Energetics and kinetics in biotechnology*, Elsevier, Amsterdam.

7

The analytical chemistry of microbial cultures

DAVID M. MOUSDALE

1. Introduction

1.1 The analytical approach to microbial fermentations

The immense potential of microbes for producing biomedical and pharmaceutical agents, enzymes, acids, flavours, and speciality chemicals has been realized in a continually increasing number of industrial fermentations. Such processes are, however, necessarily complex, both biologically and biochemically. Growth and primary and secondary metabolism are combined with the utilization (sometimes only partial) of inputs and the generation of a mixture of products and side-products, degradation products, and metabolites. The understanding of a fermentation process is therefore always an analytical challenge, whatever its commercial status, and the problems are invariably increased by the development of a microbial strain and scaling-up a fermentation process. With secondary metabolites the complex regulatory networks at the genetic level preclude beneficial changes by random mutations, which act on either growth or the supply of metabolites or cofactors to biochemical pathways (see ref. 1). Such changes can be analysed by measuring nutrient uptake and utilization, the sizes of the intracellular pools, and the fluxes through the pathways (see Chapter 9).

The aim of this chapter is to outline analytical methods which can be applied to 'demystify' fermentations with both simple and complex media (see Chapter 3) at any stage of strain development and at different scales (shake-flask, laboratory bioreactor, chemostat, or large fermenter), without the demand for high-technology equipment (such as high-field nuclear magnetic resonance (NMR) or pyrolysis mass spectrometry). Emphasis will be placed on the use of techniques that produce information on how inputs are (or are not) utilized, metabolites are accumulated, growth patterns are established, fermentations can be regulated, and the effects of mutational changes can be assessed.

1.2 General aspects of methodology

Four different types of measurement will be considered: elemental (e.g. carbon), selective (usually enzyme-based for individual compounds), group-selective (for classes of compounds), and chromatographic (for single or multiple solutes).

Fermentation broths present great technical difficulties in the use of assays. There may be compounds present which interfere with the development of absorbance in colorimetric assays, and high backgrounds often cause problems with those assays which require changes in far UV wavelengths to be accurately measured. Analytically, there are three distinct concepts to be considered here: accuracy, precision, and sensitivity. Accuracy reflects how close the measured value is to the 'true' value, while precision is a measure of how reproducible are the measured values. As an illustration of the precision obtainable, the use of the colorimetric assays described in later protocols in this chapter can give coefficients of variation (the standard deviation as a percentage of the mean) of less than 5% with only three replicate analyses. If higher degrees of precision are required, standard manuals of numerical analysis should be consulted for mathematical techniques of defining sample numbers and statistical confidence. Sensitivity is defined as the lower limit of detection of a method, and methods can be simply differentiated as being suitable for concentrations down to millimolar and those capable of accurately measuring micromolar concentrations—true 'trace' methods (in the sub-nanomolar range) are seldom necessary because fermentation media are nutritionally rich and even wild-type strains are already producing readily detectable amounts of a bioactive agent. In the protocols presented in this chapter the sensitivity of the procedure can be gauged by the concentrations of the working standard(s) used.

1.3 Sampling and sample monitoring

Whatever the accuracy and precision of any particular assay, quantitatively useful results depend on the samples which are analysed being fully representative of the fermentation at the times they are taken. The entire contents of shake flasks can be used to provide different sampling time points, but continuous vessels and fermenters must be sterile-sampled. A sample, once taken, will change if there are metabolically active cells present; these can be removed by centrifugation or by filtration through 0.2 μm filters. All the protocols for measuring inputs and metabolites described in Section 2 assume that the samples will have been processed to yield soluble or supernatant phases for analysis.

2. The utilization of inputs

2.1 Carbohydrates

The commonest carbon sources for a fermentation are carbohydrates (however, glucose often exerts a strong 'catabolic' repression on secondary metabolism (2)), usually supplied as disaccharides, oligosaccharides, or even polysaccharides (e.g. starch). Glucose may be introduced later as a feed to many fed-batch processes, in response to metabolic signals (such as oxygen uptake rate) so that glucose accumulation is avoided. A broad-specificity assay for soluble carbohydrate is the anthrone reaction (*Protocol 1*).

Protocol 1.   Determination of soluble carbohydrate with the anthrone reagent (3)

Equipment and reagents
- Anthrone
- Glucose standard (0.1% w/v in water)

A. *Preparation of assay reagent*

1. Cool 100 ml deionized or distilled water in a glass beaker in an ice–water mixture.
2. Cautiously add 250 ml concentrated sulfuric acid with constant stirring with beaker in the ice–water mixture.
3. When the acid/water mixture is cool, add 0.5 g anthrone and stir until dissolved (the solution is yellow-green and is stable for up to 7 days if stored in a dark glass bottle).

B. *Assay*

1. Add 0.1 ml of each sample in triplicate to 15 ml glass test tubes.
2. Prepare a blank with 0.1 ml deionized or distilled water and triplicate standards with up to 0.1 ml glucose standard (with sufficient water to make the volume up to 0.1 ml).
3. Add 5 ml of the anthrone reagent.
4. Place the tubes immediately in a boiling water-bath and leave for 10 min.
5. Remove the test tubes and place in a cold water-bath.
6. After 10 min read the absorbance at 620 nm in 3 ml glass cuvettes against the water blank as reference.

This method measures many hexoses other than glucose, oligo- and polysaccharides (and some pentoses) and the results are frequently referred to as 'total carbohydrate' (expressed as glucose equivalents). The anthrone assay (3) was originally described in 1946 and many variations have been devised (as discussed in ref. 4). It typifies many well-established assays in that the structure of the chromophore is complex and the mechanism of the reaction is not understood (5). Many other similar carbohydrate reagents are known (see ref. 3). *Protocol 2* (based on the procedure reported in ref. 6) describes the indoleacetic acid method for any carbohydrate that contains fructosyl residues (including sucrose, free fructose, and fructosyl polymers).

Protocol 2. Determination of fructosyl carbohydrates with the indoleacetic acid–HCl reagent

Reagents

- Indoleacetic acid (500 mg in 100 ml 25% v/v ethanol)
- Fructose standard (2 mM in water)
- Hydrochloric acid (37% w/v)

Method

1. Add 0.1 ml of each sample in triplicate to 15 ml glass test tubes.
2. Prepare a blank with 0.1 ml deionized or distilled water and triplicate standards with up to 0.1 ml fructose standard (with sufficient water to make the volume up to 0.1 ml).
3. Add 0.1 ml of the indoleacetic acid reagent to each tube.
4. Add 4 ml concentrated hydrochloric acid to each tube.
5. Place all the tubes immediately in a water-bath at 37 °C and incubate for 60 min.
6. Remove the tubes, cool to room temperature, and read the absorbance at 530 nm in 3 ml glass cuvettes against the water blank as reference.

Hydrolytic breakdown of oligosaccharides can liberate smaller oligosaccharides and monosaccharides without any change in the total assayable carbohydrate. Enzyme-based assays for several monosaccharides are included in *Table 1* (the manufacturers' instructions are themselves excellent protocols and also include historical details and literature citations). *Protocol 3* gives a straightforward high-performance liquid chromatography (HPLC) method for monosaccharides and small oligosaccharides. The analysis of carbohydrates by such a non-specific detector may require sample clean-up; solid-phase extraction cartridges offer a rapid method capable of using small sample volumes with high recoveries (7).

Protocol 3. Isocratic HPLC of carbohydrates with refractive index detection

Equipment and reagents

- HPLC pump and on-line-injector
- Aminopropyl HPLC column[a]
- Refractive index detector
- 70:30 acetonitrile:water

Method

1. Equilibrate the column with > 100 volumes of the acetonitrile:water mobile phase or until the refractive index detector shows a constant signal (at full range equivalent to $0.05 \times 1.0^{-3} \Delta RI$).

---

2. Inject 20 μl of each of a range of carbohydrate standards[b] to define the working elution times (the elution order is generally monosaccharides < disaccharides < trisaccharides[c]) and calibrate the refractive index detector for either peak higher (chart recorder) or peak area (integration).

3. Inject 20 μl of a sample at a suitable dilution to give a smaller detector response than the top of the linear range for the carbohydrate of interest.

4. Establish the identity of each solute peak[d] by accurate co-elution of the peak with standard (mix sample and standard before injection).

[a] Suitable columns can be purchased from all major HPLC suppliers and are generally available in 5 μm or 3 μm particle sizes for 4.6 × 250 mm columns.
[b] Common carbohydrates such as glucose, fructose, sucrose, lactose, maltose, and maltotriose can be separated (as the column ages its performance deteriorates and the mobile phase composition needs to be adjusted to 65:35 or 60:40 acetonitrile:water).
[c] Simple polyols elute before monosaccharides.
[d] The trisaccharide raffinose and tetrasaccharide stachyose are constituents of plant protein sources and are present in media prepared from them.

Table 1. Assay kits for fermentation substrates, metabolites, and enzymes

Compound(s) Directed	Absorbance wavelength	Enzymic method	Boehringer Mannheim catalogue number	Sigma catalogue number
Glucose	610	+	124036	
D-Glucose/D-fructose	340	+	139106	
D-Glucose/D-fructose/ Sucrose	340	+	716260	
D-Sorbitol/Xylitol	340	+	670057	
Glycerol	340	+	148270	
Citric acid	340	+	139076	
L-Malic acid	340	+	139068	
Ammonia	340	+	1112732	171-A
Urea	530	−		535-B
Urea	340	+	542946	66-20, 67-10
Uric acid	520	+		685-10
α-Amylase	405			577-3
Alkaline phosphatase	420			104-LS
Lipase	(titrimetric)			800-B
Acetic acid	340	+	148261	
Ethanol	340	+	176290	333-A
Gluconic acid	340	+	428191	
Succinic acid	340	+	176281	
Triglycerides	540	+		339-10

2.2 Oils

The use of oils as carbon sources avoids the repressive effects of carbohydrates. The utilization of the lipid is readily monitored by the sulfophosphovanillin assay (*Protocol 4*). The method is based on that described in ref. 8, and was until recently available as an assay kit for 'total lipid'. The assay is based on the reaction of lipids with sulfuric and phosphoric acids and vanillin to form a pink-coloured complex and it is important to establish that the correct chromophore is produced—carbohydrates can, for example, be 'charred' by the sulfuric acid to generate a dark-coloured solution which will contribute to the absorbance at the test wavelength (530 nm).

Protocol 4. Determination of total soluble lipid

Reagents
- Vanillin
- Lipid standard (10 mg/ml in hexane)
- Phosphoric acid

Method
1. Prepare the vanillin reagent: dissolve 200 mg vanillin in 5 ml ethanol, add 4 ml deionized or distilled water, and make up to 100 ml with phosphoric acid.
2. Add 0.05 ml of each sample in triplicate to 15 ml glass test tubes.
3. Prepare a blank with 0.05 ml deionized or distilled water and triplicate standards with 0–0.05 ml lipid standard (with sufficient water to make the volume up to 0.05 ml).
4. Add 2.0 ml sulfuric acid.
5. Place the tubes in a boiling water-bath for 10 min.
6. Remove the test tubes and place in cold water-bath.
7. Remove 0.1 ml from each tube to a fresh test tube.
8. Add 2.5 ml of the vanillin reagent, vortex, and incubate for 25 min at 25°C.
9. Measure the absorbance at 530 nm in glass cuvettes against the blank prepared in Step 3.

2.3 Nitrogen sources

The simplest nitrogen source is ammonia (or an ammonium salt), but ammonia is a powerful repressor of secondary metabolism and the expression of many enzymes of nitrogen metabolism (9). Urea is a good nitrogen source for organisms capable of expressing urease, however, it cannot be heat-sterilized because of its ready breakdown to ammonia; there are two urea assay kits available (*Table 1*). Pure amino acid are expensive for anything other than small-scale processes, but there are several commercial nitrogen sources that are mixtures of amino acids and peptides; these include yeast extracts, hydrolysed casein, and corn-steep liquor. Plant proteins such as soya bean protein are cheaper and slow-release nitrogen inputs, but are only partially solubilized during autoclaving the initial fermentation medium.

Protocol 5 is a small-scale method for the determination of total soluble nitrogen based on the Kjeldahl digestion. In this method any organic nitrogen compound is reduced to ammonia (trapped as ammonium sulfate) which is then measured by the Nessler reagent (see ref. 10).

Protocol 5. Determination of total organic nitrogen

Equipment and reagents

- Potassium iodide
- Gum acacia
- Ammonium sulfate
- Mercuric iodide
- Selenium dioxide
- Heating block (350°C)
- Pyrex test tubes (16 × 250 mm diam., 1.2 mm wall thickness)

A. *Preparation of Kjeldahl digestion catalyst*

1. Place 50 ml deionized or distilled water in a glass beaker in an ice–water mixture.
2. Cautiously add 50 ml concentrated sulfuric acid with constant stirring with the beaker in the ice–water mixture.
3. When the acid solvent is cool, add 0.1 g selenium dioxide and stir until dissolved (the solution is stable indefinitely).

B. *Preparation of Nessler reagent and nitrogen standard*

1. Dissolve 4 g potassium iodide and 4 g mercuric iodide in 25 ml of water.
2. Dissolve 3.5 g gum acacia in 750 ml deionized or distilled water.
3. Slowly add the solution of iodides to the gum acacia solution with constant stirring (this is the Nessler reagent).
4. Make up the volume of the Nessler reagent to 1000 ml and store in a dark-brown glass container (stable for several weeks at room temperature).
5. Prepare the nitrogen standard by dissolving 4.73 g ammonium sulfate in 100 ml deionized or distilled water, when completely dissolved make up to 1000 ml (this gives 1 g nitrogen/L).

C. *Assay*

1. Add 0.01 ml[a] of each sample in triplicate to the Pyrex tubes.

Protocol 5. *Continued*

2. Prepare a blank with 0.01 ml deionized or distilled water.
3. Add 0.25 ml of the Kjeldahl digestion catalyst.
4. Place the tubes immediately in the heating block at 350 °C.
5. After exactly 15 min remove each tube and leave to cool to room temperature.
6. Add 1.875 ml deionized or distilled water, 3 ml 2 M sodium hydroxide and 2 ml Nessler reagent.
7. Vortex and read the absorbance at 490 nm against the water blank prepared in Step 2.
8. Determine the nitrogen content by reference to a calibration line prepared from 0–0.01 ml ammonium sulfate standard (Step B5) (with water to final volume of 2 ml), 3 ml 2 M sodium hydroxide and 2 ml Nessler reagent.

[a] If the nitrogen content is < 0.1 g/L, add up to 1 ml and lyophilize the samples in the tubes before adding the catalyst.

Protocol 6 is a colorimetric method for the measurement of free and peptidic amino acids which uses the ninhydrin reagent of Moore and Stein (11); this procedure is particularly useful if a casein hydrolysate or other peptidic nitrogen source is used.

Protocol 6. Determination of free and peptidic amino groups

Equipment and reagents

- Citric acid
- Stannous chloride
- 2-Methoxyethanol
- Sodium hydroxide (13.5 M)
- L-leucine (1 mM)
- Sodium citrate

- Ninhydrin
- Propan-1-ol
- Acetic acid (glacial)
- 5-sulfosalicylic acid
- 10 ml polypropylene tubes
- 15 ml glass test tubes

A. *Precipitation of proteins*
1. Add equal volumes of chilled 4% sulfosalicyclic acid and the sample.
2. Leave overnight at 4 °C.
3. Centrifuge for 10 min at 10 000 *g*, 4 °C.

B. *Alkaline hydrolysis of peptides*
1. Add 0.9 ml 13.5 M sodium hydroxide to 0.1 ml of the sample in 10 ml polypropylene tubes.
2. Autoclave at 15 p.s.i. for 20 min.

3. Cool the tubes to room temperature.

4. Add 2.0 ml acetic acid.

C. *Preparation of ninhydrin reagent*

1. Dissolve 4.3 g citric acid and 8.7 g sodium citrate in 250 ml deionized or distilled water and adjust the pH to 5.0.

2. Dissolve 400 mg stannous chloride in the citrate solution (this requires gentle heating[a]).

3. Dissolve 1 g ninhydrin in 25 ml 2-methoxyethanol.[a]

4. Mix equal volumes of the ninhydrin and stannous chloride solutions.[b]

D. *Assay*

1. Add 0.5 ml of each sample in triplicate to 15 ml glass test tubes.

2. Prepare a blank with 0.5 ml water and triplicate standards with up to 0.5 ml 1 mM leucine (with sufficient water to bring the volume up to 0.5 ml).

3. Add 1.5 ml ninhydrin reagent.

4. Place the tubes in a boiling water-bath for 5 min.

5. Cool the tubes to room temperature.

6. Add 8 ml 1:1 propan-1-ol:water and stand at room temperature for 30 min.

7. Read the absorbance at 570 nm against the water blank prepared in Step 2.

[a] Prepare on the day of use.
[b] Prepare sufficient reagent for all the samples, standards, and blanks.

Protein hydrolysis requires more drastic conditions. HPLC is then used to give an accurate measurement of the liberated amino acids; a method using *o*-phthaldialdehyde pre-column derivatization (ref. 12) and fluorescence detection is given in *Protocol 7* (UV detection is also possible at 340 nm). Free amino acids are quantified by the same procedure but omitting the hydrolysis step. The utilization of a macromolecular protein can be followed with the Coomassie dye-binding method (ref. 13).

Protocol 7.   Determination of total amino acids in acid hydrolysates

Equipment and reagents

- *o*-Phthaldialdehyde (OPA)
- 2-Mercaptoethanol (MESH)
- Tetrahydrofuran (THF)
- Propanol-2-ol (IPA)

Protocol 7. *Continued*

- Hydrochloric acid[b]
- Binary gradient HPLC
- Internal standard (taurine)
- Potassium tetraborate
- Sodium acetate
- Methanol (bench grade)
- HPLC-grade methanol
- C8 HPLC column (ultracarb C8 (4.6 × 150 mm), Phenomenex UK Ltd)

- Amino acid standards[a]
- Fluorescence detector
- Hydrolysis tubes
- Oxygen-free nitrogen
- Dry ice
- Vacuum source
- Lyophilizing apparatus
- Eppendorf microcentrifuge tubes

A. *Acid hydrolysis of proteins and peptides*

1. Add 0.05 ml of the sample containing < 2 mM of any one amino acid to a hydrolysis tube.

2. Add 0.02 ml 10 mM internal standard (taurine), 0.43 ml deionized or distilled water, and 0.5 ml concentrated hydrochloric acid.

3. Flush the tube with oxygen-free nitrogen, freeze in dry ice–methanol mixture and seal the tubes under vacuum.

4. Place in heated oven at 105°C for 25 h.

5. Open the tubes and lyophilize to dryness.

6. Add 1 ml water and repeat Step 5.

7. Redissolve the tube contents in 1 ml water.

B. *Preparation of o-phthaldialdehyde derivatization reagent*

1. Dissolve 50 mg OPA in 1 ml HPLC-grade methanol.

2. Add 0.04 ml MESH.

3. Add 10 ml 0.2 mM potassium tetraborate (pH 9.5)—the reagent is fairly stable when stored in a dark glass bottle at 4°C.

C. *Gradient HPLC*

1. Prepare Solvent A: 25 mM sodium acetate (pH 5.7), 4.5% THF (v/v), and 3% IPA (v/v).

2. Prepare Solvent B: HPLC-grade methanol, 1.5% THF (v/v), and 1.5% IPA (v/v).

3. Condition the column with > 20 volumes of Solvent B and then run a gradient over 10 min to 90% Solvent A and wash with > 20 column volumes 90% Solvent A.

4. Programme the gradient profile as: 0–1 min 90–85% A, 1–25 min 85–65% A, 25–26 min 65–40% A, 26–40 min 40–30% A (reset to initial conditions over 5 min and re-equilibrate column over 10 min); flow rate 1 ml/min.

D. *Assay*

1. Add 0.02 ml of the sample to 0.02 ml OPA reagent in an Eppendorf microcentrifuge tube; leave at room temperature for exactly 60 sec.

2. Inject 0.02 ml of the reaction mixture into the HPLC column via the sample injection vial and immediately start the gradient.

3. Monitor the elution of OPA derivatives with a fluorescence detector (excitation wavelength 230 nm, emission wavelength 455 nm) at a sensitivity setting giving 50% full-scale deflection with 0.1 mM L-valine.

4. Measure the amino acid content of the sample by reference to an external standard mixture (0.1 mM amino acids[a]).

5. Correct the values for the recovery of the internal standard (taurine concentration should be 0.2 mM in the final injected sample).

[a] Aspartate, glutamate, serine, histidine, glycine, threonine, arginine, alanine, taurine, tyrosine, methionine, valine, phenylalanine, isoleucine, leucine, lysine (L-forms where appropriate).
[b] Aristar grade or better.

2.4 Phosphate and other inorganic anions

Phosphate is essential for cell growth and can have important effects on secondary metabolism; the phosphate level regulates the expression of the synthesis of several types of antibiotics (14). Inorganic salts are the usual supply of phosphate, but phytic acid (inositol hexaphosphate) is an additional and labile source present (together with inorganic phosphate) in corn-steep liquor and many plant proteins. *Protocol 8* describes the rapid and very sensitive Malachite Green technique for assaying inorganic phosphate (15).

Protocol 8.   Determination of inorganic phosphate with Malachite Green

Equipment and reagents

- Malachite Green hydrochloride
- Citric acid (34% w/v)
- Ammonium molybdate
- Potassium dihydrogen phosphate
- 5 ml polycarbonate test tubes

A. *Preparation of Malachite Green reagent*

1. Dissolve 2.1 g ammonium molybdate in 250 ml 5 M HCl.

2. Dissolve 450 mg Malachite Green in 1000 ml deionized or distilled water.[a]

3. Prepare a mixture of the Malachite Green and ammonium molybdate solutions (3:1, v/v); leave at room temperature for 30 min.

Protocol 8. *Continued*

B. *Assay*

1. Add 0.05 ml of the sample[b] to a 5 ml polycarbonate test tube.

2. Prepare a blank with 0.05 ml deionized or distilled water and triplicate standards with up to 0.05 ml 0.2 mM phosphate (with sufficient water to bring the volume up to 0.05 ml).

3. Add 0.85 ml Malachite Green reagent; mix by vortexing.

4. After 60 sec add 0.1 ml citric acid solution and mix by vortexing.

5. Read the absorbance at 645 nm against a water blank prepared in Step 2.

---

[a] Stable indefinitely in a dark-brown glass container, at room temperature.
[b] Containing < 10 nmole inorganic phosphate.

Protocol 9 describes a method for the determination of the total (free plus acid-releasable) phosphate (16). This procedure measures inorganic and organic phosphate esters; it can be applied to culture supernatants and to whole samples of fermentation broths to include any phosphate in biomass or precipitated complexes.

Protocol 9. Determination of total soluble phosphate

Equipment and reagents

- Amidol (2,4-diaminophenol HCl)
- Hydrogen peroxide (30%, w/v)
- Sodium metabisulfite
- Ammonium molybdate
- Pyrex test tubes
- Heating block

A. *Acid hydrolysis of organic phosphate esters*

1. Add 0.1 ml of the sample and 0.1 ml concentrated sulfuric acid to a Pyrex tube.

2. Place in heating block at 180°C and leave for 60 min.

3. Cool the tube to room temperature.

4. Add 0.5 ml hydrogen peroxide and continue the digestion for 30 min (if the sample is still coloured add a further 0.5 ml hydrogen peroxide and repeat the digestion step for 30 min).

B. *Preparation of ammonium molybdate and amidol reagents*

1. Dissolve 8.3 g ammonium molybdate in 100 ml deionized or distilled water with gentle heating.

2. Stir 1 g amidol vigorously into 100 ml 20% (w/v) sodium metabisulfite and filter through Whatman Number 1 paper.[a]

C. *Assay*

1. Add 4.2 ml water and 0.2 ml ammonium molybdate solution to each sample digestion tube and mix by vortexing.

2. Prepare a blank with 4.3 ml water and triplicate standards with up to 0.1 ml 10 mM phosphate (with sufficient water to bring the volume up to 0.1 ml).

3. Add 0.4 ml of the amidol reagent and leave at room temperature for 30 min.

4. Read the absorbance at 620 nm against the water blank prepared in Step 2.

[a] Prepare on the day of use.

Ion chromatography (IC) methods are very powerful techniques for accurately measuring low levels of phosphate and other inorganic ions. *Protocol 10* gives a method for assaying chloride, nitrate, phosphate, and sulfate, each of which can be determined in the same chromatographic run.

Protocol 10. Ion chromatography of chloride, nitrate, phosphate, and sulfate

Equipment and reagents

- Sodium gluconate
- Sodium tetraborate decahydrate
- Butan-1-ol
- Sodium chloride
- Potassium dihydrogen phosphate
- Conductivity detector

- Boric acid
- Glycerol
- Acetonitrile
- Sodium nitrate
- Sodium sulfate
- Waters IC-Pak[TM] [a]

A. *Preparation of mobile phase and standard solution*

1. Prepare the borate/gluconate concentrate: 16 g sodium gluconate, 18 g boric acid, 25 g sodium tetraborate, and 250 ml glycerol to 1000 ml with deionized water.

2. Prepare the working mobile phase: 20 ml concentrate (Step 1), 20 ml butan-1-ol, and 120 ml acetonitrile to 1000 ml with deionized water.

3. Prepare the anion standard concentrate 0.329 g sodium chloride, 0.548 g sodium nitrate, 0.854 g potassium dihydrogen phosphate, and 0.592 g sodium sulfate to 100 ml with deionized water.

4. Prepare the working standard solution: dilute the anion standard concentrate (Step 3) 1:10 with deionized water—this gives 200 p.p.m. (5.63 mM) chloride, 400 p.p.m. (6.45 mM) nitrate, 600 p.p.m. (6.25 mM) phosphate, and 400 p.p.m. (4.17 mM) sulfate.

Protocol 10. *Continued*

B. *Assay*

1. Set the conductivity detector to 0.01 μS sensitivity range.
2. Equilibrate the column with the mobile phase until a stable baseline is achieved (flow rate 1.2 ml/min, 40°C[b]).
3. Inject 0.02 ml of the sample (with any necessary dilution to give anions at concentrations less than those in the working standard solution).

[a] From Waters Ltd with pre-column anion Guard-Pak™ inserts and holder.
[b] Thermostatted column gives improved reproducibility and baseline stability.

3. The accumulation of fermentation metabolites

3.1 Product and side-products

Any serious study of a fermentation process requires a method for the quantitation of the product of primary interest. Chemical and/or biological assays are usually available but an HPLC method is particularly desirable if a family of products is generated (antibiotic fermentations are good examples of this—see ref. 17). Liquid chromatographic methods can be immediately developed for the isolation of putative side-products or metabolites of the product; in HPLC, for example, analytical scale separation can be readily scaled-up to preparative-size columns and, if volatile mobile phases are available, isolation of the unknown solutes is straightforward by subsequent lyophilization. This general approach is applicable to unknowns appearing in most of the HPLC protocols described in this chapter.

The genetic engineering of highly productive strains has as its goal the accumulation of the maximum amount of the desired product; this product is usually the end-product of a long biochemical pathway. Depending on how many genes have been manipulated, the accumulation of biosynthetic precursors may occur. The relatively short pathway which leads to the formation of chorismic acid (and thence the aromatic amino acids phenylalanine and tyrosine and, from these, a vast range of secondary products) illustrates the value of HPLC methods in defining the accumulation patterns of intermediates. The pre-chorismate pathway contains five alicyclic compounds, all of which are acidic but some of which are phosphorylated; a combination of three column chemistries (ion-modified partition, reverse phase, and anion exchange) was devised to measure the accumulation of the intermediates in culture filtrates of genetically manipulated *Aerobacter* strains (see ref. 18).

3.2 Products of carbohydrate metabolism

The metabolism of carbohydrates produces other carbohydrates, polyols (polyhydric alcohols), and carboxylic acids. Sugar hydrolysis and interconversion products can be detected by the methods outlined in Section 2.1. Modern developments in HPLC for carbohydrates have focused on anion-exchange methods and electrochemical detection for greatly increased separation efficiencies and low limits of detection (19). Enzyme-based assays for some polyols are available (*Table 1*) but HPLC offers much better possibilities for identification and measurement (*Protocol 11*).

Protocol 11. HPLC of sugar alcohols (polyols)

Equipment and standards

- Polyol standards[a]
- Refractive index detector
- 0.22 μm filters
- Column heater
- Sugar alcohol column (Phenomenex UK Ltd)

Method

1. Set the refractive index detector to 0.1×10^{-3} ΔRI range.
2. Equilibrate the column with water until a stable baseline is achieved (flow rate 1.0 ml/min, 60°C[b]).
3. Filter the fermentation supernatant samples through a 0.22 μm filter.
4. Inject 0.05 ml of the sample (with any necessary dilution to contain polyols at concentrations less than those in the standard solutions).
5. Determine the polyol concentration by reference to calibration lines of concentration against peak area or peak height.

[a] 5 g/L glycerol, erythritol, ribitol, mannitol, sorbitol, dulcitol.
[b] Thermostatting the column at an elevated temperature gives greatly improved column efficiencies.

Two classes of acidic metabolites are frequently encountered: sugar acids and carboxylic acids related to glycolysis and the Krebs cycle. As with polyols, diagnostic kits for some acids are commercially available (*Table 1*), but with HPLC methods many different acidic metabolites can be determined in parallel (*Protocol 12*).

Protocol 12. HPLC of carboxylic acids

Equipment and standards

- Acid standards[a]
- Aminex 87H column (Bio-Rad)
- 22 μm filters
- UV detector
- Column heater
- Fast Acid Analysis column (Bio-Rad)

A. *Assay for common aliphatic acids*

1. Set the UV detector to 210 nm (range 0.32 AUFS).

Protocol 11. *Continued*

2. Equilibrate the Aminex 87H column with 0.01 M sulfuric acid until a stable baseline is achieved (1.0 ml/min, 40°C^b).

3. Filter the fermentation supernatant samples through a 0.22 μm filter.

4. Inject 0.05 ml of the sample (with any necessary dilution to contain acids at concentrations less than those in standard solutions).

5. Determine the acid concentration by reference to calibration lines of concentration against peak area or peak height.

B. *Assay for aromatic and heterocyclic acids*

1. Set the UV detector to 254 nm (range 0.32 AUFS)

2. Equilibrate the Fast Acid Analysis column with 0.02 M sulfuric acid until a stable baseline is achieved (1.0 ml/min, 40°C^b).

3. Filter the fermentation supernatant samples through a 0.22 μm filter and inject the samples as in Step A4 above.

---

^{a} 20 mM glucuronic, gluconic, malic, lactic, and succinic acids, 10 mM citric acid, 50 mM acetic acid, 1 mM 4-hydroxymandelic, 3,4-dihydroxyphenylacetic, and 4-hydroxyphenylbenzoic acids, 0.5 mM fumaric acid.
^{b} Thermostatting the column at 40°C gives improved column efficiencies.

3.3 Amino compounds

There are three classes of amine metabolites: non-protein amino acids, aliphatic amines, and 'secondary' amino products (sugar amines, etc.). All three classes are best detected and measured by amino-acid HPLC. The method given in *Protocol 7* deliberately uses a gradient which allows 'gaps' in the elution order for the appearance of metabolites such as β-alanine, γ-aminobutyric acid, ornithine, sugar amines, and phosphoethanolamine. The *o*-phthaldialdehyde (OPA) reagent only reacts with primary amines and amino compounds (such as the amino acid proline) which contain secondary amino groups and can be derivatized with 9-fluorenylmethylchloroformate (20) after the primary amines have been reacted with OPA (21).

3.4 Ammonia

Free ammonia (as ammonium at the pH values found in most fermentations) is generated by the deamination of amino acids and by urea hydrolysis. Gaseous ammonia or ammonium hydroxide solution is also fed to medium- and large-scale fermentation processes either as a nitrogen source or for pH control. Enzymic methods can measure millimolar concentrations (or less) of ammonia (*Table 1*), but the UV blanks can be troublesomely high and unstable and protease activity in culture supernatants may interfere. Colorimetric assays (such as the Nessler reaction described in *Protocol 5*) can be useful but suffer from precipitation and side-reactions in complex fermentation media and should be used with care. Ion chromatography at low pH readily detects the ammonium cation (*Protocol 13*); this method also has the advantage of resolving potassium and sodium which are important macronutrients for microbial fermentations.

Protocol 13. Ion chromatography of sodium, ammonium, and potassium

Equipment and reagents

- Nitric acid
- Potassium chloride
- Conductivity detector
- Sodium chloride
- Ammonium chloride
- Shodex IC Y-521[a]

A. *Preparation of the mobile phase and standard solution*

1. Prepare the mobile phase: 4 mM nitric acid (0.507 ml concentrated nitric acid (70% v/v) to 2000 ml with deionized water).

2. Prepare the cation standard concentrate: 0.254 g sodium chloride, 0.297 g ammonium chloride, and 0.382 g potassium chloride to 100 ml with deionized water.

3. Prepare a working standard solution: dilute the cation standard concentrate (Step 2) 1:20 with deionized water—this gives 5 p.p.m. (0.217 mM) sodium, 5 p.p.m. (0.278 mM) ammonium, and 10 p.p.m. (0.206 mM) potassium.

B. *Assay*

1. Set the conductivity detector to 0.01 μS sensitivity range.

2. Equilibrate the column with the mobile phase until a stable baseline is achieved (flow rate 1.0 ml/min, 40 °C[b]).

3. Inject 0.05 ml of the sample (with any necessary dilution to contain cations at concentrations less than those in working standard solution).

[a] From Phenomenex UK Ltd. with guard column IC Y-521P.
[b] Thermostatted column gives improved reproducibility and baseline stability.

3.5 Peptides, proteins, and enzymes

The utilization of plant protein nitrogen sources is often incomplete and this results in the accumulation of soluble peptides (see *Protocol 6*). The microbial biomass may, however, synthesize and export proteins, and cell lysis during the fermentation (especially in the later stages) will also liberate soluble protein. With a medium containing protein inputs the kinetics of the disappearance and reappearance of protein can therefore be complex. The use of protein assays gives the overall pattern of change, but differentiating between unused inputs and biomass-derived protein requires more discriminatory methods. Gel electrophoresis in the presence of sodium dodecyl sulfate (22) is very suitable for this purpose as plant seed proteins generally give diffuse bands of subunit molecular weight < 30000, whereas biomass-derived proteins give a 'ladder' of stainable bands with a broad range of molecular weights.

Enzymes of industrial significance (such as lipases, proteases, and amyloglucosidases) are invariably produced by fermentation processes. A more general phenomenon in microbial fermentations is the synthesis of extracellular proteases if a protein nitrogen source is used. In these situations the biomass will produce a spectrum of endo- and exopeptidases. The release of dyes from collagen is a rapid and sensitive means of assaying endopeptidases (*Protocol 14*—modified from the method described in ref. 23) but is difficult to relate to absolute enzyme units; the rate of dye release also varies with the batch of Azocoll used.

Protocol 14. Determination of soluble protease with the Azocoll dye-release method

Equipment and reagents
- Azocoll (Sigma)
- 50 mM Tris-HCl buffer pH 7.2
- 0.22 μm filters
- Eppendorf microcentrifuge tubes

Method

1. Prepare the substrate by suspending 0.1 g Azocoll in 20 ml Tris buffer and stirring for 60 min at room temperature.

2. Centrifuge at 5000 *g* for 5 min and resuspend Azocoll in 20 ml Tris buffer.

3. Add 0.1 ml of the filtered (0.22 μm) supernatant sample to an Eppendorf microcentrifuge tube.

4. Add 1.4 ml of the substrate.

5. Prepare the substrate blank by mixing 1.4 ml substrate with 0.1 ml deionized or distilled water.

6. Prepare the sample blank by mixing 1.4 ml of deionized or distilled water with 0.1 ml sample.

7. Incubate the tubes at 30°C for 60 min.

8. Centrifuge the tubes at 5000 *g* for 3 min.

9. Measure the absorbance of the assay supernatant at 520 nm against a blank of 1.4 ml Tris buffer and 0.1 ml deionized or distilled water.

10. Correct the assay absorbance for any absorbance in the blanks (Steps 4 and 5).

Model low molecular weight substrates provide a reliable assay for exo- or endopeptidases; assays for leucine aminopeptidase (*Protocol 15*) and for trypsin-like endopeptidases both utilize *p*-nitroanilide esters (24, 25).

Protocol 15. Determination of leucine aminopeptidase

Reagents

- L-leucine *p*-nitroanilide
- Disodium hydrogen phosphate
- 1 M acetic acid

- Dimethysulfoxide
- *p*-Nitroaniline
- 0.2 M phosphate buffer pH 7.0

Method

1. Prepare the substrate by dissolving 25 mg leucine *p*-nitroanilide in 1 ml dimethylsufoxide and diluting to 50 ml with 0.2 M phosphate buffer.

2. Add 0.1 ml of the sample to 2.9 ml substrate solution.

3. Prepare the substrate blank by mixing 2.9 ml substrate with 0.1 ml deionized or distilled water.

4. Prepare the sample blank by mixing 2.9 ml phosphate buffer with 0.1 ml sample.

5. Incubate the assays at 30°C for 60 min.[a]

6. Terminate the reaction by adding 1 ml 1 M acetic acid.

7. Measure the absorbance at 410 nm against deionized or distilled water.[b]

8. Correct the assay absorbance for any absorbance in the blanks (Steps 3 and 4) also treated with 1 ml 1 M acetic acid.

9. Determine the *p*-nitroaniline liberated by reference to a calibration line of absorbance at 410 nm against *p*-nitroaniline dissolved in 3 ml phosphate buffer and 1 ml 1 M acetic acid.

[a] The time of incubation should be adjusted to maintain a linear rate of increase of liberated *p*-nitroaniline with time; initial screening for enzyme levels can be performed with a 60 min assay time.
[b] If any precipitate forms, remove this by centrifugation (5000 *g*).

Assay kits are commercially available for lipase, amylase, and alkaline phosphatase (*Table 1*).

3.6 Thiol compounds

Mono- and dibromobimane reagents react rapidly with thiol groups to yield highly fluorescent derivatives (26). These derivatives, with a range of biological thiols, can be resolved by reverse-phase HPLC (*Protocol 16*).

Protocol 16. HPLC of thiols as fluorescent derivatives

Equipment and reagents

- Thiol standards[a]
- Methanol[c]
- Acetonitrile[c]
- Ammonium bicarbonate
- C18 reverse-phase column[b]
- Acetic acid[c]

- Monobromobimane (Thiolyte™ from Cal-biochem, cat. no. 596105)
- Fluorescence detector
- 0.22 μm filters
- Eppendorf microcentrifuge tubes

Method

1. Prepare the derivatization reagent: dissolve 25 mg monobromobimane in 1 ml acetonitrile and mix 0.01 ml with 0.45 ml 10 mM ammonium bicarbonate (prepare fresh working reagent each day).

2. Equilibrate the column with 10% methanol/0.25% acetic acid at 1 ml/min until a stable baseline is achieved (excitation wavelength 375 nm, emission wavelength 480 nm.

3. Filter the fermentation supernatant samples through a 0.22 μm filter.

4. Mix 0.02 ml of the sample with 0.02 ml of the derivatization reagent in an Eppendorf microcentrifuge tube, cap the tube, and leave at room temperature for 3 min.

5. Inject 0.02 ml of the reaction mixture.

6. Determine the thiol concentration by reference to calibration lines of concentration against peak area or peak height.

[a] Cysteine, homocysteine, *N*-acetylcysteine, and glutathione (1 mM).
[b] Any standard 4.6 × 250 mm C18 analytical column will give satisfactory separations.
[c] HPLC grade solvents.

Thiols seldom accumulate, as such, in fermentations because they readily oxidize in aerobic environments (such as in a well-aerated fermenter). Reduction of disulfide bonds will regenerate the reactive thiols and can be accomplished by incubating in the presence of excess dithiothreitol (26).

3.7 Other common metabolites

Thousands of metabolites are potentially accumulated in a fermentation process but a major limiting factor is chemical stability. Amino acid catabolism results in the formation of short-chain fatty acids, phenylpropanoids, and some dicarboxylic acids such as fumaric acid (produced by the action of ammonia lyase on aspartate); all these acids are readily determined by organic acid HPLC (*Protocol 12*). The major technical difficulty in organic acid HPLC is that a range of other metabolites which are not acidic can elute close to common carboxylic acids, including some surprising compounds such as uridine, uracil, thymidine, and thymine. Small amounts of such hetero-cyclic compounds (at < 1 mM) give chromatographic peaks as large as tens or hundreds millimolar levels of simple carboxylic acids because of the differences in the absorbance coefficients in the far UV. Pyrimidines and their ribosides are frequently accumulated in complex media fermentations and can also be found in the batched media after heat-sterilization. Purine metabolites such as uric acid and urea can also be encountered (for assay kits see *Table 1*).

3.8 Carbon dioxide

Carbon dioxide is probably the major carbon output of all aerobic fermentations. Several CO_2 analysers are commercially available based on IR detection; on the industrial scale, mass spectrometry is the usual method (see Chapter 6).

3.9 Pigments

Secondary metabolite fermentations are frequently highly coloured, but it is only in comparatively few cases that the structure of the soluble pigment is known (for example, the polyketide-derived pigment actinorhodin synthesized by *Streptomyces coelicolor*, ref. 27). A comment frequently found in the literature is that 'melanoid' pigments are produced. True melanin is the polymeric insoluble black pigment produced by the action of tyrosinase (polyphenoloxidase) on tyrosine (28). It is likely that melanins are rarely formed in microbial fermentations, but water-soluble polymeric pigments of undefined structure are commonly accumulated (29). Another source of pigments is the reaction of carbohydrates and amino compounds during the heat-sterilization of media; this is known as the Maillard reaction and can produce a wide spectrum of heterocyclic compounds and polymers (30).

4. The insoluble phase (biomass and pelletable material)

4.1 Biomass measurements in complex media

In defined media growth is readily measured using the turbidity of the culture (see Chapter 5). When particulate material is present, however, these methods are at best approximate. An absolute measure of growth (cell increase) is by determination of the DNA content of the broth, but in complex media chemical fractionation of the pelletable material is necessary before such measurements can be undertaken. The procedure given in *Protocol 17* (derived from the methods described in refs 31 and 32) produces four fractions defined by their solubility in perchloric acid (PCA) or alkali: cold PCA fraction (metabolite pool), hot PCA fraction (nucleic acids), alkali fractions (protein and lipid), and residue fraction (cell wall polymers).

However, as stressed in Chapter 5 (*Protocol 2*) PCA is a very hazardous chemical and must be treated with respect.

Protocol 17. Chemical fractionation of biomass and pellets from complex-media fermentations

Equipment and reagents
- Perchloric acid (PCA)[a]
- Ultrasonic disintegrator (7534A Soniprobe model 250, Branson Ultrasonics)
- Sodium hydroxide
- Refrigerated centrifuge

Method

1. Centrifuge the fermentation broth sample (10 000 *g*, 30 min, 4°C).

2. Separate the supernatant and pellet.

3. Add 20 ml cold 0.2 M PCA to 1 g wet weight of the pellet and re-suspend using a glass rod; incubate at 4°C for 16 h.

4. Centrifuge (10 000 *g*, 30 min, 4°C) to yield the cold PCA-soluble fraction and the second pellet.

5. Add 20 ml 0.5 M PCA to the second pellet and resuspend using a glass rod; incubate at 70°C for 2 h.

6. Centrifuge (10 000 *g*, 30 min, 20°C) to yield the hot PCA-soluble fraction and the third pellet.

7. Add 20 ml 0.5 M sodium hydroxide to the third pellet and resuspend using a glass rod; incubate at 37°C for 16 h.

8. Centrifuge (10 000 *g*, 30 min, 20°C) to yield the alkali-soluble fraction and the fourth pellet.

9. Add 20 ml water to the fourth pellet and resuspend by ultrasonication (residual fraction).

[a] High-purity PCA is necessary (such as 'Special for spectroscopy' grades).

The composition of each of these fractions is, however, complex (33, 34). The cold PCA-soluble material will also contain any simple polysaccharides such as glycogen while the hot PCA treatment solubilizes plant cell wall polysaccharides present in protein sources as well as some biomass cell wall components. The alkali fraction is predominately cellular protein, unused input protein, and cell lipids, but it may also be highly pigmented; these insoluble pigments include any genuine melanin present and insoluble pigments generated as artefacts of medium heat-sterilization (see Section 3.9). The residual material contains varying amounts of amino acid-containing polymers such as peptidoglycan. All these fractions can be further chemically analysed and this is discussed below (Section 4.2).

4.1.1 DNA

The hot PCA fraction contains hydrolysed DNA and RNA. The 2-deoxyribose degradation product of DNA can be measured by the very selective Burton diphenylamine reagent (*Protocol 20*—from ref. 35).

Protocol 18. Measurement of DNA using the Burton reagent

Reagents

- Perchloric acid (PCA)[a]
- Diphenylamine
- Salmon sperm DNA
- Glacial acetic acid
- Paraldehyde

Method

1. Prepare the Burton reagent: dissolve 4 g diphenylamine in 100 ml acetic acid and add 0.01 ml paraldehyde (stable for a week in a brown glass container).

2. Prepare the standard DNA by incubating 20 mg in 100 ml 0.5 M PCA at 70°C for 1 h this gives a nominal standard of 0.2 mg/ml—check the actual concentration by measuring absorbance at 260 nm (*A* 260 nm for a 1 mg/ml solution is 20).

3. Add 2 ml of the Burton reagent to 15 ml glass test tubes and then add 1 ml of the sample in 0.5 M PCA (hot PCA fraction from *Protocol 20*); mix the contents of each tube immediately by vortexing.[b]

4. Prepare a blank with 1 ml 0.5 M PCA and 2 ml of the Burton reagent and triplicate standards (0.02–0.2 mg/ml).

5. Incubate at room temperature for 16–24 h.

6. Measure the absorbance at 600 nm against the assay blank.[c]

7. Determine the DNA content of the sample by reference to a calibration line.

[a] High-purity PCA is necessary (such as 'Special for spectroscopy' grades).
[b] Excessive sample or more dilute PCA will cause the diphenylamine to precipitate.
[c] If the sample is coloured, a sample blank can be prepared by incubating 1 ml of the sample with 2 ml acetic acid and subtracting the absorbance from the assay value.

4.1.2 RNA

RNA can be quantified by the reaction of the liberated ribose with the orcinol reagent (*Protocol 19*—from ref. 36). This procedure greatly overestimates the RNA content if pentose-containing polysaccharides (from plant protein sources) are also present. In this case, the best approach is to measure the total nucleic acid from the absorbance at 260 nm (ref. 37) using an absorbance coefficient of 24.0 for a 1 mg/L solution of RNA (33). The DNA content is usually small in comparison with that of RNA, and the measured RNA content can be corrected for the DNA present determined by the Burton assay of *Protocol 18*.

The base composition of nucleic acids can be determined by a variety of methods and these are discussed in ref. 38.

Protocol 19. Measurement of RNA using the orcinol reagent

Reagents
- Perchloric acid (PCA)
- Orcinol
- Ferric chloride
- RNA

Method

1. Prepare the orcinol reagent by dissolving 20 g orcinol (3,5-dihydroxy-toluene) in 100 ml ethanol (stable for several weeks in the refrigerator).

2. Prepare the standard RNA by dissolving 10 mg in 100 ml 0.5 M sodium hydroxide; this gives a nominal standard of 0.1 mg/ml—check the actual concentration by measuring absorbance at 260 nm (*A* 260 nm for a 1 mg/ml solution is 24).

3. Add 0.3 ml sample in 0.5 M PCA (hot PCA fraction from *Protocol 20*) to 2.7 ml 0.5 M PCA in a 15 ml glass test tube.

4. Add 3.0 ml 0.03% (w/v) ferric chloride and 0.2 ml of the orcinol reagent; mix by vortexing.

5. Prepare a blank with 3 ml 0.5 M PCA replacing the sample, and triplicate standards (0.01–0.1 mg/ml RNA).

6. Place all tubes in a boiling water-bath for 15 min.

7. Cool the tubes to room temperature and measure the absorbance at 665 nm against the assay blank.

8. Determine the RNA content of the sample by reference to a calibration line.

4.2 Biomass (pellet) composition

4.2.1 Cold PCA fraction

This fraction will inevitably be contaminated with the soluble components present in the fermentation broth, but the better the pellet is washed the less this contamination will be. The pelletable material which is cold PCA-soluble is predominately: free amino acid and peptides, mono- and oligosaccharides, nucleotides, and carboxylic acids. The cellular pools of low molecular weight metabolites are much greater in prokaryotic and eukaryotic organisms exhibiting secondary metabolism than in laboratory enteric bacteria such as

Escherichia coli (fermentation products and their biosynthetic precursors are also frequently detectable in the low molecular weight metabolite pool).

4.2.2 Hot PCA fraction

The majority of the material is usually carbohydrate and can be quantified by HPLC (*Protocol 3*). Any small amounts of amino acid-containing material can be acid-hydrolysed and the amino acids determined (*Protocol 7*).

4.2.3 Alkali fraction

The protein solubilized by alkali is acid-hydrolysed and the amino acids determined according to *Protocol 7*. Insoluble melanoid pigments, if present, can be estimated by absorbance at 420 nm or 500 nm by reference to a synthetic melanin dissolved in 0.5 M NaOH—during storage these pigments tend to decolorize and the measurement should be performed as soon as the fraction is prepared. Total lipid can be determined by *Protocol 4*. The composition of the biomass lipid is analysed in chloroform:methanol extracts of the pellet by thin-layer chromatography (TLC) (39).

4.2.4 Residue fraction

The carbohydrate material is estimated by the anthrone reagent (*Protocol 1*) and the amino acids by *Protocol 7* after acid hydrolysis.

4.3 Biomass compositions and elemental analyses

Complete analysis of the full biomass composition of a microbial cell is very time-consuming and has been attempted very rarely. The classic description of *E. coli* growing exponentially on glucose (described in ref. 40) shows that > 90% of the cell weight can be accounted for as protein, nucleic acid, lipids, and cell wall polymers. A study of *Streptomyces coelicolor* concluded that at least 83% of the cell weight could be similarly assessed (41). The exact cellular composition will, however, change in response to the nature of the growth medium and growth conditions; in organisms (such as *Streptomycetes*) with developmental cycles and which show morphological changes during a fermentation (42), the cell contents are also likely to be highly variable.

Microbial cells can, under appropriate conditions, accumulate large amounts of polymeric 'storage' products; these can be carbohydrate (glycogen), poly-carboxylic acids (polyhydroxybutyric acid), or inorganic (polyphosphate). Methods for the extraction and measurement of these products (and cell wall polymers such as teichoic acids) are discussed in refs. 33 and 34.

5. Carbon and nitrogen mass balances

Elemental balances in fermentations are of two kinds. In a study of the accountability of the soluble material, the partitioning of the soluble material into the various defined classes of materials is estimated at important stages of the process. The data required are (for carbon and nitrogen): supernatant phase carbon and nitrogen, the concentrations of products and any side-products, the concentrations of metabolites such as organic acids, the amounts of any unused carbohydrate or oil inputs, and the total amino acids (in acid hydrolysates). The sum of the products, metabolites, and unused inputs will fall short of the total measured because of the contribution of inorganic carbon and nitrogen. Soluble inorganic carbon comprises dissolved carbon dioxide (mostly present as bicarbonates and carbonates); this can be readily measured as the carbon dioxide driven off by acidification and moderate heat and can be routinely measured by Total Organic Carbon analysers. Inorganic nitrogen (other than ammonia) is mostly any nitrate present and this can be measured by ion chromatography (see *Protocol 10*); an alternative is to determine the total organic nitrogen directly by the digestion method given in *Protocol 5*.

Once inorganic carbon and nitrogen have been determined, the difference between the total carbon and nitrogen and that accounted for in known compounds represents 'unknowns' which can be unrecognized products or undefined metabolites; the systematic approach requires the application of an increasingly wider range of methods if the carbon and nitrogen balances are to made progressively more complete. Each individual organism presents idiosyncratic problems for fermentation analysis, but there are several useful rules which are of wider application:

(a) Secondary product-forming microorganisms frequently elaborate more than one antibiotic in the wild-type strain.

(b) Soluble pigmentation can be quantitatively important.

(c) Volatile products may be lost in the effluent gas.

(d) The production of acids and bases should be detectable by their effects on the pH.

(e) Whatever is in an aqueous supernatant is by definition water-soluble (or in colloidal solution) and this imposes quite marked limitations on the likely spectrum of accumulated materials.

(f) Accumulated side-products and metabolites may be unstable under the pH and temperature conditions in the fermentation.

Full carbon and nitrogen mass balances require, in addition to the data discussed above, sufficient information to define the full progress of the fermentation: calculated or measured inputs, evolved carbon dioxide, evolved ammonia, the volume or weight changes during the fermentation, and estimates of the loss of water by evaporation. When complex inputs are being used, the manufacturer's data can be used as a basis for calculation (but the figures are seldom exact measurements on any batch and usually represent averages about which a tolerated range of variation may or may not be specified). Evolved carbon dioxide requires gas analysis (see Section 3.8), but any evolved ammonia can be trapped in a 1 M sulfuric acid bottle connected to the exhaust gas port and analysed by a suitable colorimetric method (for example the Nessler reagent in *Protocol 5*). Laboratory-scale fermenters or bioreactors may give a continuous read-out of volume or weight; otherwise the final volume or weight must be determined at the end of the fermentation and corrected for any sample volumes taken during the course of the experiment. These data can then be used to estimate evaporative losses

References

1. Chater, K. F. (1990). *Bio/Technology*, **8**, 115.
2. Demain, A. L. (1988). In *Regulation of secondary metabolism in Actinomycetes* (ed. S. Shapiro), pp. 127–34. CRC Press, FL.
3. Shields, R. and Burnett, W. (1960). *Anal. Chem.*, **32**, 885.
4. Snell, F. D. and Snell, C. T. (1953). *Colorimetric methods of analysis*, Vol. III, pp. 195–250. D. Van Nostrand Company, NY.
5. Momose, T., Ueda, Y., Sawada, K., and Sugi, A. (1957). *Pharm. Bull.*, **5**, 31.
6. Heyrovsky, A. (1956). *Clin. Chim. Acta*, **1**, 47.
7. Bell, R. G. and Newman, K. L. (1993). *J. Chromatogr.*, **632**, 87.
8. Zöllner, N. and Kirsch, K. (1962). *Z. ges. exp. Med.*, **135**, 545.
9. Shapiro, S. (1988). In *Regulation of secondary metabolism in Actinomycetes* (ed. S Shapiro), pp. 135–211. CRC Press, FL.
10. Paul, J. (1958). *Analyst*, **83**, 37.
11. Moore, S. and Stein, W. T. (1948). *J. Biol. Chem.*, **176**, 367.
12. Simmons, S. S. S. and Johnson, D. F. (1976). *J. Am. Chem. Soc.*, **98**, 7098.
13. Bradford, M. M. (1976). *Anal. Biochem.*, **72**, 248.
14. Aharonowitz, Y. and Demain, A. L. (1977). *Arch. Microbiol.*, **115**, 169.
15. Lanzetta, P. A., Alvarez, L. J., Remack, P. S., and Candia, O. A. (1979). *Anal. Biochem.*, **100**, 95.
16. Chiba, Y. and Sugahara, K. (1957). *Arch. Biochem. Biophys.*, **71**, 367.
17. McGahren, W. J., Leese, R. A., Barbatschi, F., Morton, G. O., Kuck, N. A., and Ellestad, G. A. (1983). *J. Antibiotics*, **36**, 1671.
18. Mousdale, D. M. and Coggins, J. R. (1985). *J. Chromatogr.*, **329**, 268.
19. Hardy, M. R., Townsend, R. R., and Lee, Y. C. (1988). *Anal. Biochem.*, **170**, 54.
20. Einarsson, S., Josefson, B., and Langerkvist, S. (1983). *J. Chromatogr.*, **282**, 609.
21. Schuster, R. (1988). *J. Chromatogr.*, **431**, 271.
22. Laemmli, U. K. (1970). *Nature*, **227**, 680.
23. Chavira, R., Burnett, T. J., and Hagemann, J. H. (1984). *Anal. Biochem.*, **136**, 446.
24. Hara, I. and Matsubara, H. (1980). *Plant Cell Physiol.*, **21**, 233.
25. Mousdale, D. M. (1983). *Biochem Physiol. Pflanzen*, **178**, 373.
26. Fahey, R. C., Newton, G. L., Dorian, R., and Kosower, E. M. (1981). *Anal. Biochem.*, **111**, 357.
27. Gorst-Allman, C. P., Rudd, B. A. M., Chang, C., and Floss, H. G. (1981). *J. Org. Chem.*, **46**, 455.
28. Mencher, J. R. and Heim, A. H. (1962). *J. Gen. Microbiol.*, **28**, 665.
29. Shirling, E. B. and Gottlieb, D. (1976). In *Actinomycetes. The boundary microorganisms* (ed. R. Arai), pp. 9–41. Toppan Company, Tokyo.

30. Ellis, G. P. (1959). *Adv. Carbohyd. Chem.*, **14**, 63.
31. Ogur, M. and Rosen, G. (1950). *Arch. Biochem.*, **25**, 262.
32. Schneider, W. C., Hogeboom, G. H., and Ross, G. E. (1950). *J. Natl. Cancer Inst.*, **10**, 977.
33. Herbert, D., Phipps, P. J., and Strange, R. E. (1971). In *Methods in microbiology* (ed. J. R. Norris and D. W. Ribbons), Vol. 5B, p. 209. Academic Press, London and NY.
34. Sutherland, I. W. and Wilkinson, J. F. (1971). In *Methods in microbiology* (ed. J. R. Norris and D. W. Ribbons), Vol. 5B, p. 345. Academic Press, London and NY.
35. Burton, K. (1956). *Biochem J.*, **62**, 315.
36. Brown, A. H. (1946). *Arch. Biochem.*, **11**, 269.
37. Benthin, S., Nielsen, J., and Villadsen, J. (1991). *Biotech. Techn.*, **5**, 39.
38. Skidmore, W. D. and Duggan, E. L. (1971). In *Methods in microbiology* (ed. J. R. Norris and D. W. Ribbons), Vol. 5B, p. 631. Academic Press, London and NY.
39. Huston, C. K., Albro, P. W., and Grindley, G. B. (1965). *J. Bacteriol.*, **89**, 768.
40. Neidhardt, F. C. (1987). In Escherichia coli *and* Salmonella typhimurium *cellular and molecular biology* (ed. F. C. Neidhardt, J. L. Ingraham, K. B. Low, B. Magasanik, M. Schaechter, and H. E. Umbarger), pp. 3–6. ASM, Washington DC.
41. Davidson, A. O. (1992). PhD thesis, University of Glasgow.
42. Chater, K. F. and Merrick, M. K. (1979). In *Developmental biology of prokaryotes* (ed. J. H. Parish), pp. 93–114. Blackwell Scientific Publications, Oxford.

8

Analysis of microbial growth data

MICHAEL J. BAZIN, ANN P. WOOD, and
DAVID PAGET-BROWN

1. Introduction

In this chapter we describe some of the ways in which microbial growth kinetic data can be analysed. Most of our attention is focused on dynamic models containing the Monod growth function because it is this function that is most commonly employed to describe the kinetics of microbial growth. But first, in order to minimize ambiguity, we define some of the terms we employ.

1.1 Definitions

The term kinetics may be defined as 'the study of the rates at which chemical reactions and biological processes occur'; dynamics is 'that branch of applied mathematics which studies the way in which force produces motion' (1). Neither of these definitions has been widely applied in microbial physiology and neither is particularly useful for the purposes of this chapter. We will use the term 'microbial growth kinetics' in connection with the identification of kinetic functions which define the way in which microorganisms grow. These are usually (although not always) time-independent. By 'microbial population dynamics' we mean the way in which microbial population densities change with respect to time or, more rarely, some other independent variable such as distance. Both microbial kinetics and population dynamics involve the identification and application of mathematical equations. In the former case, these equations are most commonly used to describe the way the specific growth rate of a population is controlled by some aspect of the environment. Specific growth rate (μ) is the *per capita* rate of change in population density and may be expressed as:

$$\mu = \frac{\mathrm{d}X}{X\mathrm{d}t} = \frac{\mathrm{d}\mathrm{Ln}X}{\mathrm{d}t};$$

[1]

where X is some measure of population density and t is time. Microbial population dynamics usually involve differential or difference equations which describe the way in which populations change with respect to time and incorporate kinetic functions to define these changes. For example, the differential equation defining pure exponential growth is simply:

$$\frac{dX}{dt} = \mu X \qquad [2]$$

where μ is constant.

Before proceeding, it will be advantageous to clarify or define a few further points. In *Equation 2*, X is the dependent variable which changes with respect to the independent variable, t, and μ is a constant, i.e. for a fixed set of environmental conditions its value does not change. We may substitute a kinetic function for μ in order to express it in terms of some environmental variable. By far the most often quoted function of this sort is due to Monod (2) and depends on the concentration of a single, growth-limiting nutrient at concentration, S:

$$\mu = \frac{\mu_m S}{K_s + S}. \qquad [3]$$

Here μ_m and K_s, the maximum specific growth rate and saturation constants, respectively, are supposed to be constant but μ changes with S. The dynamics of the system are now described by two differential equations because a second dependent variable (S) has been introduced. Thus:

$$\frac{dX}{dt} = \frac{\mu_m S X}{K_s + S}, \text{ and} \qquad [4]$$

$$\frac{dS}{dt} = -\frac{\mu_m S X}{Y(K_s + S)}. \qquad [5]$$

These equations constitute a mass balance and as such both dependent variables should be measured in terms of mass *per* unit volume. For X, some estimate of biomass concentration such as dry weight should be obtained. In *Equation 5*, the term Y is the yield constant, the amount of biomass produced per unit of substrate consumed.

Equations 4 and *5* describe microbial growth in a closed system such as batch culture, i.e. one to which there is no continuous input and output of matter. In this system, substrate is consumed and biomass increases. Eventually, the nutrient concentration becomes exhausted ($S = 0$) and so $dX/dt = dS/dt = 0$. This condition is called equilibrium. The equilibrium concentration of biomass, X_e, may be obtained by dividing *Equation 4* by *Equation 5* to obtain:

$$\frac{dX}{dS} = -Y; \qquad [6]$$

so that

$$X = -YS + c; \qquad [7]$$

where c is a constant of integration. If we let $X = X_0$ and $S = S_0$ at $t = 0$, then:

$$c = X_0 + YS_0, \qquad [8]$$

and

$$X = -YS + X_0 + YS_0. \qquad [9]$$

As indicated above, at equilibrium, $S = S_e = 0$, so that:

$$X_e = X_0 + YS_0. \qquad [10]$$

Chemostats are thermodynamically open systems; there is a continuous input and output of matter. *Equations 4 and 5* can be modified to describe chemostat dynamics by including terms which reflect the openness of such systems. We let $D = F/V$, where F is the flow rate into and out of the chemostat vessel and V is its (fixed) volume and D is dilution rate, to obtain:

$$\frac{dX}{dt} = \frac{\mu_m SX}{K_s + S}, \; -DX, \text{ and} \qquad [11]$$

$$\frac{dS}{dt} = D(S_r - S) - \frac{\mu_m SX}{Y(K_s + S)}. \qquad [12]$$

where S_r is the concentration of substrate supplied to the system. Open systems may come to dynamic equilibrium called steady state. At steady state in a chemostat, the dependent variables take on fixed values, X_s and S_s, and the derivatives in *Equations 11 and 12* equate to zero. Thus:

$$D = \mu = \frac{\mu_m S_s}{K_s + S}, \qquad [13]$$

$$S_s = \frac{DK_s}{\mu_m - D}. \qquad [14]$$

and

$$X_s = Y(S_r - S_s). \qquad [15]$$

The terms D and S_r in *Equations 11 and 12* are parameters; that is to say their values can be set experimentally. This implied definition of the term 'parameter' differs from that used in statistics where 'parameter estimation' seeks to obtain values for terms we have called constants.

1.2 Kinetic functions

Several other kinetic functions other than that due to Monod have been suggested (3). Below we introduce and summarize some of them.

(a) The logistic equation (4):

$$\mu = \mu_m - \frac{\mu_m}{K} X. \qquad [16]$$

This function has been applied widely in ecology, including microbial ecology. The term, K, is called the carrying capacity of the environment and represents the maximum population density available under a given set of conditions. The specific growth rate does not depend on an abiotic variable but decreases linearly as the population increases.

(b) The Tessier equation:

$$\mu = \mu_m(1 - e^{-S/K_S}).$$ [17]

(c) The Moser equation:

$$\mu = \mu_m(1 + K_s S^{-\lambda})^{-1};$$ [18]

where λ is a constant. As pointed out by Bailey and Ollis (3), both the Tessier and the Moser equations render algebraic manipulation of microbial growth equations difficult.

(d) the Contois equation (5):

$$\mu = \frac{\mu_m S}{BX + S}.$$ [19]

This equation differs from that of Monod in that K_s is replaced by the product of a constant, B, and the biomass density, X. Thus as X increases, μ gets smaller. The Contois equation has been used to describe the growth of a microbial predator, at density P, feeding on its prey, at density H, when μ is a function of how much prey is available per predator (6,7), i.e.:

$$\mu = \frac{\mu_m H/P}{B + H/P} = \frac{\mu_m H}{BP + H}.$$ [20]

Similarly, algal growth under conditions of self-shading can be modelled using the Contois expression. If L is the incident light falling on an algal culture and growth is light-limited, then:

$$\mu = \frac{\mu_m L/X}{B + L/X} = \frac{\mu_m L}{BX + L}.$$ [21]

(e) Substrate inhibition (8):

$$\mu = \frac{\mu_m S}{K_i + S + S^2/K_p};$$ [22]

where K_i and K_p are constants. Specific growth rate functions of this sort are applicable to substrates such as phenol which, at low concentrations, are used as a source of carbon and are inhibitory at higher concentrations (9).

(f) Product inhibition (10,11):

$$\mu = \frac{\mu_m S K_p}{K_i + K_p S + C};$$ [23]

where C is the concentration of a product that inhibits growth.

1.3 Culture systems

We have already alluded to thermodynamically closed and open microbial culture systems in terms of batch and chemostat culture, respectively. In both cases the cultures are well mixed and their equations of balance can be generalized in the following form:

$$\frac{dX}{dt} = \mu X - DX,$$ [24]

$$\frac{dS}{dt} = D(S_r - S) - \frac{\mu X}{Y}.$$ [25]

Homogeneous cultures can be classified on the basis of these equations:

(a) For batch cultures, $D = 0$.

(b) In chemostat culture, D = constant.

(c) In fed-batch culture with initial volume V_0, $D = F/V_0 + Ft$, where F is the rate of nutrient addition.

The mathematical description of non-homogeneous systems usually requires the use of partial differential equations to take account of change with respect to position in space as well as time. For example, in a fixed-bed column reactor or soil column containing a constant amount of biomass (X_c) and assuming first-order utilization of substrate:

$$\frac{\delta S}{\delta t} = D^* \frac{\delta^2 S}{\delta z^2} - q \frac{\delta S}{\delta z} - kX_c;$$ [26]

where D^* is known as the dispersion coefficient, k is a first-order rate constant, and z is distance down the column. An analytical solution of this equation is given by Bazin and Menell (12). Wimpenny and Jones (13) give an account of gel-stabilized microbial systems and Prosser and Gray (14) and Theodorou *et al.* (15) derive models for column systems which do not involve partial differential equations. We refer the reader to these references for further information about non-homogeneous systems.

2. Parameter estimation

As indicated previously, in statistical terms, parameter estimation is concerned with the evaluation of what we have called constants. We now review

Table 1. Simulated chemostat data for estimating μ_m and K_s.

D	S	1/D	1/S	D/S	S/D
0.040	0.013	25.000	78.125	3.125	0.320
0.060	0.025	16.667	39.841	2.390	0.418
0.080	0.029	12.500	34.722	2.778	0.360
0.100	0.045	10.000	22.173	2.217	0.451
0.120	0.077	8.333	13.055	1.567	0.638
0.140	0.133	7.143	7.513	1.052	0.951
0.160	0.161	6.250	6.207	0.993	1.007
0.180	0.536	5.556	1.866	0.336	2.978

a few methods for determining values of such constants associated with microbial growth.

2.1 Estimation of Monod growth constants from steady-state chemostat data

It is sometimes possible to apply regression techniques to estimate μ_m and K_s from steady-state chemostat cultures using the relationship between D and S_s given in *Equation 13*. Often, however, the residual concentration of the limiting substrate is so low that it is very difficult to measure. *Table 1* shows simulated data generated using *Equation 14* with $\mu_m = 0.2$ and $K_s = 0.05$ and applying 10% random variability to represent experimental error. Linear regression analysis can be used to estimate μ_m and K_s by converting *Equation 13* to linear form in one of the following three ways:

(a) $\dfrac{1}{D} = \dfrac{1}{\mu_m} + \dfrac{K_s}{\mu_m}\dfrac{1}{S_s}$

(b) $\dfrac{S_s}{D} = \dfrac{K_s}{\mu_m} + \dfrac{1}{\mu_m} S_s;$

(c) $D = \mu_m - K_s \dfrac{D}{S_s};$

All of these equations correspond to the general equation for a straight line:

$$y = A + Bx;$$

where A is the intercept and B is the slope.

Protocol 1. Linear regression analysis to estimate μ_m and K_s

Method

1. Calculate the variables y and x from the data. For (a), $y = 1/D$ and $x = 1/S_s$; for (b), $y = S_s/D$ and $x = S_s$; for (c), $y = D$ and $x = D/S_s$.
2. Estimate A and B using linear regression.

---

3. Calculate μ_m and K_s using the following relationships:

For (a), $\mu_m = \dfrac{1}{A}$ and $K_s = B\mu_m$;

For (b), $\mu_m = \dfrac{1}{B}$ and $K_s = A\mu_m$;

For (c), $\mu_m = A$ and $K_s = B$.

With the data in *Table 1*, the following estimates for μ_m and K_s were obtained: (a), 0.27 and 0.098; (b), 0.200 and 0.0554; (c), 0.191 and 0.0490. Thus, the poorest estimate is obtained from the most widely used linear transformation, the Lineweaver–Burk method (a). This results is in agreement with that of Dowd and Rigg (16) who analysed the Michaelis–Menten equation.

Non-linear regression packages are now readily available for most micro-computers. These operate directly on the non-linear function by minimizing the sum of the squares of the residuals. Applying *Equation 13* and using a package called 'Regression', which is available for the Apple Macintosh and IBM PCs running Windows estimates of $\mu_m = 0.1981$ and $K_s = 0.0481$ were obtained from the simulated data. Regression has been reviewed by Scott (17).

2.2 The 'washout' method

When D is increased so that it greatly exceeds the specific growth rate in chemostat culture, the population will be washed out of the culture vessel since the population growth rate is less than the dilution factor. Under such conditions, the cells are saturated with substrate and μ will approach its maximum value, μ_m. Thus, *Equation 24* becomes:

$$\frac{dX}{dt} = \mu_m X - DX; \tag{27}$$

which on integration gives:

$$\ln X_t = (\mu_m - D)t + \ln X_0; \tag{28}$$

where X_0 is the biomass density just prior to the increase in D (usually after the culture has reached steady state) and X_t is the biomass t time units after the increase in D. When $\ln X$ is plotted against t, a straight line is generated with slope $= \mu_m - D$, so that $\mu_m = $ slope$+D$, or:

$$\mu_m = \frac{\ln X_t - \ln X_0}{t} + D. \tag{29}$$

To obtain suitable data for applying *Equation 29*, the dilution rate of a steady-state culture is increased, and biomass measurements (as ODs, dry weights, protein or carbon content) are made at timed intervals. It is not necessary to completely wash out the culture to obtain the required data. The following protocol includes simple examples of the calculations involved.

Protocol 2. Estimation of μ_m by the 'washout' method

Method

1. Inoculate a chemostat and incubate under batch conditions ($D = 0$) until the culture becomes turbid.

2. Switch on the nutrient flow at low D and measure the turbidity of samples at timed intervals. When the turbidity ceases to change, steady state is indicated. Increase D to a high value.

3. Continue to monitor the turbidity and plot optical density (OD) against time since the switch in D on semi-logarithmic graph paper. If the data points fall on a straight line with negative slope, washout is taking place.

4. Apply *Equation 29* or estimate the slope of the line by linear regression and use to calculate μ_m.

The following are examples of applying this method:

2.2.1

A bacterium was grown in steady-state chemostat culture and the dilution rate increased to 0.6 h^{-1} in order to determine the maximum specific growth rate. The following data were obtained:

Time (h)	OD (optical density)
0	0.64
1	0.54
2	0.46
3	0.39
4	0.33
5	0.29

$$\text{From } \textit{Equation 29, } \mu_m = \frac{\ln 0.29 - \ln 0.64}{5} + 0.6$$

$$= \frac{-1.24 - (-0.45)}{5} + 0.6$$

$$= 0.44 \text{ h}^{-1}.$$

2.2.2

An organism was grown in chemostat culture at a dilution rate of 0.35 h^{-1}. Once a steady state had been achieved, the flow rate was increased to give a dilution rate of 0.5 h^{-1}. The following data were obtained:

Time (h)	OD	ln OD
0	0.40	−0.916
1	0.37	−0.994
2	0.32	−1.139
3	0.31	−1.171
4	0.26	−1.347
5	0.25	−1.386

The slope of the line generated by plotting ln OD against time is −0.0983. Thus, μ_m = slope + D = − 0.0983 + 0.5 = 0.40 h^{-1}.

2.3 Growth yields

When carbon is the limiting nutrient, growth yields are a quantitative expression of an organism's requirement for biomass production and energy. The yield term, Y, in *Equation 5* represents substrate utilization for growth and maintenance. According to Pirt (18), the following equations can be used to analyse steady-state chemostat cultures in order to determine the 'true' growth yield (Y_{EG}), the maintenance coefficient (m) and the metabolic quotient for the energy source:

$$\frac{1}{Y} = \frac{1}{Y_{EG}} + \frac{m}{D};$$

[30]

$$q = \frac{D}{Y_{EG}} + m.$$

[31]

Protocol 3. Estimation of Y_{EG}, m, and q

Method

1. Run a chemostat culture to obtain several steady states by varying D and ensuring that the residual concentration of growth-limiting substrates is effectively zero. Sample and estimate the steady-state biomass densities.

2. Calculate for each value of D: $1/D$, $Y = X_s/S_r$, $1/Y$, and $q = D/Y$.

3. Use linear regression to calculate the slope and intercept of the straight line generated by *Equation 30*. The reciprocal of the intercept is Y_{EG} and the slope is m.

4. Similarly, calculate the regression coefficients for *Equation 31*. In this case, Y_{EG} is the reciprocal of the slope and m is the intercept.

The following is a sample calculation illustrating the application of *Protocol 3*.

2.3.1

A *Thiobacillus* species was grown in chemostat culture with thiosulfate, at a concentration of 20 mM, as the growth-limiting nutrient. At all steady states recorded, no residual thiosulfate was detected. The following data were recorded:

D (h^{-1})	Biomass density (mg dry weight L^{-1})
0.010	112.4
0.012	125.0
0.015	142.8
0.020	156.2
0.025	169.4
0.040	190.4
0.067	210.6
0.100	222.2

From these data the following variables were calculated:

1/D (h)	Y (g mol^{-1})	1/Y (mol g^{-1})	q (mmol g^{-1}/h)
100	5.62	0.178	1.779
83.33	6.25	0.16	1.92
66.67	7.14	0.14	2.10
50.00	7.81	0.128	2.56
40.00	8.47	0.118	2.95
25.00	9.52	0.105	4.20
14.92	10.53	0.095	6.36
10.00	11.11	0.09	9.00

Plotting $1/Y$ against $1/D$ gives an intercept of 8.01×10^{-2} and a slope of 9.56×10^{-4}. Thus, $Y_{EG} = 1/0.0801 = 12.48$ g mol^{-1} and $m = 0.096$ mmol g^{-1}/h. When q is plotted against D, the slope is 0.081 and the intercept, 0.945. The estimate for Y_{EG} is $1/0.807 = 12.39$ g mol^{-1} and for $m = 0.945$ mmol g^{-1}/h.

3. Simulation

Simulation is a method of studying systems by representing them in mathematical terms and processing the resulting equations, in biology often called models, on a computer. *Equation 11* and *12* constitute a model of microbial growth in chemostat culture which assumes that Monod kinetics are opera-

Table 2. Listing of Program CHEMO for simulating chemostat data assuming Monod kinetics and utilizing a fourth-order Runge–Kutta function for solving the equations numerically.

```
      PROGRAM CHEMO
      INTEGER RUNGE
      REAL MUM, KS
      DIMENSION F(2), Y(2)
C  SET VALUES FOR CONSTANTS
      MUM = 4.0
      KS = 1.0
      YLD = 0.5
C  SET VALUES FOR PARAMETERS
      D = 1.0
      SR = 10.0
C  SET INITIAL CONDITIONS
      XI = 2.0
      SI = 1.0
C  SET INTEGRATION TIME
      TMAX = 7.0
C  SET STEP SIZE
      H = 0.1
      T = 0
      Y(1) = XI
      Y(2) = SI
  9   K = RUNGE (2,Y,F,T,H)
      IF (K.NE.1) GO TO 10
      F(1) = MUM*Y(1)*Y(2).(KS 1 Y(2)) 2 D*Y(1)
      F(2) = D*(SR 2 Y(2)) 2 MUM*Y(1)*T(2)/(YLD*(KS 1 Y(2)))
  10  WRITE (*, 100)T,Y(1),Y(2)
      IF(T.LE.TMAX) GO TO 9
 100  FORMAT (1X,F8.2,2X,F8.2,2X,F8.2)
      END
      FUNCTION RUNGE (N,Y,F,X,H)
      DIMENSION Y(N),F(N),PHI(50),SAVEY(50)
      INTEGER RUNGE
      DATA M/0/
      M = M + 1
      GO TO (1,2,3,4,5)M
  1   RUNGE = 1
      RETURN
  2   DO 22 J = 1,N
      SAVEY(J) = Y(J)
      PHI(J) = F(J)
 22   Y(J) = SAVEY(J) + 0.5*H*F(J)
      X = X + 0.5*H
      RUNGE = 1
      RETURN
  3   DO 33 J = 1,N
      PHI(J) = PHI(J) + 2.0*F(J)
 33   Y(J) = SAVEY(J) + 0.5*H*F(J)
      RUNGE = 1
      RETURN
  4   DO 44 J = 1,N
      PHI(J) = PHI(J) + 2.0*F(J)
 44   Y(J) = SAVEY(J) + H&F(J)
      X = X + 0.5*H
      RUNGE = 1
      RETURN
  5   DO 55 J = 1,N
 55   Y(J) = SAVEY(J) + (PHI(J) + F(J))*H/6.0
      M = 0
      RUNGE = 0
      RETURN
      END
```

tive. Processing these equations in a computer involves determining how X and S behave with respect to time. This involves finding approximate solutions to the equations using numerical methods. Several numerical methods for doing this are available, as also are many packages specifically designed for model simulation which can be run on desktop computers. Of particular value in this respect are the Numerical Algorithm Group (NAG) library and Press *et al.* (19), both of which contain a very wide range of useful computer-based mathematical procedures.

3.1 Numerical solution of differential equations

In *Table 2* we list a simple FORTRAN program which employs the Runge–Kutta method to solve numerically *Equations 11* and *12*. In order to modify the program for other sets of differential equations, an elementary knowledge of FORTRAN is required and in *Protocol 4* we indicate how this program can be applied.

Protocol 4. Numerical simulation of dynamic models

Method

1. Write the set of differential equations:

$$\frac{dX}{dt} = \frac{\mu_m SX}{K_s + S} - DX;$$

$$\frac{dS}{dt} = D(S_r - S) - \frac{\mu_m SX}{Y(K_s - S)}.$$

In the program, F(1) and F(2) are the derivatives, Y(1) and Y(2) are the two dependent variables, X and S, and the following FORTRAN variables replace the indicated mathematical symbols: MUM $= \mu_m$, KS $= K_s$, YLD $= Y$, D $= D$ and SR $= S_r$.

2. Dimension F and Y with integer values equal to the number of differential equations.

3. Provide values for the constants in the equations.

4. Provide values for the parameters.

5. Provide FORTRAN statements for the initial conditions, i.e. the value of the dependent variables at $t = 0$. In the example these are represented as XI and SI.

6. Set the time over which the model is to be simulated (TMAX).

7. The program operates by taking small increments of time, called the step size (H), and making the appropriate calculations. Set the step size.

8. Modify Statement 9 by changing the 2 in the RUNGE function to an integer number equal to the number of differential equations.

---

9. Write FORTRAN statements for F(1), F(2),...F(N), where N is the number of equations.

10. Modify the WRITE statement (10) to include all the dependent variables, Y(1) to Y(N).

11. Modify the 100 FORMAT statement to reflect the number of variables to be written.

12. Run the program on a computer with a FORTRAN compiler.

13. If the system is expected to come to steady state, check that the simulated values match those derived analytically. In the example, X_s = 4.83 and S_s = 0.33. If steady state has not been reached in the simulation, increase the value of TMAX.

14. Reduce the step size, H, to about a tenth of its original value and repeat the simulation. Compare the two sets of simulated results. If they differ significantly, a smaller step size is indicated. The accuracy of the results depends critically on the step size employed. If H is set at 0.2 instead of 0.1 in the example, negative values for X and S may be generated which is obviously unrealistic. Some so-called 'stiff' differential equations may need very small step sizes which results in long simulation times. In such cases it is advisable to use a numerical method employing variable step sizes. Such routines can be found in the NAG library.

3.2 Dynamic parameter estimation

Simulation programs can be incorporated into routines for estimating values for the constants in differential equations by comparing the simulated results to data. The advantage of this approach is that it employs transient as well as steady-state data. The basis of the method is to minimize the sum of the squares of the differences between simulated and real data. This is accomplished by varying the values of the parameters (used in a statistical sense, i.e. what we have called 'constants') and using a minimization routine to determine the minimum. The NAG library contains several minimization routines one of which, designated E04FDF, is designed 'to find an unconstrained minimum of a sum of squares of m non-linear functions in n variables ($m \geqslant n$). It is designed for functions which are continuous and which have continuous first and second derivatives, although it will usually work even though derivatives have occasional discontinuities'. It minimizes:

$$F(x) = \sum_{i=1}^{n} [f_i(x)]^2 \qquad [32]$$

where $x = (x_1, x_2, \ldots, x_n)$ and $m \geqslant n$, that is to say it minimizes the sum of the squares of the differences between a data set and a given function by varying the values of the specified parameters. The protocol given below determines

Table 3a. Listing of a minimization program utilizing the NAG routine E04FDF for estimating μ_m and K_s by dynamic simulation

```
        PROGRAM E04FDF
        INTEGER N,M,NT,LIW,LW
        PARAMETER (N = 2,M = 100,NT = 2,LIW = 1,LW = 7*N + N* + 2*M*N + 3*M + N*(N - 1)
     +      /2)
        INTEGER NIN, NOUT
        PARAMETER (NIN = 5,NOUT = 6)
        DOUBLE PRECISION Y(M)
        DOUBLE PRECISION FSUMSQ
        INTEGER I, IFAIL, J
        DOUBLE PRECISION W(LW),X(N)
        INTEGER IW(LIW)
        EXTERNAL E04FDF
        COMMON Y
        DIMENSION R(4200)
        OPEN(21,FILE = 'DATA.DAT;',STATUS = 'UNKNOWN')
        OPEN(22,FILE = 'RESULT.DAT;',STATUS = 'UNKNOWN')
        DO 19 T = 1,100
        READ(21,*)Y(T)
  19    CONTINUE
        *Initial estimates of constants MUM and KS
        X(1) = 5.0D0
        X(2) = 1.5D0
        IFAIL = 1
        CALL E04FDF(M,N,X,FSUMSQ,IW,LIW,W,LW,IFAIL)
        IF (IFAIL.NE.0) THEN
        WRITE (22,*)
        WRITE (22,99999) 'Error exit type', IFAIL,
     +  '-see routine document'
        END IF
        IF (IFAIL.NE.1) THEN
        WRITE (22,*)
        WRITE (22,99998) 'On exit, the sum of squares is', FSUMSQ
        WRITE (22,99998) 'at the point', (X(J),J = 1,N)
        END IF
 99999  FORMAT (1X,A,13,A)
 99998  FORMAT (1X,A,3F12.4)
        END
        SUBROUTINE LSFUN1(M,N,XC,FVECC)
        INTEGER MDEC, NT
        PARAMETER (MDEC = 100,NT = 2)
        INTEGER M,N
        DOUBLE PRECISION FVECC(M),XC(N)
        DOUBLE PRECISION Y(MDEC)
        DOUBLE PRECISION FVEC(100)
        INTEGER 1
        COMMON Y
        CALL CHEMO(FVEC,XC)
        DO 20 I = 1,M
        FVECC(I) = FVEC(I) - Y(I)
  20    CONTINUE
        RETURN
        END
```

values for the constants μ_m and K_s in the CHEMO program, which is used as a function for E04FDF, described earlier. The data set was generated using CHEMO with values of $\mu_m = 4.0$ and $K_s = 1.0$ and the resulting biomass concentrations modified by adding or subtracting 30% random error to simulate experimental variability.

Table 3b. Modifications needed for CHEMO to become a sub-routine of Program E04FDF

```
SUBROUTINE CHEMO(FVEC,XC)
DOUBLE PRECISION FVEC(100),XC(2)
INTEGER I
I = 0
   .
   .
   .
MUM = XC(1)
KS = XC(2)
   .
   .
   .
FVEC(I)  5  Y(1)
I = 1 + 1
10    WRITE (*,100)T,Y(1),Y(2)
   .
   .
   .
```

Protocol 5. Utilizing a NAG minimization routine to determine μ_m and K_s

Method

Refer to the NAG manual and the example given for routine E04FDF.

1. A listing of Program E04FDF is given in *Table 3a*. Modify CHEMO as indicated in *Table 3b* so that it becomes a subroutine of this program. The first line of CHEMO now becomes:

   SUBROUTINE CHEMO (FVEC,XC)

   Employ double precision for the variables in the argument of the subroutine:

   DOUBLE PRECISION FVEC(100), XC(2)

   FVEC will contain the simulated biomass concentrations (Y(1)) and XC contains the values for MUM and KS.

2. Replace the values in MUM and KS in CHEMO with values passed from E04FDF:

   MUM = XC(1)
   KS = XC(2)
   FVEC(I) = Y(1)

3. I is a counter which determines the position of the values in the array FVEC. It is incremented by 1 after every call to the RUNGE function:

   I = I + 1

4. Assign appropriate values to the parameters in E04FDF. N and NT correspond to the number of constants being evaluated (2) and M and MDEC are the number of data points (100).

Protocol 5. *Continued*

5. Remove lines asking the user to input observed values and replace with a statement indicating the location of a data file containing these values:

```
OPEN(21,FILE = 'DATA.DAT;',STATUS = 'UNKNOWN')
```

6. Add a line which creates a file to which the results will be written:

```
OPEN(22,FILE = 'RESULT.DAT;',STATUS = 'UNKNOWN')
```

7. Provide initial estimates for X(1) (μ_m, 5.0) and X(2) (K_s, 1.5).

8. Within the subroutine LSFUN, add a line calling the subroutine CHEMO which generates the simulated values Y(1)

```
CALL CHEMO(FVEC,XC)
```

and replace the statement which contains the calculation to determine FVECC with:

```
FVECC(I) = FVEC(I) − Y(I)
```

Estimates for μ_m and K_s of 3.99 and 0.98 were obtained with standard deviations of 0.078 and 0.132, respectively.

4. Analytical methods

The methods described above depend on the acquisition of data and subsequent application to mathematical models. However, it is not always clear that a priori the models themselves are suitable descriptions of the systems under study. In many instances sets of differential equations admit to unstable solutions; *Protocol 6* describes a method for testing the stability of such systems near equilibrium or steady state. It depends on approximating the non-linear equations by linear equations and determining the nature of the eigenvalues associated with their solutions. From the eigenvalues the local stability of the system can be predicted. We illustrate the protocol using *Equations 11* and *12*, a single-species chemostat system based on Monod kinetics.

Protocol 6. Liapounov stability analysis of dynamic models

Method

1. Write the set of differential equations:

$$\frac{dX}{dt} = \mu(s)X - DX;$$

$$\frac{dS}{dt} = DS_r - \frac{\mu(s)X}{Y} - DS;$$

where $\mu(S) = \dfrac{\mu_m S}{K_s + S}$.

2. Obtain the steady-state solutions:

$$0 = \frac{\mu_m S_s X_s}{K_s + S_s} - DX_s;$$

$$0 = DS_r - \frac{\mu_m S_s X_s}{(K_s + S_s)Y} - DS_s.$$

3. Transform the dependent variables to new variables which have steady-state values of zero:

$$x = X - X_s,$$
and $$y = S - S_s.$$

4. Substitute the variable(s) in the growth function(s) with the new variables, expand in a Taylor series and drop second order terms:

$$\mu(S) = \mu(y + S_s) = \mu(S_s) + \frac{d\mu(S_s)}{d(S_s)} y + \text{second order terms}$$

$$= \frac{\mu_m S_s}{K_s + S_s} + \frac{(K_s + S_s)\mu_m - \mu_m S_s}{(K_s + S_s)^2} y$$

5. Substitute the new variables into the original equations and replace the growth function with the expanded version:

$$\frac{dX}{dt} = \frac{d(x + X_s)}{dt} = \frac{dx}{dt};$$

$$= \left[\frac{\mu_m S_s}{K_s + S_s} + \frac{(K_s + S_s)\mu_m - \mu_m S_s}{(K_s + S_s)^2} y \right](x + X_s) - D(x + X_s)$$

$$= \frac{\mu_m S_s}{K_s + S_s} x + \frac{\mu_m S_s X_s}{K_s + S_s} + \frac{(K_s + S_s)\mu_m xy}{(K_s + S_s)^2} + \frac{(K_s + S_s)\mu_m X_s}{(K_s + S_s)^2} y$$

$$- \frac{\mu_m S_s}{(K_s + S_s)^2} xy - \frac{\mu_m S_s}{(K_s + S_s)^2} X_s y - Dx - DX_s$$

$$\frac{dS}{dt} = \frac{d(y + S_s)}{dt} = \frac{dy}{dy}$$

$$= DS_r - \left[\frac{\mu_m S_s}{K_s + S_s} + \frac{(K_s + S_s)\mu_m - \mu_m S_s}{(K_s + S_s)^2} y \right]\frac{(x + X_s)}{Y} - D(y + S_s)$$

$$= DS_r - \frac{\mu_m S_s}{(K_s + S_s)Y} x - \frac{\mu_m S_s X_s}{(K_s + S_s)Y} - \frac{(K_s + S_s)\mu_m xy}{(K_s + S_s)^2 Y}$$

$$- \frac{(K_s + S_s)\mu_m X_s}{(K_s + S_s)^2 Y} y + \frac{\mu_m S_s}{(K_s + S_s)^2 Y} xy + \frac{\mu_m S_s}{(K_s + S_s)^2 Y} X_s y$$

$$- Dy - DS_s.$$

6. Eliminate steady-state terms which equate to zero and second-order terms. Note:

$$0 = \frac{\mu_m S_s}{K_s + S_s} x - Dx \text{ and } D = \frac{\mu_m S_s}{K_s + S_s};$$

Protocol 6. *Continued*

$$\frac{dx}{dt} = \frac{\mu_m X_s}{K_s + S_s}y - \frac{Dx_s}{K_s + S_s}y = (\mu_m - D)\frac{X_s}{K_s + S_s}y;$$

$$\frac{dy}{dt} = -\frac{\mu_m S_s}{(K_s + S_s)Y}x + \left[\frac{\mu_m S_s X_s}{(K_s + S_s)Y} - \frac{\mu_m X_s}{(K_s + S_s)^2} - D\right]y$$

$$= -\frac{Dx}{Y} + \left[(D - \mu_m)\frac{X_s}{(K_s + S_s)Y} - D\right]y.$$

7. Write the equations in matrix form:

$$\begin{bmatrix} \dfrac{dx}{dt} \\ \dfrac{dy}{dt} \end{bmatrix} = \begin{bmatrix} 0 & a \\ -\dfrac{D}{Y} & -\left(\dfrac{a}{Y} + D\right) \end{bmatrix} \begin{bmatrix} x \\ y \end{bmatrix}$$

where $a = \dfrac{X_s}{K_s + S_s}(\mu_m - D)$.

8. Subtract λ from each of the diagonal elements of the stability matrix, write the result as a determinant and set it equal to zero in order to obtain the characteristic equation:

$$\begin{vmatrix} 0 - \lambda & a \\ -\dfrac{D}{Y} & -\left(\dfrac{a}{Y} + D\right) - \lambda \end{vmatrix} = 0$$

i.e. $\quad \lambda^2 + \left(\dfrac{a}{Y} + D\right)\lambda + \dfrac{aD}{Y} = 0.$

9. Solve the characteristic equation to obtain the eigenvalues, λ.

$$\lambda_{1,2} = \frac{-\left(\dfrac{a}{Y} + D\right) \pm \sqrt{\left(\dfrac{a}{Y} + D\right)^2 - \dfrac{4\,a\,D}{Y}}}{2};$$

or $\quad \left(\lambda + \dfrac{a}{Y}\right)(\lambda + D) = 0.$

Thus: $\lambda_1 = -\dfrac{a}{Y}$ and $\lambda_2 = -D$.

10. Test for stability applying the following rules:
    (a) For the system to be stable all eigenvalues must be negative.
    (b) If the eigenvalues are real and negative, the system moves monotonically to steady state.
    (c) If the eigenvalues occur in complex conjugate pairs of form:
    $$\lambda = n \pm p_i;$$
    where n and p are real numbers and $i = \sqrt{-1}$, the system is

periodic. (In our example this would occur if the terms under the square-root sign had a negative value.) For $n < 0$, damped oscillations arise and the system moves to a stable steady state. For $n > 0$, oscillations of increasing amplitude occur which might give rise to sustained limit-cycle oscillations of constant amplitude independent of the initial conditions of the system. For $n = 0$, sustained oscillations also occur, but in this case their amplitudes do depend on the initial conditions.

As X_s, k_s, S_s, μ_m, and D are all positive numbers, the chemostat system is stable and moves monotonically to steady state, provided that $\mu_m > D$.

References

1. Waler, P. M. B. (ed.) (1991). *Chambers science and technology dictionary*. W. & R. Chambers, Edinburgh.
2. Monod, J. (1942). *Recherches sur la croissance bactérienne*. Herman et Cie, Paris.
3. Bailey, J. and Ollis, D. (1986). *Biochemical engineering fundamentals* (2nd edn). McGraw-Hill, NY.
4. Bazin, M. J. and Prosser, J. I. (1992). *J. Appl. Bact. Symp. Supp.*, **73**, 895.
5. Contois, D. E. (1950). *J. Gen. Microbiol.*, **66**, 95.
6. Curds, C. and Cockburn, C. R. (1968). *J. Gen. Microbiol.*, **54**, 343.
7. Bazin, M. J., Curds, C., Dauppe, A., Owen, B., and Saunders, P. T. (1983). In *Foundations in biochemical engineering* (ed. H. W. Blanch, E. Papoutsakis and G. Stephanopoulos), pp. 254–64. American Chemical Society, Washington, DC.
8. Andrews, J. F. (1968). *Biotechnol. Bioeng.*, **10**, 707.
9. Howell, J. A., Chi, C. T., and Pawlowsky, U. (1972). *Biotechnol. Bioeng.*, **14**, 253.
10. Aiba, S., Shoda, M., and Nagatani, M. (1968). *Biotechnol. Bioeng.*, **10**, 845.
11. Aiba, S. and Shoda, M. (1969). *J. Ferment. Technol. Jpn.*, **47**, 790.
12. Bazin, M. J. and Menell, A. (1990). In *Methods in microbiology* (ed. R. Grigorova and J. R. Norris), Vol. 22, pp. 123–179. Academic Press, London.
13. Wimpenny, J. W. and Jones, D. E. (1988). In *CRC handbook of laboratory model systems for microbial ecosystems* (ed. J. W. Wimpenny) Vol. 2, pp. 1–30. CRC Press, Boca Raton, FL.
14. Prosser, J. I. and Gray, T. R. G. (1977). *J. Gen. Microbiol.*, **102**, 119.
15. Theodorou, M. K., Bazin, M. J., and Trinci, A. P. J. (1984). In *Microbiological methods for environmental biotechnology* (ed. J. M. Grainger and J. M. Lynch), pp. 19–31. Academic Press, London.
16. Dowd, J. E. and Rigg, D. S. (1965). *J. Biol. Chem.*, **240**, 863.
17. Scott, E. (1992). *Binary*, **4**, 149.
18. Pirt, S. J. (1985). *Principles of microbe and cell cultivation*. Blackwell Scientific Publications, Oxford.
19. Press, W. H., Flannery, B. P., Teukolsky, S. A., and Vetterling, W. T. (1989). *Numerical recipes*. Cambridge University Press, Cambridge.

9

Metabolic flux analysis

WILLIAM H. HOLMS

1. Introduction

1.1 Basic principles

Flux analysis is a method of organizing data which shows the quantitative relationships among all the metabolic events going on in a fermentation. It is a simple description of *what* is actually happening in the fermentation and does not, in itself, consider the theory of *how* fermentations are limited or controlled. However, once the analysis is complete, it defines the ballpark within which the game is actually being played and the *interpretation* of this can often suggest what might be the factors limiting the process engineer's aspirations for his/hers defined goals. By definition, the biomass always does the best it can with what is available, unless human intervention has deliberately deranged its genetic machinery or put it into a deliberately misleading environment. An example of the first would be to delete the ability to make thymine and then transfer the biomass to a thymine-free medium where it would attempt to grow and, in so doing, kill itself because it could not make DNA. An example of the second would be to grow an organism in a glycerol, oxygen, salts medium to which a non-metabolizable inducer of β-galactosidase, such as methyl-thio-β-galactoside has been added, when the biomass would make prodigious amounts of redundant β-galactosidase. In these cases we have altered the rules and we are not surprised by the results. However, when we have not done this, we must define the game before we can think of how we wish to change it. This can only be done by flux analysis. Flux analysis organizes data so we must define what data we require:

- WHEN you measure everything that goes IN,
- WHEN you measure everything that comes OUT,
- AND you know the metabolic routes that connect these,
- THEN you can write a complete description of what the process is doing.

This description is a flux analysis (1).

1.2 Definitions and units

The basic parameter of a fermentation is the biomass which we choose to express as dry weight—usually kilogram dry weight biomass (kg dry wt). In the end, everything else is related to this. An 'input' is the amount of a feedstock which is taken up and metabolized by the biomass. Traditionally, inputs are often expressed as weights, but this causes great difficulty and confusion as 100 g of glucose is phosphorylated to give 144 g of glucose 6-phosphate and, in two more steps, a total of 198 g of glyceraldehyde 3-phosphate and dihydroxyacetone phosphate. It is much more convenient to express amounts in moles where, in the above example 1 mole of glucose becomes 1 mole of glucose 6-phosphate and eventually 1 mole of each of the triose phosphates. Relating input to the basic parameter, it becomes moles glucose/kg dry wt. When *Escherichia coli* is growing on glucose as the sole carbon source, we measure the input as the amount of glucose required to generate 1 kg dry wt. Throughputs are also amounts (in the same units) which are defined as the amount of a substrate (e.g. fructose 1,6-bisphosphate) converted to products (the triose phosphates) in generating 1 kg dry wt. A final output is the amount of a specific monomer contained in the end product (biomass) and is in the same unit. There are, of course, other products such as CO_2 and, in the particular example, acetate, which also are expressed in the same units. In the steady state the biomass generates itself at a constant rate described by the growth rate μ (per hour). The product of the amounts defined above and μ are moles/kg dry wt/h and these are fluxes which describe the rate at which an input is used, the flux by which a substrate is converted to a product, or a monomeric constituent of biomass is generated, or another product such as acetate is excreted. The last unit of possible significance in flux analysis is pool sizes, this is an amount expressed as moles of an intermediate contained as a pool within the biomass and again has the unit moles/kg dry wt in any given steady state. The rate at which the intermediate must be generated to maintain pool size is derived from μ in the same way to give moles pool intermediate/kg dry wt/h. In prokaryotes, where pool sizes are very variable and usually small relative to their throughput, this value has limited importance and the turnover of the pool is probably more significant. This is the rate of input (or output, because they are the same) divided by the pool size, i.e. (moles/kg dry wt/h)/(moles/kg dry wt) which has the dimension of a number/h and is the number of times the pool turns over every hour. It is obvious that in a linear segment of metabolism where the flux through each enzyme in the chain is the same, then the turnover of each pool of intermediates is inversely proportional to the size of the pool (this is discussed in an example below).

1.3 The central metabolic pathways (CMPs)

The CMPs (or amphibolic pathways) *do* occupy a central position in fermentations (2). Consider a fermentation where biomass is converting a single carbon

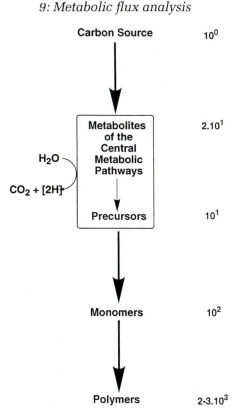

Figure 1. Flow of carbon during growth of *E. coli*.

source into biomass. Here carbon feedstock is fed into the central metabolic pathways (*Figure 1*). In this case these consist of glycolysis, the pentose phosphate pathway (PPP), PEP carboxylase, pyruvate dehydrogenase, and the Krebs cycle which altogether have 30 intermediates. All these intermediates are charged molecules—17 are phosphorylated, 18 are carboxylic acids, and 5 are both. Of these a smaller number (seven to nine depending on how you compute) are the precursors from which the monomers required (about 300) to make biomass are derived. Growth (biomass generation) is largely (but not exclusively) polymerization of these monomers to give several thousand polymers. Any one of a large number of single carbon sources (or even a combination of several) are also processed by fluxing into the CMPs, occasionally using simple variants of glycolysis, PPP, and the Krebs cycle. The main point is that catabolic routes of simple feedstocks all converge on the CMPs and all biosynthetic routes diverge from the CMPs. The CMPs therefore are the marshalling yard (contained in one box in *Figure 1*) at which fluxes of feedstocks are apportioned into fluxes to biosynthesis. Aerobically the CMPs also perform another vital function. They oxidize feedstocks to carbon dioxide and, because the oxygen input for this is water, they generate large amounts of reducing power and a relatively small amount of 'high energy' nucleoside triphosphate, principally ATP. The reducing power is trapped (NADH,H$^+$; NADPH,H$^+$; FADH$_2$) and is then fed into the electron transport system (ETS) which is, in the end, used to reduce molecular oxygen to water; some of the free energy available from this is used to phosphorylate ADP to ATP. The fluxes through the CMPs are central to flux analysis because they provide the precursors and the energy required to make all biosynthetic products.

1.4 Components of the CMPs

The CMPs contain about 30 intermediates which are interconnected by a rather larger number of enzymes, as several reactions have more than one enzyme and others have enzymes specific for one direction only. For example, in *E. coli* there are at least three enzymes which convert phosphoenolpyruvate (PEP) to pyruvate and phosphorylate another compound. There are two pyruvate kinases (one activated by fructose bisphosphate and the other by AMP) which phosphorylate ADP. In addition, the phosphotransferase systems use PEP to initiate the chain of phosphorylated compounds which take up extracellular sugars and phosphorylate them to sugar phosphates. There are other enzymes, operating in the reverse direction, which catalyse the thermodynamically unfavourable phosphorylation of pyruvate to PEP. A few of the CMP intermediates are substrates for synthesis of the monomers used to make biomass and products. We can take an example from the Krebs cycle (*Figure 2*). Citrate is isomerized to *iso*citrate, oxidatively decarboxylated to oxoglutarate (OGA), and then to succinyl coenzyme A. These four compounds are all intermediates of the CMPs. One of them (OGA) is the precursor for the synthesis of glutamate, i.e. one of the monomers required for biosynthesis. OGA is an output from the CMPs to biosynthesis. Measurement of all the outputs from the CMPs for this purpose is the key to flux analysis.

The biomass uses only a few precursors to maintain flux to many monomers, and it follows that any one precursor is the output from the CMPs for the biosynthesis of several monomers or, in other words, biosynthetic routes diverge from the CMPs. OGA is a good example of this (*Figure 3*) in that it is the precursor not only for glutamate but glutamine, proline, and arginine as well. While glutamate is amidated to glutamine in one step, there are four reactions required to convert glutamate to proline and eight to make it into arginine. The flux through each of the eight enzymes on the route to arginine is the same and is defined by the amount of arginine required to make biomass. It follows that, if we measure (1) the amount of arginine in biomass (which, for *E. coli*, is 0.252 moles arginine/kg dry wt), we know that 0.252 moles of glutamate must be made to supply the arginine for 1 kg dry wt biomass. In the same way, it happens that the proline content of biomass is also 0.252 moles and for glutamine is 0.201 moles and for glutamate itself is 0.353 (all per kg dry wt). Thus in order to supply this family of amino acids

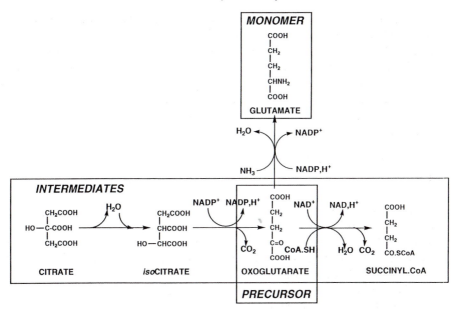

Figure 2. Functions of components of the central metabolic pathways.

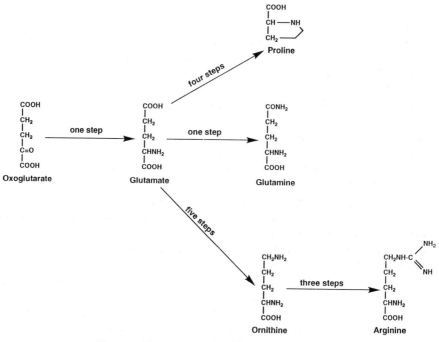

Figure 3. Monomers derived from oxoglutarate.

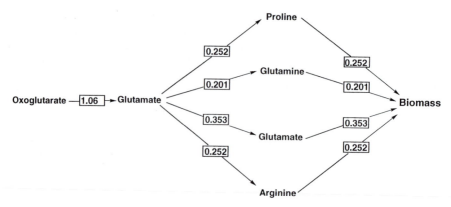

Figure 4. Throughputs from oxoglutarate to *E. coli* ML308 (moles/kg dry wt biomass).

for 1 kg dry wt biomass, a total of 1.058 moles glutamate must be made and, to do this, 1.058 moles of OGA must be taken from CMPs and it is this number which is important for flux analysis. We clearly need a simple method of organizing these data. The fluxes through all the enzymes of a linear chain are the same and we can, therefore, ignore these and show only where fluxes are divided at diverging junctions (*Figure 4*) and thus derive the net output of OGA required for biosynthesis. (It is significant, that, while outputs to monomers are diverging routes, these routes ultimately converge to make biomass, but that is another story.) It must be stressed that these are net fluxes or throughputs and that other metabolites are involved. These are taken from pools which are regenerated. This can easily be explained by looking at the segment of the route to arginine which converts glutamate to ornithine (*Figure 5*). The throughput of every reaction in *Figure 5* is 0.252 moles/kg dry wt biomass. 0.252 moles Glu provides the carbon for 0.252 moles Orn but 0.504 moles OGA are aminated to Glu, this allows the second amination to occur. However, in order to maintain the pools of OGA and Glu, the OGA thus generated is reductively reaminated to Glu. In the same way the acetyl residue of AcCoA is used to protect the amino group of Glu during the phosphorylation, reduction, and amination reactions to *N*-acetylornithine and is then shed as acetate. The AcCoA pool is regenerated, but this requires a prior phosphorylation of the acetate by ATP. The overall reaction is thus:

$$0.252 \text{ moles OGA} + 0.504 \text{ moles NH3} \rightarrow 0.252 \text{ moles Orn}$$
$$0.504 \text{ moles ATP} \rightarrow 0.504 \text{ moles ADP} + 0.504 \text{ moles P}_i \text{ OH}$$
$$0.756 \text{ moles NADPH,H}^+ \rightarrow 0.756 \text{ moles NADP}^+$$

The pools of NADPH,H$^+$ are maintained by oxidative metabolism of intermediates of the CMPs and oxidative phosphorylation in which oxygen is reduced to H$_2$O by the electron transport system. The pool of OGA is maintained by the primary carbon input. This is a good example of the dual func-

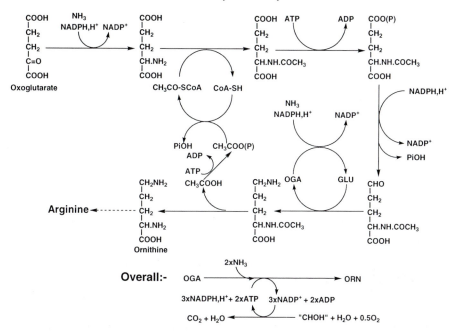

Figure 5. Regeneration of pools during conversion of oxoglutarate to ornithine.

tion of the CMPs which supply the carbon flux from OGA to Orn and the energy input required to drive these reactions. From the point of view of analysing flux of carbon to biosynthesis the important measurement is the flux of OGA-carbon to Orn-carbon and subsequently to Arg-carbon. As we have already shown, the output of OGA to Arg from the CMPs can be quantified by measuring the Arg content of the ultimate product (biomass). The total output derived from OGA carbon to biosynthesis is the sum of the outputs to all the monomers required for the generation of 1 kg dry wt biomass. But this is only one of the outputs of carbon-precursors from the CMPs. How do we measure all of them and how do we handle the data thus obtained? This will be illustrated by three examples.

2. Flux analysis of *E. coli* ML308 growing on glucose, pyruvate, or fumarate as sole sources of carbon

2.1 The data

Flux analysis uses data and, for this system, these are:

- 11.24 moles glucose are used to make 1 kg dry wt biomass and 5.20 moles acetate at a growth rate (μ) of about 0.94 with carbon dioxide as the only other product containing carbon (1).

- 56.12 moles pyruvate are used to make 1 kg dry wt biomass, 26.10 moles acetate, and 0.08 moles lactate in batch (1) or turbidostat culture (3) at a growth rate (μ) of about 0.70.
- 26.23 moles fumarate are used to make 1 kg dry wt biomass with carbon dioxide as the only other output (1) at growth rate (μ) of about 0.63.

The first task is to calculate the outputs to biosynthesis of the monomers in 1 kg dry wt biomass and the excretion of acetate. We have already shown how this is done for the glutamate family of amino acids and we will consider only one more example, the monomers derived from pyruvate. Any standard text book of biochemistry contains the biosynthetic routes but, for *E. coli*, the layout in Mandelstam and McQuillen (2) is particularly user-friendly. Pyruvate (*Figure 6*) is the CMP precursor of alanine, valine, and leucine. Each of these monomers is ultimately made by amination of a keto-acid but, because the amino donors are regenerated by oxidative catabolism, we can ignore these as well as the reduction, dehydration, and oxidation reactions also involved. The precursors required from the CMPs are:

- alanine: one pyruvate
- valine: two pyruvates
- leucine: two pyruvates, one AcCoA

In the same way we now calculate the provision of precursors for all the monomers and acetate excretion as moles of precursor required to make one mole monomer.

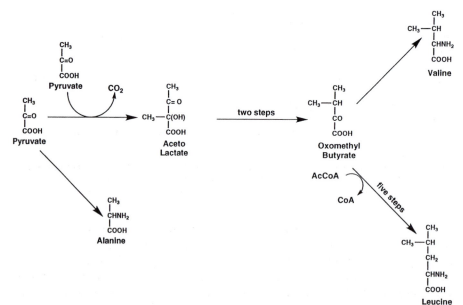

Figure 6. Monomers derived from pyruvate.

Table 1. Synthesis of monomers from amphibolic precursors in *E. coli* ML308[a]

Monomer content		Precursors used for biosynthesis							
		G6P[b]	TP	PG	PEP	PYR	OAA	OGA	AcCoA
Ala	0.454					0.454			
Arg	0.252							0.252	
Asp	0.201						0.201		
Asn	0.101						0.101		
Cys	0.101			0.302					
Glu	0.353							0.353	
Gln	0.201							0.201	
Gly	0.430			0.430					
His	0.050	0.050							
Ile	0.252					0.252	0.252		
Leu	0.403					0.806			0.403
Lys	0.403					0.403	0.403		
Met	0.201					−0.201	0.201		
Phe	0.151		0.151		0.302				
Pro	0.252							0.252	
Ser	0.302			0.302					
Thr	0.252						0.252		
Trp	0.050		0.100	0.050	0.050				
Tyr	0.101		0.101		0.202				
Val	0.302					0.604			
AMP	0.115		0.115	0.115					
dAMP	0.024		0.024	0.024					
GMP	0.115		0.115	0.115					
dGMP	0.024		0.024	0.024					
CMP	0.115		0.115				0.115		
dCMP	0.024		0.024				0.024		
UMP	0.115		0.115				0.115		
dTMP	0.024		0.024				0.024		
C_{16} fatty acid	0.280								2.240
Glycerophosphate	0.140			0.140					
Carbohydrate as glucose	1.026	1.026							
Total		1.98	0.14	1.36	0.55	2.32	1.69	1.06	2.64

[a]All numbers are mol/kg dry weight biomass.
[b]G6P, glucose 6-phosphate; TP, triose-phosphate; PG, phosphoglycerate; PEP, phosphenolpyruvate; PYR, pyruvate; OAA, oxalacetate; OGA, oxoglutarate; AcCoA, acetyl-coenzyme A.

The greatest amount of measurement now required is the monomeric content of the biomass and this is dealt with, in general, in Chapter 7 and, for *E. coli* in particular, in refs 1 and 4. Lipid is taken to be phospholipid of C_{16} fatty acids and all the carbohydrates (e.g. sugars and amino sugars of the cell wall) are presumed to be derived from glucose 6-phosphate while pentose and tetroses are also taken from this precursor via the PPP. These data can now be collected (*Table 1*) and the precursors required to make 1 kg dry wt *E. coli* calculated by summation of the moles of each precursor required to make the measured amount in moles of each monomer contained in 1 kg dry wt biomass.

2.2 Construction of a flux or throughput diagram

We must first construct a diagram which relates the provision of precursors from the CMPs (*Figure 7*). Each conversion of substrate to product is indicated by an arrow with a box in the middle which will eventually contain the flux (or throughput) of this particular enzymatic conversion. Every output of precursors to biosynthesis is similarly accommodated. There are five further points worthy of comment.

- The uptake of glucose (in *E. coli*) is by the specific glucose phosphotransferase system which delivers glucose 6-phosphate into the CMPs. The original phosphate donor to the phosphoenolpyruvate-dependent phosphotransferase system (PTS) is phosphoenolpyruvate (PEP) which is shown to generate pyruvate by this mechanism. Any other PEP converted to pyruvate is by pyruvate kinase which is also shown.

- In glycolysis, aldolase generates one mole of each of the two triose phosphates (therefore two boxes) which are then interconverted by triose phosphate isomerase and thus enter one pool.

- AcCoA enters the Krebs cycle to participate in flux to oxoglutarate, but the bulk is completely oxidized to CO_2.

- The other carbon drawn from the cycle to generate precursors comes from the anaplerotic provision of oxalacetate from PEP by PEP carboxylase and this also is accommodated.

- Finally, acetate is excreted by reversal of the mechanism employed to take it up when it is acting as sole source of carbon. That is, the thiol-ester of AcCoA is exchanged with inorganic phosphate to give acetyl phosphate which phosphorylates ADP to generate acetate which is excreted (by a proton symport) and this also is shown.

Figure 7 contains all the reactions of the CMPs to convert glucose into precursors for the biosynthesis of *E. coli* and acetate excretion. As we will see below it also will accommodate the total oxidation of the remainder of the glucose input to CO_2. It must be stressed that this diagram has been constructed for *E. coli* growing on glucose. For other carbon sources or organisms, modification of this diagram is required. For example, in eukaryotes the anaplerotic provision to the Krebs cycle is by pyruvate carboxylase and for *E. coli* growing on fumarate no such provision is needed, but oxalacetate is decarboxylated to PEP which then reverses glycolysis for gluconeogensis. When we construct a diagram of this kind specific to the particular case we have satisfied the three criteria required for flux analysis:

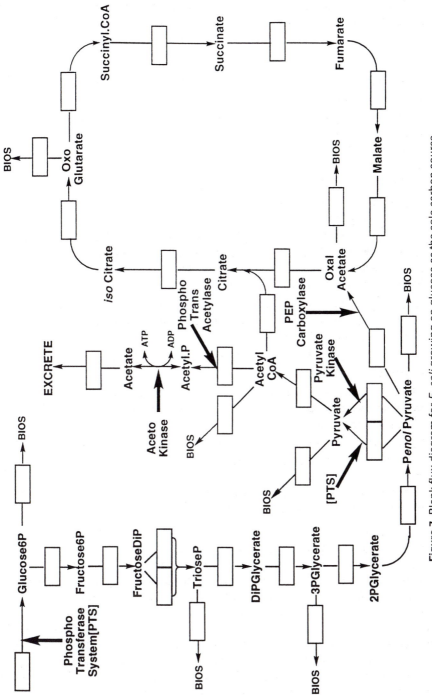

Figure 7. Blank flux diagram for *E. coli* growing on glucose as the sole carbon source.

- WHEN you measure everything that goes IN,
- WHEN you measure everything that comes OUT,
- AND you know the metabolic routes that connect these,
- THEN you can compute a flux analysis

How is this done?

2.2.1 Analysis of the flux of glucose, pyruvate, and fumarate to E. coli (and acetate)

We will consider glucose in detail.

First we enter our inputs and outputs into a throughput diagram (*Figure 8*) and then enter the immediate consequences of these events. When 11.24 moles glucose are taken up, the same amount of PEP is used as the phosphate-donor and converted to pyruvate. The sum of the outputs of oxalacetate and oxoglutarate to biosynthesis requires the anaplerotic provision of 2.75 moles oxaloacetate from PEP. Excretion of acetate removes 5.20 moles AcCoA from the CMPs. The rest is simple arithmetic (*Figure 9*). 11.24 moles glucose are delivered as glucose 6-phosphate of which 1.98 moles are used for biosynthesis and the remainder (9.26 moles) phosphorylated again and delivered into the triose phosphate pool (2 × 9.26 = 18.52) of which 0.14 mole is used for biosynthesis and the remainder is oxidized to 18.38 moles diphosphoglycerate. After 1.34 moles 3-phosphoglycerate are used for biosynthesis, 17.04 moles PEP are available. 11.24 moles of this pool are already committed to the PTS, 0.55 mole is required for biosynthesis, and 2.75 moles for anaplerotic provision to the Krebs cycle. The balance (2.50 moles) is available for pyruvate kinase and thus converted to pyruvate, of which a total of 13.74 moles are available. Of this amount 2.32 moles are used for biosynthesis and 11.42 moles decarboxylated to AcCoA. 2.64 moles AcCoA are used for biosynthesis and 5.20 moles deviated to acetate excretion, leaving 3.58 moles to enter the Krebs cycle for which the same amount (3.58 moles) oxalacetate must be available and eventually 3.58 moles oxoglutarate generated, 1.06 moles oxoglutarate are used for biosynthesis leaving 2.52 moles to be decarboxylated and oxidized to oxalacetate. Together with the anaplerotic provision 5.27 moles oxalacetate are available of which 1.69 moles are used for biosynthesis and the balance (3.58 moles) recycled.

Figure 9 is a complete description of glucose throughput by the CMPs to precursors, acetate, and CO_2 production during conversion of 11.24 moles glucose to 1 kg dry wt biomass. This is a diagram of throughputs but it is easily converted to a flux diagram by multiplying every number by the growth rate constant for this system ($\mu = 0.94$/h) which converts the throughputs to fluxes (moles/kg dry wt/h). Furthermore, it can also be expanded to show the throughputs or fluxes through every biosynthetic enzyme, as was previously shown for the glutamate family (*Figure 4*).

It is important to realize that these are net carbon fluxes or throughputs,

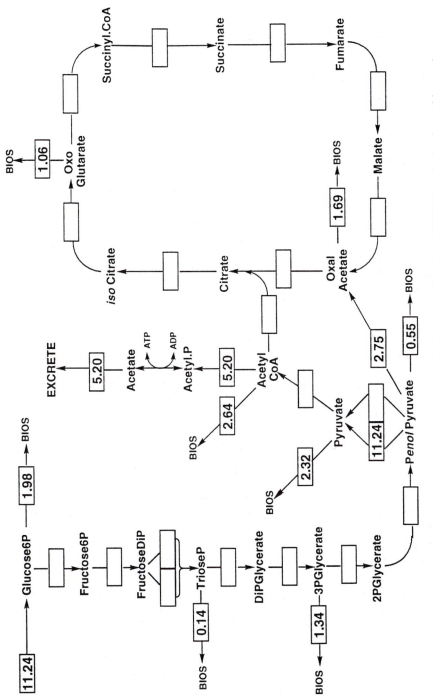

Figure 8. Uptake of glucose and provision of precursors for biosynthesis in *E. coli* ML308 (moles/kg dry wt biomass).

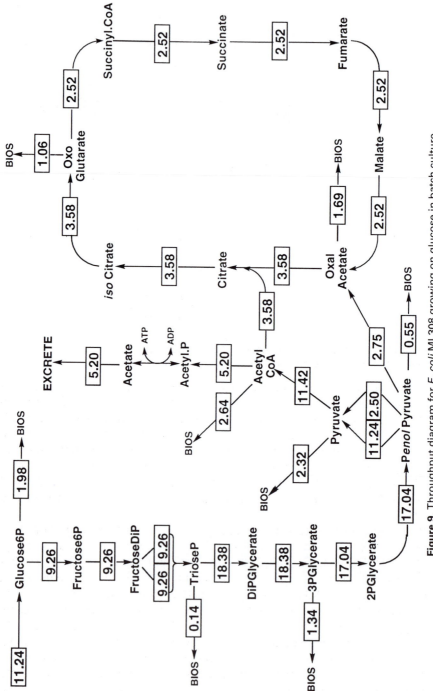

Figure 9. Throughput diagram for *E. coli* ML308 growing on glucose in batch culture.

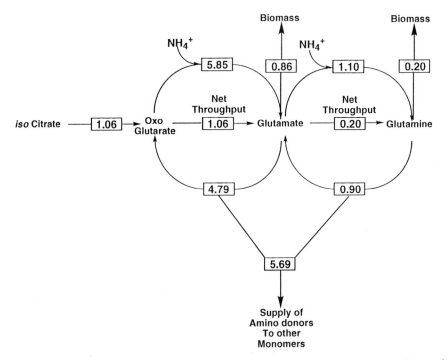

Figure 10. Throughputs for monomers derived from oxoglutarate and provision of amino donors to other reactions (moles/kg dry wt biomass) in *E. coli* ML308.

and if some of the intermediates or monomers are used for other purposes the additional load must be balanced by cyclic regeneration. This can be shown in a number of ways, but the utilization of glutamate and glutamine is a particularly good example in *Figure 10*, modified from ref. 1, because these are the primary amino-donors for many reactions. The throughput of OGA to biosynthesis is 1.06 (0.86 to Glu, Pro, and Arg and 0.20 to Gln), but considerably more Glu and Gln are used as amino donors regenerating OGA and Glu which are re-aminated by ammonia using energy input from oxidative metabolism.

It is also important to realize that *Figure 9* is only a true description if we have measured all the outputs and if the balance of carbon is oxidized to CO_2.

The PTS for the uptake of glucose is also used for some of the sugars, but other carbon sources do not use this mechanism and enter metabolism at other parts of the CMPs. This requires modification to the diagrams used to describe what happens in the CMPs but the principles are exactly the same. For pyruvate (*Figure 11*), PEP is made by PEP synthase, which is the substrate for gluconeogenesis, and there is a very large excretion of acetate and a small amount of lactate. Fumarate (*Figure 12*), on the other hand, enters directly into the Krebs cycle and provides all other precursors via malate enzyme to pyruvate or PEP carboxykinase to PEP (2), without any acetate

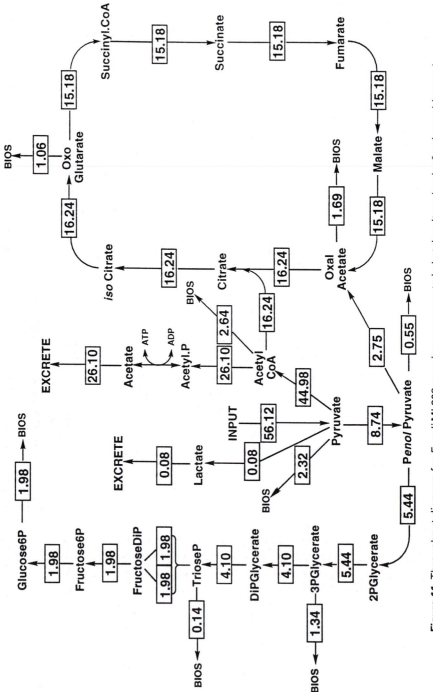

Figure 11. Throughput diagram for *E. coli* ML308 growing on pyruvate in batch culture (moles/kg dry wt biomass).

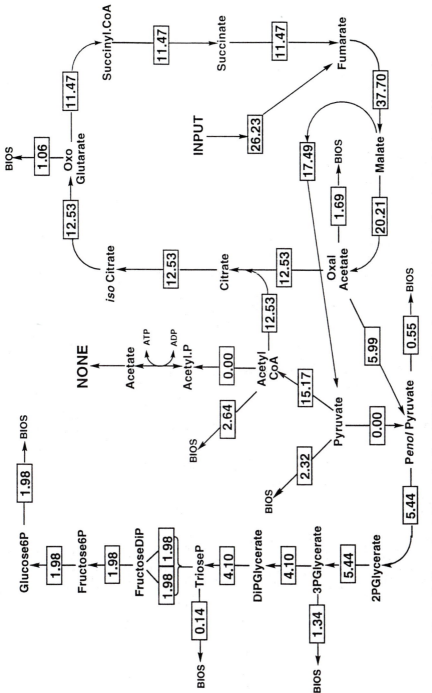

Figure 12. Throughput diagram for *E. coli* ML308 growing on fumarate in batch culture (moles/kg dry wt biomass).

excretion. This illustrates a potential problem in flux analysis. Throughputs from Krebs cycle C_4-acids to glycolysis must always total 23.48 moles/kg dry wt and both malate enzyme and oxalacetate decarboxylase are available for this purpose. *Figure 12* shows both these enzymes working to give a pyruvate/PEP provision in such a way that further interconversion of PEP and pyruvate is not required. However, there is no way of knowing if the distribution between the two $C_4 \rightarrow C_3$ enzymes is as shown. All the throughput could be by malate enzyme, in which case 5.99 moles PEP would need to be made by PEP synthase. Alternatively, oxalacetate decarboxylase could operate exclusively, in which case 17.49 moles pyruvate would need to be made from PEP by pyruvate kinase. Indeed, intermediate distributions of throughput between the two enzymes (other than that shown in *Figure 12*) are also possible, with pyruvate kinase or PEP synthase balancing the requirements for pyruvate and PEP. What is absolutely certain is that there is a net conversion of 23.48 moles malate to 5.99 moles PEP and 17.49 moles pyruvate, and *Figure 12* chooses the simplest way to accomplish this.

The technique of flux analysis is summarized in *Protocol 1*.

Protocol 1. Technique of flux analysis

Data required
- Uptake of feedstock(s) (moles/kg dry wt biomass)
- Biomass growth rate, μ (per hour)
- Monomeric composition of biomass (moles/kg dry wt biomass)
- Other outputs (moles/kg dry wt biomass)

Method

1. Calculate the outputs of precursors from CMPs to outputs and monomers in biomass.

2. Construct a diagram of the CMPs appropriate to the uptake of inputs and provision of precursors to biomass monomers and other outputs.

3. Enter the uptake of feedstock(s) and outputs of precursors into the basic diagram.

4. Calculate and enter the consequences of uptake and anaplerosis.

5. Complete the throughput diagram by calculating throughputs (moles/kg dry wt biomass) through each enzyme of the CMPs from input(s) to outputs of precursors.

6. Convert the throughput diagram to a flux (moles/kg dry wt biomass/h) diagram by multiplying each throughput by the growth rate constant (μ).

7. Use the flux diagram to devise strategies for intervention.

The interpretation of flux analysis and how to use this technique to intervene in a fermentation are dealt with below (Sections 3 and 4) as are its significance for control theory (Section 5) and commercial application (Section 6).

3. Interpretation of flux analysis

3.1 Fluxes in CMPs must balance one another

The fluxes into, through and from the CMPs must balance one another. In our example, where glucose carbon is converted into biomass carbon, this means that the flux of carbon *in* must be distributed into the flux of precursors *out*, and to sufficient oxidation to CO_2 to provide the reducing power and ATP required to convert these precursors into monomers and biomass. This is a stoichiometric relationship determined by the genome. For example, the requirement for phosphoglycerate to generate the serine family of amino acids is precisely determined by the amounts of serine, cysteine, and glycine needed to make biomass. The same is true for all the other precursors, and it follows that the relative fluxes to precursors are predetermined by the DNA. In other words, the demand for precursors are fixed relative to each other. Clearly the uptake of glucose by *E. coli* generates more intermediates in the CMPs than required to satisfy this demand. This situation cannot be accommodated by the accumulation of CMP intermediates or other low molecular weight compounds because the transmembrane osmotic pressure differential is limited by the strength of the cell wall (1). Broadly speaking, there are three mechanisms by which this potentially fatal situation can be avoided:

(a) Intermediates in excess of requirements can be polymerized, e.g. to glycogen (5, 6).

(b) The mechanism which couples oxidative metabolism to energy generation may 'slip' so that excess carbon is dissipated as CO_2 and excess energy is liberated as heat (7–10).

(c) Surplus intermediates of the CMPs can be excreted as low molecular weight compounds (1, 11, 12).

Clearly, it is the last of these three strategies which *E. coli* adopts when growing aerobically on glucose or pyruvate.

3.2 What does acetate excretion tell us?

If we look at *Figures 9* and *11*, we can ask the question: Why is acetate excreted? There are some obvious answers:

• too much feedstock is taken up;
• too much AcCoA is generated;
• there is an 'open door' for acetate excretion;
• probably the flux to oxalacetate and oxoglutarate, during growth on glucose, is too small relative to other precursors.

The first three of these are obvious (*Figures 9* and *11*), but the last needs some explanation. The flux through the pools of all the precursors from glucose 6-phosphate to AcCoA, during growth on glucose, exceeds the demands made upon them in that more could be drawn out at the expense of acetate excretion. This suggests that the flux to the anaplerotic provision of the Krebs cycle limits biosynthesis and thus the utilization of all precursors. If the availability of precursors from the Krebs cycle were increased, the availability of the other precursors would be sufficient to meet demand.

The throughput diagram for fumarate (*Figure 12*) tells a completely different story. With this substrate, uptake of feedstock into the CMPs exactly matches the outputs to precursors and oxidation to CO_2. Either uptake limits μ or is balanced to the ability to generate precursors or, if there is an oversupply of carbon uptake into the CMPs, it is dissipated as CO_2.

The descriptions of the processes by flux analysis suggests ways in which acetate excretion can be modulated for both glucose and pyruvate feedstocks.

4. Intervention to modulate acetate excretion

4.1 Intervention by restriction of feedstock uptake

One solution to the excess flux from glucose to AcCoA would simply be to restrict it, and the easiest way to achieve that is by continuous culture in a chemostat. The technique is quite simple—reduce the dilution rate and measure acetate excretion. As the dilution rate is lowered μ_{max} of 0.94 is restricted, acetate excretion is diminished and eventually falls to zero at μ of 0.71 (1). Analysis of this steady state shows that 8.64 moles of glucose are required to make 1 kg dry wt biomass (*Figure 13*). At this dilution rate, the flux of carbon through the CMPs is in perfect balance with the requirements for precursors and energy generation. There are several interesting comparisons to be made between the glucose-limited and glucose excess steady states (*Figures 9* and *13*):

- the outputs to precursors are identical;
- the throughputs in the Krebs cycle are identical;
- the throughputs in glycolysis are lowered;
- the conversion of PEP to pyruvate is exclusively dedicated to the phosphotransferase system for glucose uptake and none goes by pyruvate kinase.

Exactly the same technique gives a similar result with pyruvate (3) but, in this case as μ_{max} of 0.7 is lowered, acetate excretion is diminished, but is not totally abolished until a μ of about 0.3. This proportionally larger requirement for the restriction of feedstock reflects the enormously excessive uptake of pyruvate in batch or turbidostat culture.

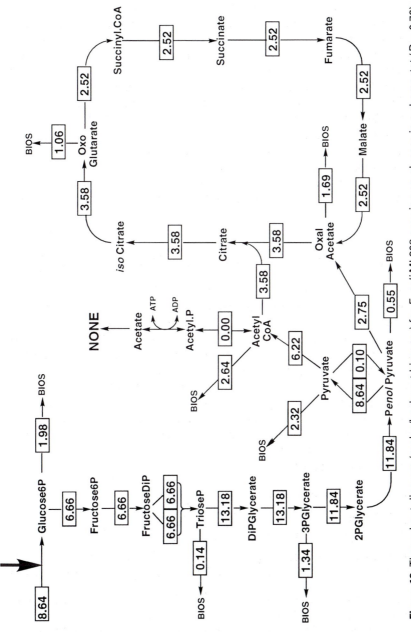
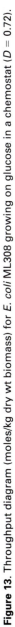

Figure 13. Throughput diagram (moles/kg dry wt biomass) for *E. coli* ML308 growing on glucose in a chemostat ($D = 0.72$).

4.2 Intervention by enzyme inhibition

The immediate cause of acetate excretion is oversupply of AcCoA by pyruvate dehydrogenase. This enzyme is inhibited by bromopyruvate (13, 14) and can prevent acetate excretion during growth of *E. coli* on pyruvate (3). At a concentration (50 μM) which totally prevents acetate excretion in pyruvate batch cultures, there is also a profound inhibition of growth (3). The growth rate (0.3) is the same as the dilution rate ($D = 0.3$) required to stop acetate excretion in the chemostat. The coincidence is probably significant because both interventions are achieving the same result—diminution of carbon intake to the CMPs.

4.3 Intervention by deletion of acetate excretion mechanism

Acetate is excreted by reversal of the pathway used for acetate uptake: this requires phosphorylation by ATP catalysed by acetokinase and then conversion of acetyl phosphate to AcCoA by a phosphotransacetylase. The mechanism does not distinguish between acetate and fluoroacetate which is taken up and converted to fluorocitrate; fluorocitrate cannot be metabolized further and is toxic. Selection under the appropriate conditions (3, 15) for fluoroacetate-resistant mutants yields strains which have lost the ability to take up (or excrete) acetate. Such strains do not excrete acetate when grown in batch culture on pyruvate (*Figure 14*).

Briefly:

- The outputs of precursors are the same.
- The uptake of pyruvate falls by 30% or, in other words, acetate excretion stimulates pyruvate uptake.
- There is no acetate excretion, whereas 47% of the input pyruvate is excreted by this route in the wild type.
- There is a very large stimulation of lactate excretion (14% of pyruvate uptake).
- There is an increase in AcCoA oxidized in the Krebs cycle. This presumably compensates for the reducing power required to reduce pyruvate to lactate, the loss of ADP phosphorylation by acetyl phosphate and the loss of contribution to the proton motive force by the excretion of acetate via a proton symport.

4.4 Intervention to improve provision of precursors

All precursors must be provided in the exact proportion demanded by biosynthetic demand and, as described in Section 3.2, it is possible that the throughput of PEP carboxylase limits the provision of oxalacetate and oxoglutarate. Chao and Liao (16) have varied the activity of this enzyme in

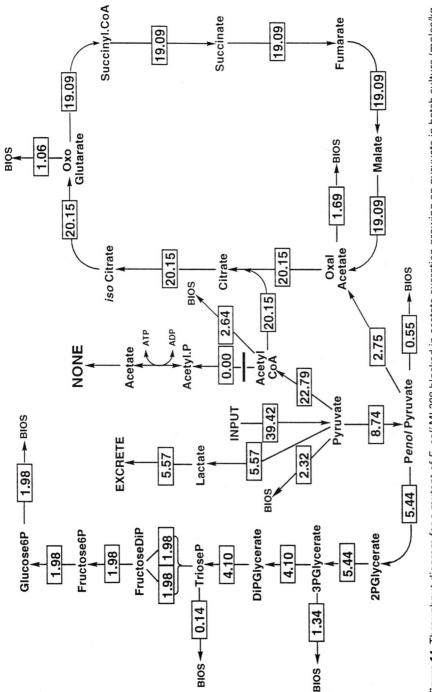
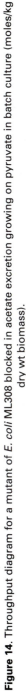

Figure 14. Throughput diagram for a mutant of *E. coli* ML308 blocked in acetate excretion growing on pyruvate in batch culture (moles/kg dry wt biomass).

another strain (*E. coli*, K12) and shown that increasing the dose of this enzyme decreases acetate excretion. Unfortunately, this strain is quite different from ML308 in that it grows much more slowly and excretes much less acetate. Okungbowa (17) has increased the dose of PEP carboxylase in *E. coli* ML308, this gives an improved conversion of either glucose or pyruvate to biomass with a diminished acetate excretion and is directly comparable with our references strain.

The comparison of *E. coli* ML308 with the PEP-carboxylase enhanced recombinant (JOE4) is very interesting and will be discussed for growth on glucose. This strain uses 8.74 moles glucose/kg dry wt biomass and excretes 2.30 moles acetate at a growth rate of 0.87/h. The throughput diagram (*Figure 15*) is directly comparable with *Figure 9* (ML308). Enhancing the capacity of PEP carboxylase does not increase the throughput because that is determined by the outputs of oxoglutarate and oxalacetate to biosynthesis which are unchanged. However, glucose uptake (and therefore PTS activity) is reduced by 22%, pyruvate kinase is eliminated (zero), and acetate excretion is reduced by 56%. The supply of AcCoA is reduced by 46% compared to that found in the wild-type, but the allocation of outputs from this pool are profoundly different (*Table 2*). Proportionally, in the recombinant much more of the available AcCoA is used for biosynthesis (lipid and anaplerosis), somewhat less is excreted as acetate, and *very* much less is oxidized to CO_2 in the Krebs cycle. Clearly, there is a fundamental difference in the steady states between the two strains when growing on glucose. The mechanism by which partition of flux at PEP is altered has not been studied but the results of flux analysis suggest possibilities which could be examined (*Table 3*). The larger glucose uptake in the wild-type batch delivers excess carbon into the pool of PEP which is usefully dephosphorylated to pyruvate by pyruvate kinase. This is directly comparable with the uptake of glucose in the chemostat (*Figure 13*) when the flux through glycolysis is restricted, so that the available supply of PEP is exactly equal to the demands for glucose uptake and biosynthesis. (This was achieved by lowering the dilution rate until acetate excretion fell to zero.) The recombinant, with enhanced PEP carboxylase activity, also restricts glucose uptake to eliminate the need for pyruvate kinase, but it does this in the presence of excess extracellular glucose. Clearly the recombinant restricts uptake through the glucose PTS. Now the increased activity of PEP carboxylase does not increase the throughput of this enzyme, so it presumably exerts its effect by altering pool sizes of intermediates significant for the glucose-PTS. There are two possibilities. Either the pool size of the initial PTS phosphate donor (PEP) is reduced and PTS is limited by its ability to access this lowered pool, or there are changes in pools of effectors of the glucose-PTS which regulate its activity. (Exactly the same holds for the pyruvate dehydrogenase inhibited system, Section 4.2.) Glycolytic throughputs in glucose are virtually identical in the wild-type chemostat and the recombinant batch. However, the disposition of the AcCoA pools is quite different (*Table 2*).

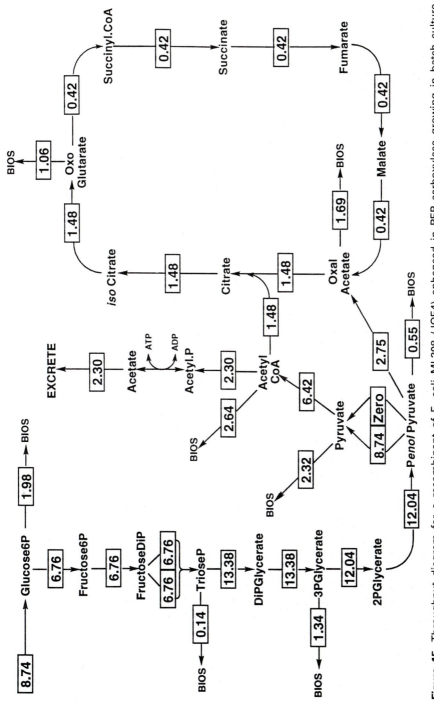

Figure 15. Throughput diagram for a recombinant of E. coli ML308 (JOE4) enhanced in PEP carboxylase growing in batch culture (moles/kg dry wt biomass).

Table 2. Throughputs of the AcCoA pool in *E. coli* growing on glucose

Throughputs (moles/kg)	ML308 Batch Moles/kg	%	ML308 Chemostat Moles/kg	%	JOE4 Batch Moles/kg	%
To AcCoA	11.4	100	6.22	100	6.42	100
To biosynthesis (including OGA)	3.70	32.4	3.70	59.5	3.70	57.6
To acetate excretion	5.20	45.5	0.00	0.00	2.30	35.8
To oxidation	2.52	22.1	2.52	40.5	0.42	6.5

Table 3. Throughputs of phosphoenolpyruvate pool in *E. coli* growing on glucose

Throughputs	*Escherichia* coli ML308 Batch Moles/kg	%	Chemostat Moles/kg	%	JOE4 Batch Moles/kg	%
To PEP	17.04	100	11.84	100	12.04	100
To PTS	11.24	66	8.64	73	8.74	73
To pyruvate kinase	2.50	15	−0.10	−<1	0.00	0
Total to pyruvate	13.74	81	8.54	72	8.74	73
To PEP carboxylase	2.75	16	2.75	23	2.75	23
To biosynthesis	0.55	3	0.55	5	0.55	5
Total to biosynthesis	3.30	19	3.30	28	3.30	28

The supply of AcCoA exceeds the requirement for biosynthesis in the recombinant (2.72 moles/kg dry wt) but is only slightly greater than in the wild-type chemostat (2.52 moles/kg dry wt). In the recombinant, 85% of the excess AcCoA is excreted as acetate and the balance (15%) is oxidized in the Krebs cycle. In the wild-type chemostat none of the AcCoA is excreted as acetate and what is not used for biosynthesis is oxidized in the Krebs cycle. Why do virtually identical throughputs from glucose to AcCoA result in such different outputs from this pool? The answer probably lies in different pool sizes of intermediates at the different growth rates observed (0.3 for the wild-type in the chemostat and 0.87 for the recombinant in batch). Regulation of the Krebs cycle is brought about by effectors of citrate synthase which is inhibited by high $NADH,H^+/NAD^+$ ratios and by oxoglutarate (2). The fluxes to $NADH^+$ and to oxoglutarate are obviously higher in the recombinant ($\mu = 0.87$) than the wild-type in the chemostat ($\mu = 0.3$), and this could limit citrate synthase so that relief from AcCoA generation can only obtained by acetate excretion. A necessary corollary of this hypothesis is that excretion of 2.30 moles acetate/kg dry wt is in some way equivalent to oxidation of 2.10 moles (2.52–0.42) AcCoA in the Krebs cycle. Of course, a fraction of the reducing power could 'slip' and be released as heat (Section 3.1). Perhaps some day there will be calorimeters available to measure this but, in the shorter term, careful measurements of $NADH,H^+/NAD^+$ ratios and oxo-glutarate pools in the various steady states found during growth on glucose would be very interesting!

4.5 Other means of diminishing acetate excretion

There are other obvious means of intervention, made obvious by flux analysis, which have not so far been tested.

- If *E. coli* could be encouraged to grow on glucose and a Krebs cycle intermediate simultaneously, the increased supply of oxalacetate would demand more AcCoA to give oxoglutarate and the requirements of all other precursors would be increased. A likely system would be a continuous culture fed with glucose and fumarate (in relatively small amounts). The approach would be a turbidostat with a relatively small excess of glucose and increasing concentrations of fumarate added to the feed until acetate excretion was eliminated. At low excess glucose concentrations it is unlikely that co-utilization of fumarate would be a problem but, if there were, it might be necessary to raise a mutant in which the dicarboxylic acid uptake mechanism was expressed constitutively. Such a turbidostat would not necessarily grow faster but would sustain a higher cell density than on glucose alone.

- If another 'sink' were introduced to utilized intermediates, acetate excretion would diminish. One such mechanism would be to induce glycogen synthesis which does not normally occur when *E. coli* is growing at maximum rate.

4.6 Conclusions

- Flux analysis of a system makes obvious the strategy for intervention. There can be several such opportunities.

- Uptake of primary C-source is always related to outputs, including excreted products.

- Excretion of acetate can be a very large fraction of output and can indeed stimulate uptake.

- Intervention does not always give the expected results, and the modified system must be analysed to determine what factors other than the target have been changed.

- When you know what a system is actually doing, you can change it by any of several means to achieve a desired result.

5. What controls flux?

5.1 Theories

Flux analysis describes the metabolic activity of the biomass, in particular the distribution of fluxes at metabolic junctions. It does not tell you how these are controlled. There is no shortage of speculation to answer this question. Basically, there are two theories which are usually presented in opposition to each other and have generated a vast literature which can best be summarized by two short reviews (18,19) published simultaneously.

Kacser and Porteous (18) have proposed a mathematical model of control theory, in which the basic assumption is that there is a finite amount of control in any system and the sum of the control coefficients of all the enzymes in any system is defined as 1 (100%). When the effects of very small perturbations in steady states are examined experimentally, the conclusion is that 'control', defined in this way, is distributed throughout the system and it is rare to find any one enzyme reaction with a very high control coefficient. Even if a reaction with a control coefficient close to 1 is found it does not follow that this reaction is the 'pacemaker' for the whole system, because the theory includes negative control coefficients. The significance of these cannot be overemphasized. If, for example, we are looking at control of flux to a product we might find that one enzyme on the route has a high control coefficient, and we might be tempted to conclude that this is significant for control of flux to product. However, if 'upstream' from this there is a junction at which flux is diverted to a product that we have not yet discovered, then that flux could well be the determinant, by a large negative control coefficient, of flux to product. The conclusion is obvious. If you do not know everything that the system is doing, you cannot start to work out how it is controlled. The solution is also obvious. You must analyse flux, i.e. measure everything that goes in and everything that comes out, before you can consider how the system is controlled.

Crabtree and Newsholme (19) have called attention to the powerful allosteric controls exerted on irreversible enzymes in the CMPs. The supporters of Kacser's control theory have pointed out that, in the steady state, these enzymes do not seem to exert any degree of control much greater than other enzymes. It seems to me that both sides in the confrontation offer experimentally variable facts, and it would be more sensible to reconcile them rather than express them in opposition to each other; I think this can be done very simply. In the steady state, fluxes through all pools and the sizes of these pools remain constant. For example, the excretion of acetate when *E. coli* is growing on glucose is a very good mechanism to achieve this. There is no need for any one enzyme in the whole system to be rigidly controlled and that is what is observed. In other words, the flux through glycolysis to precursors and to PEP is balanced with the subsequent flux to the non-phosphorylated precursors by the excretion of acetate. Pyruvate dehydrogenase is the fulcrum of this balance. If acetate excretion has a large negative control coefficient it means that the glycolytic system itself does not require much control elsewhere. However, a sudden perturbation to this steady state (such as shutting of an input like carbon source or oxygen) could be catastrophic. If glycolysis continued (e.g. without oxidative generation of ATP), then the

ATP pool would be depleted by generation of phosphorylated intermediates. When oxygen again became available, the biomass would not be able to resume normal activity because of the unavailability of ATP and the biomass would be 'dead'. The intervention of allosteric control of irreversible enzymes (in this case, fructose bisphosphate kinase) prevents this, and this type of control has evolved to protect the pools of essential cofactors (ATP/ADP; $NADPH,H^+/NADP^+$) from sudden perturbations in the flow of metabolites. In the steady state there is no need for these emergency controls and the pools sizes of their effectors are such that these controls are not operative.

Both Kacser and Newsholme are 'right' in the sense that their theories are valid explanations of metabolic control. These theories are not mutually exclusive, but the mechanisms operate in different circumstances.

5.2 Determination of flux—a statement of the obvious

What does decide flux? *E. coli* can grow on a number of different single carbon sources with growth rates from 0.32 to almost 1.0/h (1), and is essentially doing the same thing over this three-fold range of all the fluxes in the biomass. It seems obvious that the determinant of fluxes through the CMPs is the rate of delivery of carbon into the CMPs and the problem of distribution of fluxes to precursors. If the uptake is excessive or if the problem of distribution is difficult then fluxes are balanced, in *E. coli* at least, by the excretion of acetate (*Table 4*). The enzymes used to excrete acetate are constitutive, in that they are expressed during growth on all carbon sources (*Table 5*) as shown by Brown *et al.* (15). While the same enzymes are used to take up acetate when this is the sole source of carbon, they have been selected not for this purpose but for acetate excretion. This is the only possible explanation for the constitutive expression of this mechanism. It operates as a safety valve, compensating for a flux of carbon into the CMPs which exceeds the demands for fluxes of precursors to biosynthesis and oxidation to provide reducing power and ATP. Bacteria have been selected to survive wildly fluctuating availability of feedstocks, and the ability to excrete acetate is one of the principal mechanisms which allows *E. coli* ML308 to do this. This is why it is always available even when it is not needed, but when exceptional demands are placed upon it (such as steady-state growth on pyruvate or gluconate) the activity of the acetate excretion mechanism is increased even more (*Table 4*) to allow balance within the CMPs.

This facility has been selected to balance the provision of precursors to biosynthesis and, being strategically placed at the fulcrum of the CMPs, it fulfils this purpose. It follows that, when this facility is not required, the flow of carbon into and through the CMPs is balanced to the flow of carbon from the CMPs. It is, therefore, extremely probable that carbon sources which do achieve this balance through the CMPs do so because their rate of uptake or delivery into the CMPs is rate-limiting *per se* or controlled to be so. This is presumably why comparable substrates, such as glucose and fructose, show

Table 4. Uptake of various carbon sources and acetate excretion by E. coli ML308

Carbon source	Growth rate μ	Uptake Moles/kg	Moles/kg	Acetate excretion Moles/kg	Reference Moles/kg	
Glucose	0.94	11.24	10.57	5.20	4.89	(1)
Glucose (Chemostat)	0.72	8.64	6.22	0	0	(1)
Glucose (JOE.4)	0.87	8.84	7.6	2.30	2.00	(17)
Glucose 6-phosphate	0.95	12.38	11.76	4.21	4.00	(1)
Fructose	0.72	10.58	7.62	0	0	(1)
Glycerol	0.70	20.00	14.00	0	0	(1)
Gluconate	0.90	12.76	11.48	7.20	6.48	(1)
Glucuronate	0.87	13.49	11.74	10.43	9.07	(1)
Lactate	0.60	39.44	23.66	6.77	4.06	(1)
Pyruvate	0.70	56.12	39.29	26.10	18.27	(3)
Acetate	0.43	46.88	20.16	−46.88	−20.16	(21)
Fumarate	0.63	26.23	16.53	0	0	(1)
Oxoglutarate	0.32	20.77	6.65	0	0	(1)

Table 5. Acetokinase and phosphotransacetylase activities in *E. coli* K12PA309 grown on various carbon sources

Carbon source	Acetokinase μmols/min/mg protein	Phosphotransacetylase μmol/min/mg protein
Glucose	1.5	1.2
Glycerol	1.3	1.3
Ribose	1.3	1.2
L-Malate	1.7	1.5
Acetate	1.8	1.3
Pyruvate	4.1	2.6
DL-Lactate	3.7	2.8
Gluconate	3.6	2.5

faster growth rates (glucose, $\mu = 0.94$) if they excrete acetate than if they balance input to the CMPs (fructose, $\mu = 0.72$) so that there is no need to excrete acetate. However, the uptake of glucose can be controlled, as shown in the recombinant (JOE4) where the uptake (8.74 moles/kg dry wt/h) is much less than in ML308 (10.57 moles/kg dry wt/h). In the case of glycerol ($\mu = 0.70$), the precise mechanism which controls uptake is feedback inhibition of the enzyme (glycerokinase) which determines the rate at which glycerol both enters the cell and delivers it into the CMPs (20).

The hypothesis proposed here is that, for *E. coli* at least, uptake is limiting or acetate is excreted. The result is a steady state or precursor provision and growth with no obvious controlling function for any one enzyme in the CMPs. If the resulting tranquillity is suddenly perturbed, catastrophic changes in the pool-sizes of intermediates essential for later resumption of growth are preserved by the intervention of the allosterically responsive irreversible enzymes.

Control by limitation of uptake is more efficient, at least from an anthropocentric viewpoint, but this generally results in slower growth. Preservation of pools by acetate excretion might be thought to be less efficient, but it does permit faster growth and the excreted product can subsequently be recycled. In both strategies, steady states are established where there is no need for draconian control intervention *within* the CMPs. There is, however, at least one example where these general principals do not apply and that is growth of *E. coli* ML308 on acetate as the sole source of carbon (21). In this steady state, growth is rather slow ($\mu = 0.43$) and the precursors for biosynthesis (other than AcCoA) are generated by flux through the glyoxylate bypass (*Figure 16*). This creates a unique junction in the CMPs where *iso*citrate lyase (ICL) and *iso*citrate dehydrogenase (ICDH) compete for a common substrate. This creates a problem in that ICDH has a much greater affinity for *iso*citrate than does ICL, which is resolved by phosphorylation of a very large part of the ICDH enzyme to give an inactive form. This is achieved by a bifunctional kinase/phosphatase using ATP to phosphorylate and inactivate

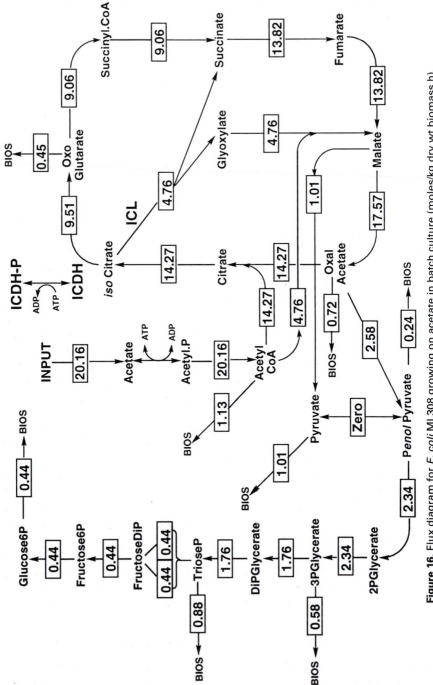

Figure 16. Flux diagram for *E. coli* ML308 growing on acetate in batch culture (moles/kg dry wt biomass.h).

Table 6. Flux through *iso*citrate dehydrogenase relative to enzyme activity in *E. coli* ML308 growing on various carbon sources

Carbon source	ICDH flux[a] (mol/kg/h)	ICDH activity[b] (mol/kg/h)	Activity/ flux
Glucose	3.36	60.7	18.1
Fructose	5.65	53.0	9.4
Glycerol	4.68	66.2	14.1
Gluconate	4.12	81.2	12.4
Pyruvate	11.63	72.8	6.3
Oxoglutarate	2.36	135.6	57.5
Fumarate	8.12	92.6	11.4
Acetate	9.84	10.0	1.02

[a] From flux diagrams.
[b] By *in vitro* assay (21).

and hydrolysing off inorganic phosphate to reactivate (22). The restraint on ICDH allows the intracellular concentration of *iso*citrate to be increased from <20 μM to 570 μM, a level at which ICL can operate efficiently (23). The significance of this control can be seen (21) by comparing the flux through ICDH with the activity of the enzyme in the biomass (*Table 6*) during growth on several carbon sources. In all cases examined, except acetate, the activity of ICDH in the biomass exceeds the actual flux of *iso*citrate to oxoglutarate. During growth on acetate, there is still a very large amount of ICDH present, but exactly the correct proportion is inactivated by phosphorylation to maintain the fluxes through both ICDH and ICL required of the steady state when growing on acetate. It is the *balance* of these two fluxes which decides (controls ?) the steady state.

Finally, we should consider the turnover of the *iso*citrate pool. The flux through the pool is 3.37 moles/kg dry wt/h in the glucose steady state and more than four times as much (14.27) in acetate. However because the pool on acetate is so much bigger (1.54 compared to <0.05 moles/kg dry wt) the turnover is less. On glucose the *iso*citrate pool turns over at least 1.87 times/sec (and perhaps ten times as fast), while on acetate it turns over only 2.6 times/sec. The only purpose of the increase in the *iso*citrate pool is to overcome the low affinity shown to it by *iso*citrate lyase.

There may well be other systems where control of CMP enzymes are significant for achieving junctions specific to particular carbon sources. Furthermore, it is very likely that it will depend on covalent modification of one of the 'normal' CMP enzymes at the junction.

6. Applications for flux analysis in the real world

This chapter has illustrated the practical importance of flux analysis in a particular strain of *E. coli* which selected itself for the particular amusement of microbial physiologists. However, flux analysis is a very practical tool which can be used to define the physiological behaviour of any microbial system. Many of these have been developed to make useful products such as antibiotics.

With my colleagues at Bioflux, I have been actively engaged in this field for almost thirteen years. Unfortunately, the results of this work are of commercial value and specific publication of the results is restricted by confidentiality agreements, although some short and very general papers have appeared (24). However, very occasionally, some of this applied work enters the public domain. One such example is the production of clavulanic acid (made by *Streptomyces clavuligerus*) which is a potent inhibitor of penicillinase. Originally, this was thought to be made from ornithine but, when flux analysis showed that the fermentation also generated urea, it was realized that the precursor was arginine and this was subsequently proved by experiment (25–27).

It is not surprising that flux analysis is helpful in improving industrial fermentations which share one major objective, i.e. to encourage a biomass to increase flux to a particular product. All microbial species have survived by selection of mechanisms which give advantage to the survival of their genome for which the biomass is only a vector. The fluxes to this purpose are invariably much greater in the wild, than the fluxes to the products which we want them to make. When we impose unnatural selective pressures on them to make more of a particular product we distort the physiological machine which they have evolved. Flux analysis describes how these deliberately selected strains actually work and is the blueprint which allows further intervention to make even greater amounts of desirable products.

7. Conclusions

7.1 General

- Flux analysis is a practical tool which provides a complete description of a steady state.
- Flux diagrams suggest how to intervene to move a biomass into a different steady state.
- Steady states do not necessarily operate at maximum attainable growth rates or give optimal conversion of feedstock to biomass.

7.2 *E. coli* ML308

- In this reference strain, entry of primary feedstock into the CMPs is balanced to the provision of precursors of monomers and the generation of energy to convert these into biomass.
- Balance is generally achieved by the restriction of uptake of carbon feedstock or excretion of intermediates of the CMPs.

- In one case, a specific enzyme of the CMPs is tightly regulated to achieve balance. This solution is unique to the particular problems involved in balancing the CMPs in growth on acetate.

- It is possible that balance can be achieved by 'slip', through uncoupling oxidative phosphorylation, to oxidize excess AcCoA to CO_2 and heat.

7.3 Control of CMPs

- Generally, steady states are determined by the uptake of the carbon source. This is why measurement of control coefficients within the CMPs show little evidence of control.

- When steady states are perturbed, pools of intermediates, essential for transition to a new steady state, are reserved by the intervention of allosterically controlled irreversible enzymes.

Note added in proof. Since this chapter was written a review (28) has appeared which compliments this chapter in that it deals more fully with the theoretical implications of flux analysis. In particular it covers energy balances, maintenance energy, pool turnover, control of the CMPs, control theories and the fundamental limitation to growth rate.

References

1. Holms, W. H. (1986). *Curr. Topics Cell. Regul.* **28**, 59.
2. Mandelstam, J. and McQuilllen, K. (ed.) (1982). *Biochemistry of bacterial growth* (3rd edn). Blackwell Scientific Publications, Oxford.
3. El-Mansi, E. M. T. and Holms, W. H. (1989). *J. Gen. Microbiol.*, **135**, 2875.
4. Neidhardt, F. C. (1987). In E. coli *and* S. Typhimurium: *Cellular and molecular biology* (ed. J. L. Ingraham, K. Brooks Low, B. Magasanik, M. Schaechter and H. E. Umbarger), Vol. 1, p. 3. American Society for Microbiology, Washington, D.C.
5. Dawes. E. A. and Senior, P. J. (1973). *Adv. Microbiol. Phys.*, **10**, 135.
6. Dietzler, D. N., Leckie, M. P., Sternhein, W. L., Ungar, J. M., Crimmins, D. L. and Lewis, J. W. (1979). *J. Biol. Chem.*, **254**, 8276.
7. Neijssel, O. M. and Tempest, D. W. (1979). *Symp. Soc. Gen. Microbiol.*, **29**, 53.
8. Stouthamer, A. H. (1979). *Microbial biochemistry* (ed. J. R. Quayle), pp. 1–47. University Park Press, Baltimore, MD.
9. Roels, J. A. (1980). *Biotech. Bioeng.*, **22**, 2457.
10. Tempest, D. W. and Neijssel, O. M. (1984). *Annu. Rev. Microbiol.*, **38**, 459.
11. Demain, A. L. (1972). *J. Appl. Chem. Biotech.*, **22**, 345.
12. Meyer, H. P., Leist, C. and Fiechter, A. (1984). *J. Biotech.*, **1**, 355.
13. Bisswagner, H. (1981) *J. Biol. Chem.*, **256**, 815.
14. Lowe, P. N. and Perham, R. N. (1984). *Biochem.*, **23**, 91.
15. Brown, T. D. K., Jones-Mortimer, M.C. and Kornberg, H. L. (1977). *J. Gen. Microbiol.*, **102**, 327.
16. Chao, Y.-P. and Liao, J. C. (1993). *Appl. and Environ. Microbiol.*, **59**, 4261.

17. Okungbowa, J. (1991). In *Genetic manipulation of metabolite fluxes in* Escherichia coli. PhD thesis. University of Glasgow, Glasgow.
18. Kacser, H. and Porteus, J. W. (1987). *TIBS*, **12**, 5.
19. Crabtree, B. and Newsholme, E. A. (1987). *TIBS*, **12**, 4.
20. Novotny, M. J., Frederickson, W. L., Waygood, E. B. and Saier, Jr., M. H. (1985). *J. Bacteriol.*, **162**, 810.
21. Holms, W. H. (1987). *Biochem. Soc. Symp.*, **54**, 17.
22. Nimmo, H. G., Borthwick, A. C., El-Mansi, E. M. T., Holms, W. H., Mackintosh, C. and Nimmo, G. A. (1987(). *Biochem. Soc. Symp.*, **54**, 93.
23. El-mansi, E. M. T., Nimmo, H. G. and Holms, W. H. (1985). *FEBS Lett.*, **183**, 251.
24. Holms, W. H., Hamilton, I. D. and Mousdale, D. (1991). *J. Chem. Tech. Biotechnol.*, **50**, 139.
25. Elson, S. W., Baggaley, K. H., Davison, M., Fulston, M., Nicholson, N. H., Risbridger, G. D. *et al.* (1993). *J. Chem. Soc., Chem. Commun.*, **1993**, 1212.
26. Valentine, B. P., Bailey, C. R. The late Andrew Doherty, Morris, J., Elson, S. W., Baggaley, K. H. *et al.* (1993). *J. Chem. Soc., Chem. Commun.*, **1993**, 1210.
27. Elson, S. W., Baggaley, K. H., Fulston, M., Nicholson, N. H., Tyler, J. W. Edwards., J. *et al.* (1993). *J. Chem. Soc., Chem. Commun.*, **1993**, 1211.
28. Holms, W. H. (1996). *FEMS Microbiology Reviews*, **19**, 85.

List of suppliers

Culture preservation

Anchor Glass Co. Ltd, Brent Cross Works, North Circular Road, London NW4 1JS, UK.

API-bioMerieux, 69280 Marcy l'Etoile, France.

Denley Instruments Ltd, Billingshurst, Sussex RH14 9EY, UK.

Edwards High Vacuum International, Manor Royal, Crawley, West Sussex RH10 2LW, UK.

LabM, Tapley House, PO Box 10, Bury, Lancs BL9 6AU, UK.

Planer Products Ltd, Windmill Road, Sunbury-upon-Thames, Middlesex TW16 7HD, UK.

Statebourne (Cryogenics) Ltd, Paison Industrial Estate, Washington, Tyne and Wear NE37 1EZ, UK.

UNIPATH Ltd, Wade Road, Basingstoke, Hants RG24 0PW, UK.

Vacuum Industrial Products Ltd, Unit 11, Sheddingdean Industrial Estate, Marchants Way, Burgess Hill, West Sussex RH15 8QY, UK.

Growth of hyperthermophiles

Aldrich Ltd, The Old Brickyard, New Road, Gillingham, Dorset SP8 4JL, UK.

Becton Dickinson UK Ltd, Between Towns Road, Cowley, Oxford OX4 3LY, UK.

Bioengineering AG, Sagenrainstrasse 7, CH-8636 Wald, Switzerland.

Difco Laboratories, PO Box 14B, Central Avenue, East Molesley, Surrey KT8 0SE, UK.

Fisher Scientific UK, Bishop Meadow Road, Loughborough, Leics LE11 0RG, UK.

FT Applikon Ltd, Station Drive, Bredon, near Tewkesbury, Gloucs GL20 7HH, UK.

Gelman Sciences, 600 South Wagner Road, Ann Arbor, Michigan 48103-9019, USA.

Inceltech (UK) Ltd, 10, Nimrod Industrial Estate, Elgar Road South, Reading, Berks RG2 0EB, UK.

Kelco, Merck Ltd, Hunter Boulevard, Magna Park, Lutterworth, Leics LE17 4XN, UK.

Mettler-Toledo Ltd, 64, Boston Road, Beaumont Leys, Leics LE4 1AW, UK.
Nalgene (Europe) Ltd, Rotherwas, Hereford HR2 6JQ, UK.
Sartorius Ltd, Longmead Business Centre, Blenheim Road, Epsom, Surrey KT19 9QN, UK.
Sigma Chemical Company, Fancy Road, Poole, Dorset BH17 7NH, UK.
Sorvall, Du Pont (UK) Ltd, Wedgewood Way, Stevenage, Herts SG1 4QN, UK.
Sterilin Ltd, 43–45 Broad Street, Teddington, Middlesex TW1 3QT, UK.
Thermoelectric International Ltd, Unit 17E, Eurolink Industrial Estate, Sittingbourne, Kent ME10 3RN, UK.
Watson Marlow Ltd, Falmouth, Cornwall TR11 4RU, UK.
Weber Scientific International Ltd, 40 Udney Park Road, Teddington, Middlesex TW11 9BG, UK.

Laboratory fermenters and associated equipment

Laboratory fermenters
FT Applikon Ltd, Station Drive, Bredon, near Tewkesbury, Gloucs GL20 7HH, UK.
Bioengineering AG, Sagenrainstrasse 7, CH-8636 Wald, Switzerland.
Braun Biotechnology Ltd, B. M. Browne (UK) Ltd, Unit 2, Tincent's Kiln Industrial Park, Calcot, Reading, Berks RH 31 7SB, UK.
Inceltech (UK) Ltd, 10, Nimrod Industrial Estate, Elgar Road South, Reading, Berks RG2 0EB, UK.
Life Science Laboratories Ltd, Luton, Beds LU4 9DT, UK.
New Brunswick Scientific (UK) Ltd, Edison House, 163 Dixons Hill Road, North Mymms, Hatfield, Herts AL9 7JE, UK.

Oxygen and pH electrodes
Dr W. Ingold AG, c/o Mettler-Toledo Ltd, 64 Boston Road, Beaumont Leys, Leics LE4 1AW, UK.
Kent Industrial Measurement Ltd, Stonehouse, Gloucs GL10 3TA, UK.
Russell pH Ltd, Auchtermuchty, Fife KY14 7DP, Scotland, UK.
Uniprobe Instruments Ltd, Cardiff CF5 1HG, Wales, UK.

Peristaltic pumps
Watson Marlow Ltd, Falmouth, Cornwall TR11 4RU, UK.

Biomass measurement

BioOrbit kit
Labsystems (UK) Ltd, Unit 5, The Ringway Centre, Edison Road, Basingstoke, UK.

BioOrbit Luminometer, Scientific Laboratory Supplies Ltd., Unit 27, Wilford Ind. Estate, Ruddington Lane, Nottingham NG11 7EP.

Dielectric permittivity
Aber Instruments Ltd, Science Park, Aberystwyth, Dyfed SY23 3AH, Wales, UK.
Hewlett Packard, Heathside Park Road, Cheadle Heath, Stockport, Cheshire, SK3 0RB.

Electrical counting and sizing
Coulter Electronics, Northwell Drive, Luton, Beds, UK.

Flow cytometry
Becton Dickinson UK Ltd, Between Towns Road, Cowley, Oxford OX4 3LY, UK.

Fluorescence probes
Biochem Technology Inc., 66 Great Valley Parkway, Malvern, Pennsylvania 19355, USA.

Image analysis
Applied Imaging, Unit 3A, Hylton Park, Wessington Way, Sunderland, Tyne and Wear SR2 3HD, UK.

NIR spectroscopy
Perstop Analytical Ltd, Cooper Road, Thornbury, Bristol BS12 2UW, UK.
Perkin Elmer Ltd, Maxwell Road, High Wycombe, Berks HP9 1QA, UK.

Turbidity measurement probes
Mettler-Toledo Ltd, 64 Boston Road, Beaumont Leys, Leics LE4 1AW, UK.

Analysis of microbial cultures
Boehringer-Mannheim UK (Diagnostics and Biochemicals) Ltd, Bell Lane, Lewes, East Sussex BN7 1LG, UK.
Sigma-Aldrich Co. Ltd, Fancy Road, Poole, Dorset BH12 4QH, UK.

HPLC
Phenomenex UK Ltd, Queens Avenue, Macclesfield, Cheshire SK10 2YF, UK.
Bio-Rad Laboratories Ltd, Bio-Rad House, Maylands Avenue, Hemel Hempstead, Hertfordshire HP2 7TD, UK.
Calbiochem-Novabiochem (U.K.) Ltd, Boulevard Industrial Park, Padge Road, Beeston, NOttingham NG9 2JR, UK.

Ion chromatography
Waters Ltd, Blackmoor Lane, Watford, Hertfordshire WD1 8YW, UK.

Fractionation equipment
Branson Ultrasonics, Clayton Road, Hayes, Middlesex UB3 1AN, UK.

Gas chromatography
Microsensor Technology Inc., 41762 Christy Street, Fremont, California, 94538, USA.

Electrochemical sensors
International Sensor Technology, 3 Whatney, Irvine, CA 92718, USA.

Ion separation
VG Gas Analysis Systems Ltd, Aston Way, Middlewich, Cheshire CW10 0HT, UK.

Thermoelectric coolers
Universal Analyzers Inc., 1771 South Satro Terrace, Carson City, NV 89706, USA.

Sample manifolds
Balzers AG, FL-9496 Balzers, Fürstentum, Liechtenstein.

Pressure and Flow Instruments
MKS Instruments, 6 Shattuck Road, Andover, MA 01810, USA.

Infra-red and Paramagnetic analysers
Siemens PLC, Siemens House, Oldbury, Bracknell RG12 8FZ, UK.

Statistical software
SAS Institute Inc., SAS Campus Drive, Cary, NC 27513, USA.

Culture
Becton Dickinson Microbiology Systems, PO Box 243, 250 Schilling Circle, Cockeysville, MD 21030, USA.
Unipath Ltd, Wade Road, Basingstoke, Hampshire RG24 0PW, UK.

Addresses of culture collections, microbial databases, and national and international culture collection organizations

Addresses of the larger culture collections listed in the World Directory of Collections of Cultures of Microorganisms (1) serving the major groups of organisms

Organism	Collection	Number of of strains	Contact address
Algae	National Centre for Medical Culture Collections [CMCC(B)]	4000	Temple of Heaven, Beijing 100050, China. Tel: 701 7755 429
	Culture Collection of Algae at the University of Texas at Austin [UTEX]	2089	Department of Botany, Austin, Texas TX78713-7640, USA. Tel. 512 471 4019
	Algensammlung am Institut fur Botanik [ASIB]	1570	Sternwartestrasse 15, Innsbruck A-6060, Austria. Tel: 512 507 5939
	Sammlung von Algenkulturen [SAG]	1400	Nikolausberger Weg 18, D-3400 Gottingen, Germany. Tel: 49 551390
	Culture Collection of Algae and Protozoa [CCAP]	1273	Far Sawrey, Ambleside, Cumbria, LA22 0LP, UK. Tel: 44 5394 42468

Organism	Collection	Number of of strains	Contact address
	Provasoli-Guilland Centre for Culture of Marine Phytoplankton [CCMP]	1000	McKown Point, West Boothby Harbor, Maine 04575, USA. Tel: 207 633 2173
	Peterhof Genetic Collection of Microalgae [PGC]	700	Universiteskaya Nab. 7/9, Leningrad, Leningrad V34 199034, Russia. Tel: 812 4278851
	Collection of Algal Cultures, Leningrad University [CALU]	600	Oranienbaumskoye sch.2, Leningrad-Stary Peterhof 198904, Russia. Tel: 812 2182000
	Collection of Microalgae of the Institute of Plant Physiology [IPPAS]	600	35 Botanich, st. Moscow, 127276, Russia. Tel: 7 095 4822904
	Culture Collection of Autotrophic Organisms [CCALA	523	Dukelska 145, Trebon, CS 379 82 CS, Czechoslovakia. Tel: 333 2522
Animal cell lines	American Type Culture Collection [ATCC]	2300	12301 Parklawn Drive, Rockville, Maryland 2052 USA. Tel: 301 881 2600
	European Collection of Animal Cell Cultures [ECACC]	1500	Porton Down, Salisbury, Wiltshire SP4 0JG, UK. Tel: 44 980 610391
	Collection Nationale de Cultures de Microorganismes [CNCM]	332	25 Rue de Docteur Roux, F-75724 Paris Cedex 15, France. Tel: 33 1 45688251
	Institute for Fermentation Osaka [IFO]	233	17-85 Juso- Honmachi 2-chome Yodoawa-ku, Osaka 532, Japan. Tel: 06 302 7281
	Centro Substrati Cellulari: Cell Lines Collection and Hybridomas [CSC-CLCH]	170	A.Bianchi 7, Brescia 25100, Italy. Tel: 030 2290 248
	Rio de Janeiro Cell Bank (Banco de Celulas do Rio de Janeiro) [BCRJ]	109	PO Box 68201, Rio de Janeiro, Rio de Janeiro 21944, Brazil. Tel: 55 21 5908736

Organism	Collection	Number of of strains	Contact address
Bacteria	Culture Collection, University of Goteborg [CCUG]	27 600	Guldhedsg 10, Goteborg, S-413 46 Sweden. Tel: 46 31 604625
	American Type Culture Collection [ATCC]	14 400	12301 Parklawn Drive, Rockville, Maryland 20852, USA. Tel: 301 881 2600
	Agricultural Research Service, US Dept of Agriculture [NRRL]	10 300	1815 North University St., Peoria, Illinois 61604, USA. Tel: 309 685 4011 ext. 385
	Laboratorium voor Microbiologie Universiteit Ghent [LMG]	9000	Faculteit der Wetenschappen, K.L. Ledganckstraat 35, Ghent B-9000, Belgium. Tel: 32 91 645108
	Centre des Yersinia [CY]	8990	25 Rue de Docteur Roux, Paris 75724, Cedex 15, France. Tel: 33 1 45688251
	Collection of Marine Microorganisms [KMM]	8000	Pr. 100-let Vladivostoku, 159 Vladivostok, Primorsky Krai 690022, Russia. Tel: 423 22 33 81
	Salmonella Genetic Stock Centre [SGSC]	8000	2500 University Drive, NW Calgary, Alberta T2N 1N4, Canada. Tel: 403 220 6792
	The Wellcome Bacterial Collection [WRL] available through National Collection of Type Cultures [NCTC]	6800 11 800 (total holding)	61 Colindale Avenue, London NW9 5HT, UK. Tel: 801 200 4400
	National Collections of Industrial and Marine Bacteria Limited [NCIMB]	6000	23 St Machar Drive, Aberdeen AB2 1RY, Scotland, UK. Tel: 44 224 273332
	Czechoslovak National Collection of Type Cultures [CNCTC]	5500	Srobarova 48, Prague 10 CS-100 42, Czechoslovakia. Tel: 42 2 731 241 8
Fungi	Agricultural Research Service, US Dept of	44 000	1815 North University St. Peoria, Illinois 61604,

Organism	Collection	Number of of strains	Contact address
	Agriculture [NRRL] Centraalbureau voor Schimmelcultures [CBS]	32 000	USA. Tel: 309 685 4011 PO Box 273, Oosterstraat 1, NL-3740AG Baarn, Netherlands. Tel: 31 2154 81 211
	American Type Culture Collection [ATCC]	20 200	12301 Parklawn Drive, Rockville, Maryland 20852, USA. Tel: 301 881 2600
	International Mycological Institute [IMI]	18 000	Bakeham Lane, Egham, Surrey TW20 9TY, UK. Tel: 44 784 470111
	Mycoteque de l'Universite, Catholique de Louvain [MUCL]	14 500	Place Croix du Sud 3, Bte 6, Louvain-la-Neuve, B 1348, Belgium. Tel: 32 10 473742
	Canadian Collection of Fungus Cultures [CCFC]	10 000	K.W. Neatby Bldg. #20, Ottawa, Ontario K1A 0C6, Canada. Tel: 613 9961665
	Fungal Cultures, University of Goteborg [FCUG]	9000	Carl Skottsberga Gata 22, Goteborg S-413 19, Sweden. Tel: 46 18 182794
	Fungal Genetics Stock Center [FGSC]	8000	Dept. of Microbiology, University of Kansas, Medical Center, 3901 Rainbow Blvd, Kansas City, K66160-7420, USA. Tel: 913 588 7044
	Institute for Fermentation Osaka [IFO]	7093	17-85 Juso- Honmachi 2-chome Yodoawa-ku, Osaka 532, Japan. Tel: 06 302 7281
	Institute of Hygiene and Epidemiology— Mycology Laboratory [IHEM	5000	Rue Juliette Wytsman 14, Brussels B-1050, Belgium. Tel: 32 2 6425630
Plant cell lines	Deutsche Sammlung von Mikroorganismen und Zelkulturen GmbH	750	Mascheroder Weg 1b, D-38124 Braunschweig, Germany.

Organism	Collection	Number of of strains	Contact address
	[DSM]		Tel: 49 531 26160
	Culture Collection of Autotrophic Organisms [CCALA]	169	Dukelska 145, Trebon, CS 379 82, Czechoslovakia. Tel: 333 2522
	Korean Collection for Type Cultures [KCTC]	31	PO Box 131, Cheongryang, Seoul 131, Korea. Tel: 962 8801
	American Type Culture Collection [ATCC]	25	12301 Parklawn Drive, Rockville, Maryland 20852, USA. Tel: 301 881 2600
	Biotechnology Culture Collection [BTCC]	25	Jl.Ir. H Juanda 18, PO Box 323, Bogor, 16122, Indonesia. Tel: 0251 21038/21039
	Collection de genomes d'organismes symbiotiques [CRBF]	20	Cite Universitaire, Quebec G1K 7P4, Canada. Tel: 418 656 2384
Plasmids	Laboratory of Molecular Biology— Plasmid Collection University Ghent [LMBP]	2500	K.L. Ledeganckstraat 35, Ghent, B-9000, Belgium. Tel: 32 91 645131
	Centraalbureau voor Schimmelcultures [CBS]	800	PO Box 273, Oostertraat 1, NL-3740AG Baarn, Netherlands. Tel: 31 2154 81211
	National Collection of Type Cultures [NCTC]	600	61 Colindale Avenue, London NW9 5HT, UK. Tel: 801 200 4400
	Dept of Microbiology [DMPMC]	500	Queen Elizabeth II Medical Centre, Nedlands, Western Australia 6009. Tel: 09 389 2286
	Culture Collection and Research Center [CCRC]	363	PO Box 246, Hsinchu, Taiwan 30099, Republic of China. Tel: 886 35 223191
	China Centre for Type Culture Collection [CCTCC]	337	Lou Jia Shan, Wuhan, Hubei 430072, The People's Republic of China. Tel: 027 722157

Organism	Collection	Number of of strains	Contact address
	The Upjohn Culture Collection [UC(UPJOHN)]	310	301 Henrietta Street, Kalamazoo, Michigan 49001, USA. Tel: 616 385 7158
	National Bank for Industrial Microorganisms and Cellular Cultures [NBIMCC]	156	125 Tsarigradsko chaussee blvd., Bl.2, Sofia, BG-1113, Bulgaria. Tel: 359 2 720865
	Korean Federation of Culture Collection [KFCC]	114	Shinchondong Sodaemunku, Seoul 120-749, Korea. Tel: 02 392 0950
	School of Medical Technology Western Australia [SMTWA]	100	GPO Box U1987, Perth, Western Australia 6001, Australia. Tel: 09 350 7374
Viruses	American Type Culture Collection [ATCC]	1350 animal 590 plant 400 bacteria	12301 Parklawn Drive, Rockville, Maryland 20852, USA. Tel: 301 881 2600
	Medical Microbiological Laboratory [MML]	1884 animal	Oslo, Norway. Tel: 47 22118080
	Russian Collection of Industrial Microorganisms [VKPM]	880 bacteria	1 Dorozhny proezd. 1 Moscow 113545, Russia. Tel: 7 095 3153774
	Czechoslovak National Collection of Type Cultures [CNCTC]	550 animal 200 bacteria	Srobarova 48, Prague 10, CS-100 42, Czechoslovakia. Tel: 42 2 7312418
	Yale Aebovirus Research Unit [YARU]	700+ animal	Box 3333, New Haven, Connecticut 06510, USA. Tel: 203 932 5711
	JII Plant Virus Collection [JII]	650 Plant	John Innes Centre, Norwich Research Park, Colney Lane, Norwich, Norfolk NR4 7OH, UK. Tel: 0603 52571
	Centre for General Viruses Culture Collection [CGVCC]	105 animal 130 plant 85 bacteria 180 insect	Wuhan, Hubei 430071, The People's Republic of China. Tel: 027 723712 385

Organism	Collection	Number of of strains	Contact address
	National Institute of Animal Health [NIAH]	385 animal	Kannondai 3-1-1, Tsukuba, Ibaraki-ken 305, Japan. Tel: 0298 38 7835
	Division Vector-Borne Viral Diseases [DVBVD]	335 animal	PO Box 2087, Fort Collins, Colorado 4811, USA. Tel: 303 221 6400
	Plant Virus Collection [GCRI]	325 plant	Worthing Road, Littlehampton, Sussex, BN17 6LP, UK. Tel: 0903 716123
Yeasts	Agricultural Research Service, US Dept of Agriculture [NRRL]	14 500	1815 North University St., ts Peoria, Illinois 61604, USA. Tel: 309 685 4011
	Centraalbureau voor Schimmelcultures [CBS]	5000	PO Box 273, Oostertraat 1, NL-3740AG Baarn, Netherlands. Tel: 31 2154 81211
	American Type Culture Collection [ATCC]	4300	12301 Parklawn Drive, Rockville, Maryland 20852, USA. Tel: 301 881 2600
	Czechoslovak Collection of Yeasts [CCY]	3600	Dubravska cesta 9, CS-842 38 Bratislava, Czechoslovakia. Tel: 42 7 3782625
	Collezione dei Lieviti Industriali [DBVPG]	3000	Borgo 20, Giugno 74, Perugia I-06100, Italy. Tel: 39 75 5856300
	Institute for Fermentation, Osaka [IFO]	2677	17-85 Juso- Honmachi 2-chome, Yodoawa-ku, Osaka 532, Japan. Tel: 06 302 7281
	Department of Plant Sciences [UWO]	2500	London, Ontario N6A 5B7, Canada. Tel: 519 679 2838
	All-Russian Collection of Microorganisms [VKM]	2498	Pushchino, Moscow Region 142292, Russia. Tel: 7 095 9257448
	Institute of Hygiene and Epidemiology— Mycology Laboratory [IHEM]	2000	Rue Juliette Wytsman 14, Brussels B-1050, Belgium. Tel: 32 2 6425630

Organism	Collection	Number of of strains	Contact address
	Labatt Culture Collection Production Research Department [LCC]	2000	150 Simcoe Street, London, Ontario, N6A 4M3, Canada. Tel: 519 667 7354
	National Collection of Yeast Cultures [NCYC]	2000	Norwich Research Park, Colney Lane, Norwich, Norfolk, NR4 7UA, UK. Tel: 0603 255000

Addresses of national and international organizations

ECCO, European Culture Collections Organization, E. Falsen, Culture Collection of Goteborg, Dept of Clinical Bacteriology, Guldhedsg 10, S-41346 Goteborg, Sweden.

JFCC, Japan Federation for Culture Collections, K. Yamasato, Institute of Applied Microbiology, University of Tokyo, 1-1-1 Yayoi, Bunkyo-ku, Tokyo 113, Japan.

MIRCEN, The Microbial Resource Centre Secretariat, Division of Scientific Research and Higher Education, United Nations Educational and Cultural Organization (UNESCO), 7 Place de Fontenoy, 75700, Paris, France.

UKFCC, The United Kingdom Federation for Culture Collections, F. G. Priest, Dept Biological Sciences, Heriot Watt University, Edinburgh, EH14 4AS, Scotland, UK.

USFCC, The United States Federation of Culture Collections, M. Jackson, Dept 47P, Building AP9A, Abbott Laboratories, Abbott Park, IL 60064, USA.

WFCC, World Federation for Culture Collections, D. Fritze, Deutsche Sammlung von Mikroorganismen und Zelkulturen GmbH (DSM), Mascheroder Weg 1b, D-3300 Braunschweig, Germany.

Addresses of microbial databases

MINE, MINE Coordinating Secretariat, CBS, Oosterstraat 1, NL - 3740 AG Baarn, Netherlands.

MSDN, Microbial Strain Data Network Secretariat, 307 Huntingdon Road, Cambridge, CB3 0JX, UK. INTERNET:MSDN@CGNET.COM.

WDCM, World Data Center on Microorganisms, Riken, Saitama, Japan. INTERNET: "Gopher fragrans.riken.go.jp70''.

Reference

1. Sugawara, H., Ma, J., Miyazaki, S., Shimura, J., and Takishima, Y. (ed.) (1993). *World directory of collections of cultures of microorganisms*: *Bacteria, fungi and yeasts* (4th edn), World Federation for Culture Collections World Data Center on Microorganisms, Saimata, Japan.

Index

absorber in vent gas 147–8
acetate 220–30, 231, 241–5
  deletion of excretion mechanism 234
  determination of flux 241–5
  excretion 232–4
  inhibition 234
  intervention 234–9
acetyl coenzyme A 218–37
actinomycetes 11
ADP 105
aeration of fermenter 81
Aerobacter 178
aerotolerant hyperthermophiles 27
agar 62
  for hyperthermophiles 28–9
agitation of fermenter 81
air-drying microorganisms 8
alarm on fermenter 97
algae 7, 17, 20
Alicyclobacillus acidocaldarius 29
allosteric control 240–1, 243
American Type Culture Collections (ATCC)
  6–7, 54
amino acid 59, 63, 216–19, 219–22, 227–30
  assay 172–5
  compound 180
  pH 90
ammonia 170
  assay 180–1
ammonium salt 59, 86, 89–90
AMP 105
amphibolic pathway 214–19
anaerobic incubation 41, 44
  of hyperthermophiles 43
analyser system for vent gas 150–1
analysis of inputs for fermenters 166–88; *see*
   assay
  of growth data 193–11; *see also* growth data
  of mass balance 189–91
  of metabolic flux 213–47
analytical methods for growth data 208–11
animal cell line 7, 20
antibiotic 59, 60
antifoam 63, 80, 93
APIZYM testing system 3
Archaea 23–50
arginine 217–19
aseptic connections 81–3
Aspergillus niger 16
assay
  amino acid, total 173–5
  ammonium 181
  biomass 186

carbohydrate 166–9
carboxylic acid 179–80
chloride 177–8
DNA 187
free amino group 172–3
kit list 169
leucine aminopeptidase 183
lipid, soluble 170
nitrite 177–8
nitrogen, organic 171–2
oil, lipid 170
pellet composition 186, 188–9
peptidic amino group 172–3
perchloric acid (PCA) 188–9
phosphate 175–8
pigment 185
potassium 181
protease, soluble 182
RNA 187–8
sideproduct 178
sodium 181
sugar alcohol 179
sulfate 177–8
thiol 183–4
ATP 57, 60, 104–6, 216–17, 234, 240–1
autoclave 77, 78, 84
  modified 41
avermectin 55
Azomonas insignis 14

Bacillus 23
  stearothermophilus 29
  subtilis 109
bacteria 7, 9, 10–12, 17, 20, 23–50
  plant pathogen 11
  strain 7
baffle 81
barophilic hyperthermophile 41–2
bioluminescence 104–6
biomass
  bicarbonate 154–5
  measurement in complex media 185–6
  yield 40–1, 94, 345
biomass, determination of
  bioluminescence 104–6
  capacitance 122–3, 124
  chemiluminescence 104–6
  composition 189
  definition 103–4, 214
  dielectric permittivity 121–5
  direct count microscopy 110–11

DNA analysis 107–8
dryweight method 114–17
electrical counting and sizing 120–1
epifluorescence 113
fermenter 94
filtration probe 125
flow cytometry 121
fluorescence 108–9
image analysis 113–14
mass balance analysis 125
mass spectrometry 125–6
mathematical modelling 125–6
near infrared spectroscopy 109–10
nephelometry 120
off-line measurement 104
on-line measurement 104
packed cell volume 117–18
pellet composition 188–9
probe 123–4
specific rate 104
turbidimetry 118–20
viable cell count 111–13
bioreactor, *see* fermenter
Biotechnology Action Programme (BAP) 3,
    5, 6–7
Biotechnology Research for Innovation
    Development and Growth in Europe
    (BRIDGE) 3, 5, 7
biotin 57
Box–Behnken design 68–9
brewing 124
Burton reagent 187

calcium 59
calculation of
    gas consumption rate 152–6
    calculation of gas evolution rate 152–6
Candida 109
capacitance measurement of biomass 122–3
carbohydrate assay 166–9
    fructosyl 168
    HPLC 168–9
    soluble 167
carbon dioxide in metabolism 222–39
    analysis 185, 190–1
    in bioreactors 93, 100
    vent gas 131–2, 137, 139, 154–6
carbon
    mass balance 189–91
    in nutrition 57–9, 86, 219–46
    pH 90
carboxylic acid assay 179–80
cations in media 29–30
Centraalbureau voor Schimmelcultures (CBS)
    6, 7
central metabolic pathway 214–19, 222–45

centrifugal freeze-drying 15–16
cephamycin C 58, 60
characterization of microorganisms 2–3
chemically defined media 55–7
chemiluminescence 104–6
chemoorganotroph 53–63
chemostat 94, 236–8
chloride assay 177–8
chorismic acid 178
citrate 216, 243–5
clavulanic acid 246
collection, microbial 7
Commission of the European Community
    (CEC) 5, 6
complex media 54–5, 185–6
computer data logging 80, 96–101
contamination, microbial 8, 86
continuous
    growth 8, 9–11
    culture 32, 94–6
Contois equation 196
cooler in vent gas 147–8
corrosion of equipment 32
Corynebacterium glutamicum 109
Coulter Counter 120–1
cryopreservation 8, 18–20
    cooling rate 19
    hyperthermophile 42–5
    storage temperature 19
    warming rate 21
cryoprotection 19, 43
culture 57–64; *see also* media
    collection of 3–4
    collections, addresses for 253–60
    for hyperthermophile 45–50
curation 4
cyanobacteria 17

data
    analysis, mass spectrometer 144
    collection, vent gas 151–2
    retrieval 3
    growth 193–210; *see also* growth data
    storage 3
database
    address for 253–60
    list of 6–8
    microbial 4–7
dehydration 1, 8
    techniques 11–17
desiccant 147
desiccation 8
desiccator 11–13
design of growth media 53–7
Deutsche Sammlung von Mikroorganismen
    und Zelkulturen (DSM) 5, 42–3

Deutsches Institu für Medizinsche
　　Dokumentation und Information
　　(DIMDI) 7
dielectric permittivity 121–5
differential equation 193, 204–5
dimethyl sulfoxide 19, 43
direct count microscopy 110–11
dissolved carbon dioxide in
　　fermenter 93, 100
dissolved oxygen
　　in fermenter 151
　　tension 90–2, 100
DNA 113, 121, 231
　　analysis 107–8, 187
　　hybridization 3
dryer in vent gas 147–8
drying in
　　desiccator 11–13
　　support medium 11–13
dry weight of biomass
　　Eppendorf method 115
　　filtration method 116–17
　　glass tube method 115–16
dynamic parameter estimation 205–8

EDTA 61
efrotomycin 55
eigenvalue 208–11
electrical
　　counting of biomass 120–1
　　sizing of biomass 120–1
electrochemical sensor in vent gas analysis
　　133–4
electrophoresis 3
environmental factors in microbial growth
　　62–3
enzyme 216–19
　　activity 3
　　allosteric 240, 243–5
　　assay 181–3
　　production 2
epifluorescence 113
Escherichia coli 61, 62, 72, 109, 121, 189,
　　214–17, 219–31, 233–46
ethanol 159, 161
eukaryotic
　　metabolism 222
　　microalgae 17
European Culture Collection Organization
　　(ECCO) 4, 5, 260
exponential growth equation 194

factorial design in media optimization 67–9
Faraday cup detector 143–4

fed-batch process 98–9, 125
Federation of the European Microbiological
　　Societies (FEMS) 5
fermentation process efficiency 56
fermenter 63
　　aeration and agitation 81
　　alarm 97
　　aseptic connections 81–3
　　biomass 94
　　choice of 76–8
　　computer data logging 96–101
　　continuous culture 94–6
　　control 87–96
　　dissolved carbon dioxide 93
　　fed-batch process 98–9
　　flow 95
　　foam 93
　　gas-lift 32–3, 35–41
　　hood 84
　　hyperthermophiles 31–42
　　inoculation 83–4
　　line connection 82–3
　　measurement 87–96
　　media 86–7
　　oxygen tension 90–2,
　　　100
　　redox 93–4
　　remote access 97
　　requirements for 76
　　sample value 85–6
　　sampling 84–6
　　septum ports 82
　　software 97
　　sterilization 78–80, 94
　　storage 94
　　syringe 84
　　temperature 41, 92–3, 98
　　vent gas analysis 94
　　volume 95–6
filamentous fungi 2–3, 20
filter in vent gas 147–8
filtration probe 125
flame ionization detector 132
flow
　　measurement 95
　　control 95, 149–151
flow-cytometry 121
fluorescence 108–9
　　amino acid 173–5
flux analysis 213–47
　　interpretation 231–2
　　intervention 232–9
　　technique 230
　　throughput diagram 222–4
foam formation 63
　　control 93
　　detection 93, 146
FORTRAN program 204–5

freeze-drying 14–17
  shelf 16–17
  spin method 15–16
frozen storage 8
full factorial search (in media optimization) 65
fumarate 219–30, 232, 239
fungi 7, 9, 10, 11
  filamentous 2–3, 20
  freezing of 19
  phytopathogenic 10

galactose 61
gas chromatography of vent gas 132–3
  phase, calculated 152–60
  vent analysis, *see* vent gas analysis
gas-lift reactor 32–3
  construction and operation of 35–41
gel electrophoresis 182
gelrite media for hyperthermophiles 29–31
gene 1
  probes 2
genetic marker 2
geothermal
  environment 23–4
  sampling in 24–6
glass vessel 32, 77–9
gluconeogenesis 222, 227
glucose 58, 61, 167
  metabolism 219–39
glutamate 216–9
glycerol 19, 43
glycolysis 215, 222–38
glyoxylate bypass 243
Gram-negative bacteria 121
growth
  continuous 8, 9–11
  culture system 197–8
  data 193–211
  analytical method 208–11
  definition 193–5
  differential equation 204–5
  dynamic parameter estimation 205–8
  kinetic function 195–7
  Monod parameter estimation constant 198–9
  simulation 202–4
  washout method 199–201
  yield 201–2
  factor 61
  hyperthermophile 31–41
  with inhibitors 3
  logarithmic 10
  manipulation 8
  media 53–72
  rate specific 193
  of variant cells 10

high performance liquid chromatography 3, 110, 168–9, 178, 184, 189
  carboxylic acid 179–80
  sugar alcohol 179
  thiol 183–4
honey 12
hood on fermenter 84
hyperthermophile 18
  barophilic 41–2
  cryopreservation 42–5
  culture procedure 45–50
  fermenters for 31–41
  growth of 31–41
  isolation of 23–6
  liquid media 26–8
  solid media 28–31
  suppliers 249–50
  transport of 25
Hyperthermus butylicus 30

image analysis of biomass 113–14
impeller 81
independent variable optimization 64–72
inducers in media 61
inert gas 150
ingredients of media, consistency 54
inoculation of fermenters 83–4
inorganic ion 60
inositol 12
International Mycological Institute (IMI) 6, 19
internet site 6, 7, 261
ion
  chromatography 177–8, 181
  separation in mass spectrometer 141–2
iron 59
*iso*citrate 216, 243–5
isoenzyme pattern 2, 3
isolation of hyperthermophiles 23–6
isopropylthio-β-D-galactoside 61
isotope 131

Japan Federation for Culture Collections (JFCC) 5, 260

kanamycin 62
kinetics 193–208
  function of growth data 195–7

Index

Kjedahl digestion 171–2
knock-out pot 147–8
Krebs cycle 215–38
Laboritorium voor Microbiologie Universiteit (LMG) 7
L-drying 11, 20
  method 13–14
Lentinus edodes 19
leucine aminopeptidase assay 183
Leuconostoc paramesenteroides 61
Liapounov stability analysis 208–11
limiting nutrient 94
  equation 194
line connection to fermenter 82–3
liquid media
  for hyperthermophiles 26–8
  for *Pyrobaculum islandicum* 48
  for *Sulfolobus* 46–7
  for *Thermatoga maritima* 49–50
liquid phase calculation 152–60
logarithmic growth 10
luciferin 105
Luft-type infrared analyser 135, 138

magnetic sector analyser 141–2
magnetodynamic analyser 137–8
Maillard reaction 185
maintaining collections 2
Malachite Green 175–6
manganese 59
mass balance analysis 125
mass spectrometer 125–6
  applicability 144–5
  data analysis 144
  detectors 142–4
  ionization 140–1
  ion separation 141–2
  sample inlet 139–40
  vacuum system 139
media
  chemically defined 55–7
  complex 54–5, 185–6
  fermenter 86–7
  hyperthermophiles 26–31
    agar 28–9
    gelrite 29–31
    liquid 26–8
    polyacrylamide 29
    silica gel 29
    solid 28–31
    starch 30–1
  optimization 64–72
  silica gel 11–12, 20
metabolic flux analysis 213–47
Methanococcus
  jannaschii 42
  thermolithotrophicus 41

mathematical model
  of biomass 125–6
  control efficiency 240
methylene blue 110–11
Methobacterium thermoautotrophicum 25
mevinolin 55
microaerophilic hyperthermophiles 27
microbe identity 54
microbial
  database 4–7
  pH 3, 30
  resource collections 7
Microbial Information Network Europe (MINE) 3, 6, 7, 260
Microbial Resource Centres (MIRCEN) 4, 6, 260
Microbial Strain Data Network (MSDN) 6, 261
microorganism
  characterization of 2–3
  sources of 4–7, 253–60
microscopy, direct count 110–12
moisture content in storage 16
Monod
  growth constant 198–9
  kinetics 202–4, 208–11
Moser equation 196
most probable number technique 25
multistream sample manifold 148–9

NADH 108, 216–19, 238–9
NADPH 108, 216–19, 241
National Collection of Industrial and Marine Bacteria (NCIMB) 13, 14
National Collection of Yeast Cultures 13
near infrared spectrometry 109–10
nephelometry 120
neutral red 110
nitrogen
  assay 171–2
  mass balance 189–91
  nutrition 58–9
  in vent gas 133, 134
nitrate 59, 90
  assay 177–8
Nocardia lactamdurons 58
noise in data 152
non-filamentous organism 11
Numerical Algorithm Group 204
  minimization routine 205–7
nutrient, limiting 94
nutritional requirements
  carbon source 57–9
  growth factors 61
  inorganic ion 60
  nitrogen source 58–9
  oxygen 60, 81

off-line measurement of biomass 104
oil assay 170
  soluble lipid 170
oil storage 9–10, 20
on-line measurement of biomass 104
optimization of media 64–72
organic acid analysis 184–5
organic compounds, volatile 131, 139, 146, 149, 157–60
ornithine 217–19
osmoregulatory chemicals 19
oxaloacetate 224–30, 234–8
oxoglutarate 216–19, 224–30, 234–8
oxygen 132, 133
  dissolved 151
  measurement 136–9
  in nutrition 60, 81
  tension in fermenter 90–2, 100

packed cell volume 117–18
paraffin storage 9–10, 20
paramagnetism 136–9
penicillin 59
Penicillium
  chrysogenum 109, 114, 124, 125
  ochrochloron 16
pentose phosphate pathway 215
peptide assay 181–3
perchloric acid 107–8, 185–9
peristaltic pump 95
  suppliers 250
pH
  control agents 89–90
  in cultivation 59, 60, 62, 98
  measurement 87–9
  microbial culture 3, 30
phenolphthalein 110
phosphate 60–1
  assay 175–8
phosphoenol pyruvate (PEP) 215–19, 222–30, 234–8, 241
  carboxylase 215
phosphotransferase system 222–30, 236–8
phytopathogenic fungi 10
P.I.D. controller 87
pigment analysis 185
Plackett–Burman design 65–9
plant cell line 8, 20
  pathogenic bacteria 11
plasmid 7, 20
polyacrylamide, for hyperthermophiles 29
polyol assay 179
polypropylene glycol 93
population dynamics 193
potassium 59
  assay 181

preservation
  long-term 10
  of microorganisms 1–21
  techniques 8–9
pressure of vent gas 149–50, 151
proportional integral differentiation 87
protease assay 182
protein assay 173–5, 181–3
protozoa 17
Pseudomonas
  aeruginosa 114
  fluorescens 114
  putida 109, 124
Pyrobaculum
  aerophylum 27
  culture of 48
  islandicum 30, 35, 46
    media for 48
Pyrococcus 26, 40
  abyssi 30
  furiosus 25, 27, 30–1, 32–5, 43, 45
  medium for 27–8
  woesei 25, 30, 35
Pyrodictum
  brockii 25
  occultum 25
pyruvate 219–30
  dehydrogenase 215, 240

quadruple analysis 141–2
quarantine 4
Quincke-type analyser 138

redox in fermenters 93–4
regression data 199
remote access of fermenter 97
re-preservation 10
respiration 57
respiratory quotient 99–100, 160–1
response surface, exploration 67–9
Rhizobium 6
RNA 113, 121
  analysis 187–8
Runge–Kutta function 203–4

Saccharomyces cerevisiae 61, 99, 109, 114, 121, 124
safety 4
salt requirements 60, 87
sample
  inlet in mass spectrometer 139–40
  probe position 145–6
  transport 146–7
  valves in fermenter 85–6

sampling in
fermenters 84–6
geothermal environments 25–6
media 166
secondary electron suppressor 143–4
security 97
of collections 4
selective agents 61
septum port in fermenter 82
serial dilution count 112–13
shelf-freeze drying 16–17, 20
shelf-life 21
shiitake mushroom 19
silica gel 132
growth in 29
storage in 11–12, 20
silicone emulsion 93
simplex optimization 64, 69–72
simulation growth data 202–4
skimmed milk 12
sodium assay 181
software fermenter 84–6
solid media for
hyperthermophiles 28–31
Pyrobaculum islandicum 48
Sulfolobus 47
Thermotoga maritima 49
solidifying agent 62
source of microorganisms 4–7, 253–60
sparger 81
Sphingomonas 29
spin freeze-drying 15–16, 20
sporulating fungi 9, 10–11, 13, 17
staining of cell 110–11
stainless steel 31–2, 77–9
starch media, for hyperthermophiles 30–1
statistical search (in media optimization) 65–7
steady-state, interruption of 96
sterilization 78–80, 83, 94
large volumes 86
medium alterations 63
storage 94
cryopreservation method 18–20
frozen 8
hyperthermophiles 43
L-drying method 13–14, 20
shelf-freeze drying method 16–17, 20
silica gel method 11–13, 20
spin freeze-drying 15–16, 20
under paraffin 9–10, 20
water method 10–11, 20
strain, bacterial 7
Streptomyces 61, 109, 124
coelicolor 185, 189
clavuligerus 114, 246
tendae 114
Streptomycetes 189
sugar alcohol 179

sulfate 60–1
assay 177–8
Sulfolobus 29, 30
cultivation of 46–7
sulfur 24, 26–7, 35, 47
suppliers of equipment 249–52
support medium 11–13
syringe 84
pressurized 41

temperature 3
cryopreservation 17, 19–21
in cultivation 62–3
drying of fungi 16
fermenter 41, 92–3, 98
hyperthermophiles 24–5, 31
lowering 1
vent gas 149–50
Tessier equation 196
thermoacidophile 25, 30, 43–4
Thermococcus litoralis 35
thermoelectric cooler 147
thermomagnetic analyser 136–7
Thermoplasma
acidophilum 30
volcanium 30
Thermoproteus tenax 29
Thermotoga maritima 46
culture of 49–50
Thermus 23
aquaticus 29
thermophilus 29
Thiobacillus 202
thiol assay 183–4
trace element 59
turbidimetry 118–20
turbidostat 94, 232, 239

United Kingdom Federation for Culture
Collections (UKFCC) 5, 260
urea 170

vacuum
drying 11, 13–14
system in mass spectrometer 139
variable independent (nutrition factors)
64–72
vent gas analysis 94, 125–6
absorber 147–8
analyser system 150–1
cooler 147–8
data collection 151–2
dissolved oxygen 151
dryer 147–8
electrochemical sensors 133–4

filter 147–8
flame ionization 132
flow 149–50, 151
gas chromatography 132–3
infrared absorption 134–6
knock-out pots 147–8
mass spectrometry 139–45
multistream sample manifold 148–9
paramagnetism 136–9
pressure 149–50, 151
respiratory quotient 160–1
sample probes 145–6
sample transport 146–7
temperature control 149–50
thermal conductivity 131–2
volatile organic compounds 157–60
well-mixed liquid and gas phases 152–6
vesicular arbuscular mycorrhizal fungi 13
vessel, *see* fermenter
viability 1, 13, 14, 16
determination of 121–5
viable cell counts 111–13
virus 7, 20
vitamin 61, 63

volatile organic compound 131, 139, 146, 149, 157–60
volume control, continuous culture 95–6

washout method of growth data 199–201
water storage 10–11, 20
weir 95–6
wet weight of biomass 117
World Data Center 6, 7
World Federation of Culture Collections (WFCC) 3, 4, 5–6, 260

xylose 61

yeast 7, 11, 12, 17, 20, 98–9, 161
yield
biomass 34–5
growth data 201–2

zinc 59
Zymomonas mobilis 109